Periodization of Strength Training for Sports

Fourth Edition

Tudor O. Bompa, PhD
Carlo A. Buzzichelli

HUMAN
KINETICS

Library of Congress Cataloging-in-Publication Data

Names: Bompa, Tudor O., author. | Buzzichelli, Carlo, 1973- author.
Title: Periodization of strength training for sports / Tudor O. Bompa, Carlo A. Buzzichelli.
Other titles: Periodization training for sports
Description: Fourth Edition. | Champaign : Human Kinetics, 2022. | Third edition published: Champaign : Human Kinetics, [2015], under title Periodization training for sports. | Includes bibliographical references and index.
Identifiers: LCCN 2020038406 (print) | LCCN 2020038407 (ebook) | ISBN 9781718203082 (Paperback) | ISBN 9781718203099 (ePub) | ISBN 9781718203105 (PDF)
Subjects: LCSH: Periodization training. | Weight training.
Classification: LCC GV546 .B546 2022 (print) | LCC GV546 (ebook) | DDC 613.7--dc23
LC record available at https://lccn.loc.gov/2020038406
LC ebook record available at https://lccn.loc.gov/2020038407

ISBN: 978-1-7182-0308-2 (print)

Senior Acquisitions Editor: Roger W. Earle; **Managing Editor:** Shawn Donnelly; **Copyeditor:** Rodelinde Albrecht; **Indexer:** Kevin Campbell; **Proofreader:** Lisa Himes; **Permissions Manager:** Martha Gullo; **Graphic Designer:** Dawn Sills; **Cover Designer:** Keri Evans; **Cover Design Specialist:** Susan Rothermel Allen; **Photograph (cover):** © Human Kinetics; **Photographs (interior):** © Human Kinetics, unless otherwise noted; **Photo Asset Manager:** Laura Fitch; **Photo Production Manager:** Jason Allen; **Senior Art Manager:** Kelly Hendren; **Illustrations:** © Human Kinetics, unless otherwise noted; **Printer:** Sheridan Books

Human Kinetics books are available at special discounts for bulk purchase. Special editions or book excerpts can also be created to specification. For details, contact the Special Sales Manager at Human Kinetics.

Printed in the United States of America   10 9 8 7 6 5 4 3 2 1

The paper in this book is certified under a sustainable forestry program.

Human Kinetics
1607 N. Market Street
Champaign, IL 61820
USA

United States and International
Website: **US.HumanKinetics.com**
Email: info@hkusa.com
Phone: 1-800-747-4457

Canada
Website: **Canada.HumanKinetics.com**
Email: info@hkcanada.com

E8282

Tell us what you think!
Human Kinetics would love to hear what we can do to improve the customer experience. Use this QR code to take our brief survey.

Periodization of Strength Training for Sports

Fourth Edition

Contents

Preface

This fourth edition of *Periodization of Strength Training for Sports* is visibly and contextually different from past editions. Even the title has been changed slightly to reflect a more simplified and straightforward focus on the two major methodological elements of training for sport: *periodization* and the *science and methodology of strength training*. We felt this change was needed for two important reasons.

1. Although *periodization* as a training system has existed for almost 2,800 years—since the ancient Olympic Games (776 BC)—some contemporary training concepts are based on unclear or misleading theories and are influenced by fads and commercialized training equipment gimmicks. The result is that training programs today are often based on pseudoscience rather than on research reinforced by decades of insight and expertise.

2. Despite a strong body of scientific information and reinforced investigative findings, the *science of strength training for sports* did not make the expected inroads into the daily training programs of some coaches and fitness instructors. That is why we are sharing with you, our readers, scientific information and expertise in the methodology of strength training that will help you improve the quality of your training plans and programs, and ultimately enhance your athletes' performance. To this end, we have given particular attention to two primary scientific concepts—*neuromuscular physiology* and *Newton's laws of motion*—and added clear, relatable explanations so you can justify the use of strength training and apply the concepts to improve athletic performance. The improvement of athletic standards, from speed-power sports to long-distance sporting events, occurs only with the improvement of *sport-specific strength*.

This fourth edition is specifically designed for the strength and conditioning experts of the future and for athletes who want to invest in their own success through an improved scientific–theoretical understanding of strength training and its effective application to maximize sport performance.

We strongly suggest that you base your training decisions on *science*, not on myths, anecdotal opinions, or guessing games.

Train smart.

Acknowledgments

A book is the outcome of the work of authors who wish to share specific information and know-how calculated to attract many interested readers. Although the names of the authors are always shown on the cover, the names of the many other people responsible for the final form of a book are rarely shared with readers. As a show of respect for the contributions of these professionals, we want to share with you the names of the individuals who have been directly involved in the compilation of this book.

To complete this book, we worked together as a team, the Human Kinetics team. This team was led by Roger Earle, senior acquisitions editor, and Shawn Donnelly, managing editor. The overall content and structure of this book is the result of a persistent and patient effort by Roger over several years, and Shawn's literary talent and familiarity with the content is evident on almost every page.

We would also like to show our deepest respect for the contributions of Rodelinde Albrecht, copyeditor; Kevin Campbell, indexer; and Martha Gullo, permissions manager. Their perseverance and diligent work have significantly increased the quality of this book.

The artwork of a book often represents the vision of incredible professionals. We would like to honor the contributions of all of these individuals, including Dawn Sills, graphic designer; Keri Evans, cover designer; Susan Allen, cover design specialist; Laura Fitch, photo asset manager; Jason Allen, photo production manager; Kelly Hendren, senior art manager; and Susan Sumner, director of print production.

We dedicate this book to the coaches, instructors, trainers, health and fitness professionals, and students, in recognition of their quest to bridge the gap between science and the practice of sports training.

Part

I

Foundations of Strength Training

The stronger the foundation,
the higher the peak performance!

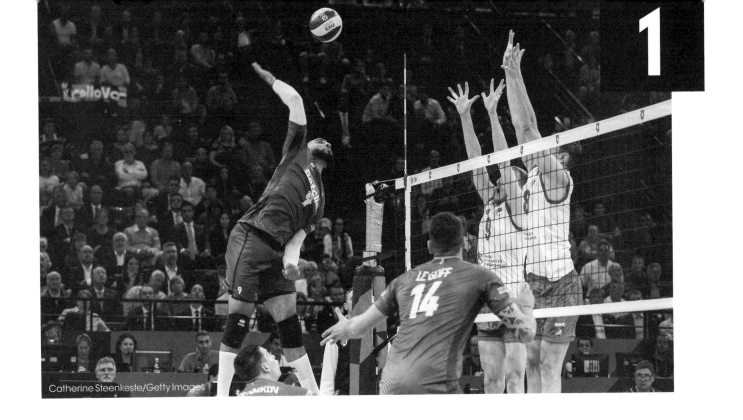

Catherine Steenkeste/Getty Images

Strength, Power, and Muscular Endurance in Sports

Most sporting activities incorporate either strength (force or F), speed (S), endurance (E), flexibility, or a combination of these. Strength exercises involve overcoming resistance (water, gravity, opponents); speed exercises maximize quickness and high frequency; endurance exercises involve long distance, long duration nonstop activity, or many repetitions; flexibility exercises maximize range of motion. Finally, coordination exercises involve complex movements.

Obviously, the ability to perform certain exercises varies from athlete to athlete, and an athlete's ability to perform at a high level is influenced by genetics: the inherited abilities in strength, speed, endurance, and flexibility. These abilities may be called conditional motor capacities, general physical qualities, or biomotor abilities. *Motor* refers to movement, and the prefix *bio* indicates the biological (bodily) nature of these abilities. The term *ability* implies the role of the nervous system, as the expression of each kind of physical performance happens with a certain degree of skill.

Success in training and competition is not determined solely by an athlete's genetic potential, however. Athletes who strive for perfection in their training—through determination and methodical planning of periodization—can reach the podium or help their team win a major tournament. Although talent is extremely important, an athlete's ability to focus on training and to relax in competition can make the difference in his or her ultimate achievement. To move beyond inherited strength or other genetic potential, an athlete must focus on physiological adaptation in training.

Strength, in our opinion, is a significant ability because it can be beneficial to increase athletic potential beyond present standards. Even in long distance, aerobic-dominant sports, such as marathon, strength can have visible benefits for a runner. Just consider that during a marathon race a runner needs approximately 55,000 strides to cover a distance of 26.2 miles (42.2 km). An athlete who follows a specific strength training for this event can apply a slightly higher force against the ground and as a result increase stride length by nearly a half inch (1 cm). With this improvement, the runner can reduce the duration of the race by 48 seconds to 2 minutes. Isn't it worth spending the time to increase the propulsion force, the push-off phase of the running step, against the gravitational force?

In other sports, especially speed-power dominant sports, athletes can visibly improve performance by applying training methods intended to increase maximum strength (MxS) and power (P).

The Aeneas Story: A Prelude to Contemporary Strength Training for Sports

Have you ever asked yourself since when strength training has been used to improve athletic performance? You will find out from the story of Aeneas. Do you remember the Aeneid, the epic story of the Trojan hero Aeneas, written by the Roman poet Virgilius Maro (Virgil, 70-19 BC)? As you may recall, Paris, the son of Priam, the king of Troy, went to visit Menelaus, the king of Sparta. During a party in honor of the Trojan visitors, Paris met Helen, Menelaus's spouse. He fell in love with her and decided to take her home to Troy. The furious Menelaus incited his fellow Greeks to invade Troy and take Helen back to Sparta. But Helen refused to return to Menelaus, so he and his compatriots decided to take her back by force. The Trojan War (1200 BC) between the Greeks and the Trojans lasted for 10 years, with no side having the chance of winning it.

Losing any desire to continue the war, the Greeks decided to return home. However, Ulysses, the trickiest Greek around, proposed leaving a gift for the Trojans: the mythical Trojan horse. After building a huge wooden horse, the Greeks retreated. During the night, a group of Greek warriors hid inside the horse. The next day, the Trojans were so happy to finally see the end of the war that they decided to bring the gift left by the Greeks into the fortress. The following night the Greek warriors came out of the horse, attacked the guards, and opened the gate for the Greek army to invade the fortress. The Trojans' confusion and chaos led to their defeat, and the fortress was destroyed forever.

Among the few survivors of the war was Aeneas, a Trojan hero. He decided to take a few warriors with him and leave for Italy. During his trip to Italy, Aeneas had to stop on some Mediterranean islands for supplies. Virgil wrote that Aeneas was welcome on every island and received supplies, but with one condition: a rowing race against the crew from the island (figure 1.1a). Here is how the Roman poet described the Trojans' daily preparation for the race:

- First, the rowers did some exercises; this is like the warm-ups we do nowadays.
- They rowed for a while; this is what we now call the main part, the most important activity, of the session.
- They lifted some stones (figure 1.1*b*); this is the strength training we now do after some training sessions.
- Finally, they had a relaxing hot bath and a massage; these are the regeneration and compensation activities after training we use today.

Amazingly, what Aeneas knew 3,200 years ago is still questioned today! Some coaches in swimming, Nordic skiing, team and racket sports, and martial arts still cannot accept and recognize the positive effect strength training has on athletic performance.

How is it possible that Aeneas—just an ordinary warrior with no knowledge of the science and methodology of training—knew 3,200 years ago that if rowers increase their strength, the force applied against the water also increases and the speed of the boat improves?

Interestingly, some of the training concepts and training plans we use now were used in simplistic form by our ancestors. How is it possible that Aeneas, without knowing Isaac Newton's third law of motion—for the simple reason that Newton (1643-1727) had not been born yet—could know that for every action there is a reaction of equal magnitude, but in the opposite direction? Aeneas had the common sense to realize that in order for the boat to travel faster, the rowers must apply greater force against water resistance, and that an athlete can overcome water resistance or the force of gravity only if he or she increases the force applied against the water resistance or the force of gravity on the terrain.

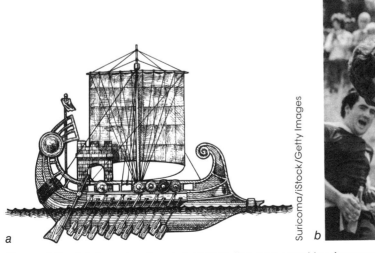

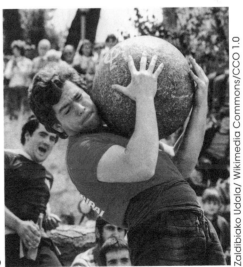

Suricoma/iStock/Getty Images

Zaldibiako Udala/ Wikimedia Commons/CCO 1.0

Figure 1.1 (*a*) A rowing boat similar to the one used by Aeneas to travel to Italy. (*b*) A man lifts a heavy stone to improve his strength, much like rowers did during the time of Aeneas.

Let us take a practical example. Speed is a highly regarded quality for soccer players and other athletes. Coaches constantly look for fast players. However, high-velocity running, swimming, and so on are possible under only two conditions:

- If the athlete has a good genetic inheritance, such as a high percentage of fast-twitch muscle fibers. The higher the number of fast-twitch fibers (say 53%), the faster the player.
- Strength training is essential for all athletes, especially for those who did not inherit a high percentage of fast-twitch muscle fibers. When an athlete improves strength, the force applied against the ground is increased and the athlete can run faster. Imagine how fast a player can be if he or she has inherited a higher number of fast-twitch muscle fibers and attempts to improve strength training in addition!

Six Strength Training Programs

Athletes and coaches in various sports use six main programs for strength training: bodybuilding, high-intensity training, weightlifting, power training throughout the year, powerlifting, and periodization of strength. Overall, periodization of strength is the most influential methodology in sport training.

Bodybuilding

The training programs used in bodybuilding manipulate training variables (such as sets, reps, rest periods, and speed of execution) to increase hypertrophy (muscle size). The increase of muscle hypertrophy is possible because of adaptations in the form of energy substrate overcompensation and muscle protein accretion. To that end, bodybuilders perform sets of 6 to 12 reps to exhaustion.

Increased muscle size is rarely beneficial, however, to athletic performance. (The few exceptions may include younger or lower-level musculature athletes, American football players—particularly linebackers—scrum players in rugby, and some performers in track-and-field throwing events.) More specifically, the slow, repetitive contractions in bodybuilding offer only limited positive transfer to the explosive athletic movements in many other sports. For instance, whereas athletic skills are performed quickly, taking from 100 to 180 milliseconds, leg extensions in bodybuilding take 600 milliseconds, and the time to catch position in weightlifting takes about 1200 milliseconds (table 1.1).

Table 1.1 Duration of Contact Phase

Event	Duration (millisec)
100 m dash (contact phase)	90-250
Long jump (takeoff)	105-150
High jump (takeoff)	150-180
Gymnastics vault (takeoff)	100-120
Time to catch position in weightlifting	1,150-1,200

Data from C.B. Tucker, A. Bissas, and S. Merlino, *Biomechanical Report for the IAAF World Indoor Championships 2018: Long Jump Men* (Birmingham, UK: International Association of Athletics Federations, 2019); G. Nicholson, T.D. Bennett, A. Bissas, and S. Merlino, *Biomechanical Report for the IAAF World Indoor Championships 2018: High Jump Men* (Birmingham, UK: International Association of Athletics Federations, 2019); and E. Hall, D.C. Bishop, and T.I. Gee, "Effect of Plyometric Training on Handspring Vault Performance and Functional Power in Youth Female Gymnasts," *PLoS ONE* 11, no. 2 (2016): e0148790, https://doi.org/10.1371/journal.pone.0148790.

There are exceptions. Selected bodybuilding techniques, such as supersets and drop sets, are used during the hypertrophy phase of training for certain sports where the main objective is to increase muscle size. Because neuromuscular adaptations are not vital to bodybuilding, however, it does not usually include explosive concentric or high loads with long rest periods. That is why bodybuilding is rarely recommended in strength training for sports.

High-Intensity Training

High-intensity training (HIT) involves using high training loads throughout the year and performing all working sets to at least positive failure. Firm believers in HIT claim that strength development can be achieved in 20 to 30 minutes; they disregard high-volume strength training for events of long, continuous duration (such as mid- and long-distance swimming, rowing, canoeing, and cross-country skiing). HIT programs are not organized according to the competition schedule. For sports, strength is periodized according to the physiological needs of the sport in a given phase of training and the date for reaching peak performance. Athletes who use HIT training often gain strength very quickly but tend to lose strength and endurance as their competitive season progresses. Furthermore, the high level of muscle soreness and neural fatigue caused by the intensification methods (such as forced reps or negative reps) used in HIT programs interferes with the more specific physical work as well as the athlete's technical or tactical work throughout his or her weekly training.

Weightlifting

Weightlifting exerted important influence in the early days of strength training. Even now, some coaches and trainers use traditional weightlifting moves (such as the clean and jerk, the snatch, and the power clean) despite the fact that they might or might not target prime movers (the actual muscles used in specific sport skills), they might not be force-vector-specific for the sport, or they do not train the elastic-reactive component of strength because they lack the stretch–shortening cycle often present in running sports. Because the prime movers, the direction of the application of force, and the presence or lack of the stretch–shortening cycle in the very sporting activity should always be considered in the design of a strength training program, coaches should closely analyze the primary movements in their sport to decide whether weightlifting exercises would be beneficial. For example, American football linemen might benefit from the lifts while rowers and swimmers would not.

In order to avoid injury, it is also essential to carefully assess the ins and outs of weightlifting techniques, especially for young athletes and those with no strength training background. Indeed, it is a time-consuming process to master weightlifting techniques, but the athlete must achieve sufficient technical proficiency to use loads that generate a training effect. In summary, although weightlifting can be a good way to improve overall body strength and power, strength and conditioning coaches must evaluate both its specificity and its efficiency.

Power Training Throughout the Year

Power training throughout the year is characterized by the use of explosive bounding exercises, medicine ball throws, and strength exercises regardless of the yearly training cycle. Some coaches and trainers, especially in track and field and certain team sports, believe that power training should be the main focus of training from the first day of preparation through the major championship. They theorize that if power is the dominant ability, it must be trained for throughout the year, except during the transition phase (the off-season).

Power capability certainly does improve by doing power training throughout the year. The key element, however, is not just whether the athlete improves but rather the athlete's rate of improvement, both throughout the year and especially from year to year. Strength training has been shown to lead to far better results than power training, in terms of improvements in sprinting and jumping capabilities, especially with athletes with a limited strength training background and even more so, at every level of athletic development, when the athletes use periodization of strength, where the emphasis of strength training changes throughout the phases of the annual training plan in an optimal sequence. For instance, because power is a function of maximum strength, improving one's power requires improving one's maximum strength. As a result, strength training results in faster power improvement and allows athletes to reach higher levels.

Powerlifting

Individuals who participate in powerlifting train to maximize their strength in the squat, bench press, and deadlift. Many powerlifting training methods have emerged in the last two decades, some of which are very specific to geared powerlifting (in which lifters wear knee wraps, a bench shirt, and squat and deadlift suits to increase their lifts).

The key point, however, is that powerlifters train to maximize one biomotor ability: strength. In contrast, an athlete usually needs to train all biomotor abilities, and more precisely their subqualities, in a sport-specific combination. As a result, a sport coach usually cannot devote the same amount of time to strength training that powerlifters do in terms of both weekly frequency and workout duration.

Furthermore, though the squat, bench press, and deadlift are the bread and butter exercises for general strength, an athlete needs to perform exercises that have a higher biomechanical correspondence to the specific motor skill, especially during the specific preparation and competitive phase. We are particularly referring to the squat stance used in powerlifting, where the feet are rotated outward and very distant from one another. For most sports, the squat stance used in powerlifting is inappropriate because the biomechanics of the application of force is very different from what happens on the field or on the track, and therefore athletes cannot maximize their potential when they use it. For example, what happens when you train the bench press with a wide grip or the squat with a wide stance, and suddenly you start using a narrower grip or stance? You are weaker than in the grip or stance that you have been training at. The neuromuscular adaptations had a higher degree of specificity to the points of application of force, body posture, and kinetic chain dynamics that happened in the trained grip or stance than in the new one. Do you go from being a very strong wide-stance squatter to a very weak narrow-stance squatter? No. You have only lost a certain percentage of maximum strength, and that explains the difference between general strength transfer and specific strength transfer, and why at a certain moment of the annual plan and also during your career as an athlete, you have to switch to more biomechanically specific exercise.

Periodization of Strength

Periodization of strength must be based on the specific physiological requirements of a given sport and, again, must result in the highest development of either power, power endurance, or muscular endurance. Furthermore, strength training must revolve around the needs of periodization for the chosen sport and employ training methods specific to a given training phase. The goal is to reach peak performance at the time of major competitions.

All periodization of strength programs begin with a general anatomical adaptation phase that prepares the body for the phases to follow. One of the goals of periodization of strength is to bring the athlete to the highest possible level of maximum strength within the annual plan so that gains in strength can be converted into gains in power, power endurance, or muscular endurance. By *highest possible*, we mean within the time constraints of the weekly training volume devoted to general physical training, and more specifically to strength training.

The planning of phases is unique to each sport and also depends on the individual athlete's physical maturity, competition schedule, and peaking dates.

The concept of periodization of strength training for sports has evolved from two basic needs:

1. To integrate strength training into the annual plan and its training phases

2. To increase sport-specific strength development from year to year

The first athletic experiment using periodization of strength was organized for Mihaela Penes, a gold medalist in the javelin throw at the 1964 Tokyo Olympic Games. The results of applying periodization of strength were presented in 1965 in Bucharest and Moscow (Bompa 1965a, 1965b).

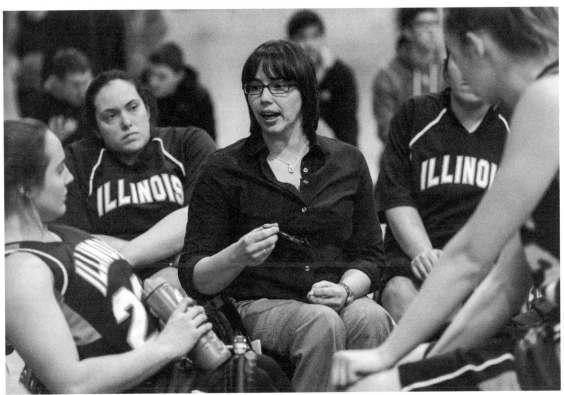

© Human Kinetics

Strength training programs must revolve around the needs of periodization for the chosen sport.

The original periodization of strength model was altered in 1968 to suit the needs of endurance sports that require muscular endurance (Bompa 1977). This current book discusses periodization of strength models, as well as training methods, for both power and endurance sports.

The basic periodization of strength model also appears in *Periodization: Theory and Methodology of Training* (Bompa 1983; Bompa 1993; Bompa 1999). In 1982, Stone et al. presented a theoretical model of strength training in which periodization of strength started with hypertrophy and included four phases: hypertrophy, basic strength, strength and power, and peaking and maintenance. A comprehensive book on periodization, *Periodization of Strength: The New Wave in Strength Training* (Bompa 1993), was followed by *Periodization Breakthrough* (Fleck and Kraemer 1996), which again demonstrated that periodization of strength is the most scientifically justified method for optimizing strength and sport performance.

The Relationships Between Strength Training and Energy Systems

If you want to improve your ability to diagnose the deficiencies of your athletes and to best organize your training, you should also consider the relationships between the dominant energy system in your sport and the type of strength training you need to use. Table 1.2 clearly illustrates that there is a physiological relationship between strength training and energy systems: the shorter the duration of an athletic activity, the more important maximum strength is.

Throughout the energy system continuum, from the phosphagen to the oxidative system, MxS is a determinant in or has an important contribution to the final performance. In the first few seconds of an athletic activity, the energy is supplied by the phosphagen energy system. For sports falling into this category (such as throwing events in track and field, weightlifting, and sprinting), MxS has to be constantly developed and improved.

For longer duration sports (oxidative system), such as rowing, Nordic skiing, and triathlon, MxS also has some importance, especially during the preparatory phase, because it improves movement economy, but it is not as determinant as in the power sports dominated by the phosphagen and glycolytic systems. Furthermore, as slow-twitch fibers increase in size, not only does MxS increase their force-generating capacity, it also provides greater surface area for capillarization and mitochondrial density.

Table 1.2   Relationships Between Strength Training and Energy Systems

Energy system	ANAEROBIC (OXYGEN INDEPENDENT)				OXIDATIVE (OXYGEN DEPENDENT)		
	Phosphagen		Glycolytic				
Duration	1-6 seconds	7-8 seconds	8-20 seconds	20-60 seconds	1-2 minutes	2-8 minutes	8-120+ minutes
Type of strength training needed	MxS P		MxS P PE	MxS P PE MES	MxS P PE MEM	MxS PE MEM	MxS (<80% of 1RM) PE MEL

Key: MxS = maximum strength; P = power; PE = power endurance; MES = muscle endurance short; MEM = muscle endurance medium; MEL = muscle endurance long

For sports where energy is supplied by the phosphagen system, MxS has an additional importance: to increase the size of fast-twitch muscle fibers and to improve motor unit recruitment ability. Finally, a strong development of MxS is also essential for other power-dominant sports (from team sports to martial arts and sprinting events in track and field), where energy is supplied by glycolytic energy system. For sports belonging to this category, MxS along with power training, contributes to improve the speed of contraction, increasing the discharge rate of muscle contraction.

Sport-Specific Combinations of Strength, Speed, and Endurance

Strength, speed, and endurance are the important physical abilities for successful athletic performance. The *dominant* ability is the one from which the sport requires a higher contribution. (For instance, endurance is the dominant ability in long-distance running.) Most sports require peak performance in at least two abilities. The interrelationships of strength, speed, and endurance create crucial physical athletic qualities. A better understanding of these relationships will help both athletes and coaches understand power and muscular endurance and plan sport-specific strength training programs.

As illustrated in figure 1.2, combining strength and endurance creates *muscular endurance*, the ability to perform many repetitions against a given resistance for a prolonged period. *Power*, the ability to perform an explosive movement in the shortest time possible, results from the integration of maximum strength and maximum speed. The combination of endurance and speed is called *speed-endurance*. *Agility* is the product of a complex combination of speed, coordination, flexibility, and power as demonstrated in gymnastics, wrestling, American football, soccer, volleyball, baseball, boxing, diving, and figure skating. *Flexibility*, or the range of motion of a joint, is very important in training. Different sports require varying degrees of flexibility to prevent injury and to promote

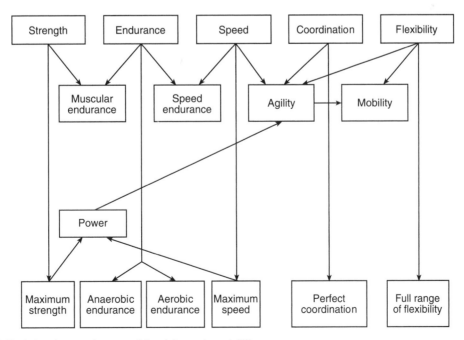

Figure 1.2 Interdependence of the biomotor abilities.

optimal sport performance. When agility and flexibility combine, the result is (field) *mobility*, the ability to cover a playing area quickly with good timing and coordination. Agility is improved through adaptations in maximum strength.

The sport-specific phase of specialized training that occurs following the initial years of training, characterized by multilateral training, is crucial for all national-level and elite athletes who aim for precise training effects. Specific exercises during this period allow athletes to adapt to their specializations. For an elite athlete, the interrelationship of strength, speed, and endurance depends on the sport and the athlete's needs.

Figure 1.3 shows three examples in which strength, speed, and endurance are dominant. In each case, when one biomotor ability dominates, the other two do not participate to a similar extent. This example, however, is pure theory and applies to few sports. In the vast majority of sports, each ability has a given input. Figure 1.4 shows the dominant composition of strength, speed, and endurance in several sports. Coaches and athletes can use figure 1.4 to determine the dominant biomotor abilities used in their sports.

Each sport has its own specific physiological profile and characteristics. Understanding the energy systems and how they apply to sport training is vital for all coaches who design and implement sport-specific training programs. Although the purpose of this book is to discuss in specific terms the science, methodology, and objectives of strength training for sports, the physiological complexity of each sport also requires a very good understanding of the energy systems dominant in that sport, and how they relate to training.

Energy required for strength and aerobic training is produced in the body through the breakdown and conversion of food into a usable form of fuel known as ATP (adenosine triphosphate). Because ATP has to be constantly replenished and reused, the body relies on three main systems of energy replenishment to facilitate ongoing training: the anaerobic alactic (ATP-CP) system, the anaerobic lactic system, and the aerobic system. The three systems are not independent of each other but collaborate based on the physiological requirements of the sport. Sport-specific program development should always be focused on training the dominant energy system of the sport.

Specific development of a biomotor ability must be methodical. A developed dominant ability directly or indirectly affects the other abilities; the extent to which it does depends strictly on the similarity between the methods employed and the specifics of the sport. Thus, development of a dominant biomotor ability may have a positive or, rarely, a negative transfer. When an athlete develops strength, they may experience a positive transfer to speed and endurance. On the other hand, a strength training program designed only to develop maximum strength may negatively affect the development of aerobic endurance. Similarly, a training program aimed exclusively at developing aerobic endurance may transfer negatively to strength and speed. *Because strength is a crucial athletic ability, it must always be trained along with the other abilities.*

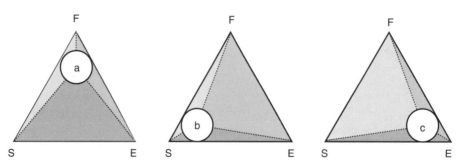

Figure 1.3 Relationships between the main biomotor abilities where *(a)* strength (F), *(b)* speed (S), or *(c)* endurance (E) is dominant.

Misleading, unfounded theories have suggested that strength training slows down athletes and affects the development of endurance and flexibility. Research discredits such theories (Atha 1984; Dudley and Fleck 1987; Hickson et al. 1988; MacDougall et al. 1985; Micheli 1988; Nelson et al. 1990; Sale et al. 1990). One study that specifically looked at cross-country skiers found that maximum strength training alone not only improved maximum strength and the rate of force development of skiers but also had a positive transfer to work economy by increasing the time to exhaustion (Hoff, Gran, and Helgerud 2002). Another study of runners and cyclists also found an improvement in both running and cycling economy and power output with the combination of endurance training and heavy resistance training (Rønnestad and Mujika 2013).

Combined strength and endurance training with sport-specific loading parameters does not affect the improvement of aerobic power or muscular strength (i.e., no negative transfer results). Similarly, strength programs pose no risk to flexibility if stretching routines are integrated into the overall training program. Endurance athletes in sports such as cycling, rowing, cross-country skiing, and canoeing can safely use strength and endurance training concurrently with their other training. The same is true for athletes in sports requiring strength and flexibility.

For speed sports, power represents a great source of speed improvement. A fast sprinter is also strong. High acceleration, fast limb movement, and high frequency are possible when strong muscles contract quickly and powerfully. In extreme situations, however, maximum loads may momentarily affect speed—for example, when speed training is scheduled after an exhausting training session with maximum loads. Fatigue at both the nervous system and the muscular level will impede the neural drive and performance.

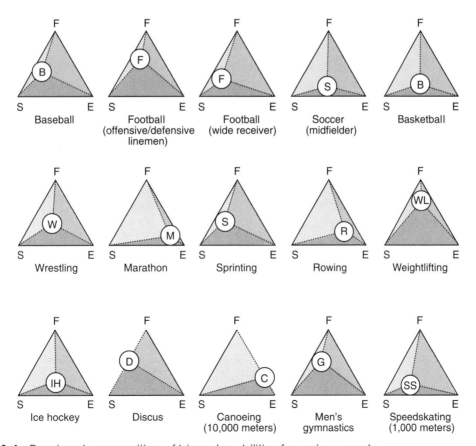

Figure 1.4 Dominant composition of biomotor abilities for various sports.

For this reason, macrocycles aimed at the development of maximum strength should include acceleration development and submaximal speed, whereas maximum speed is better developed in conjunction with power. At training unit level, speed training should always be performed before strength training.

Most actions and movements are more complex than previously discussed. Strength in sports should be viewed as the mechanism required to perform skills and athletic actions. Athletes do not develop strength just for the sake of being strong. The goal of strength development is to meet the specific needs of a given sport, to develop specific strength or combinations of strength, and to increase athletic performance to the highest possible level.

Combining force (F) and endurance (E) results in *muscular endurance* (ME). Sports may require muscular endurance of long, medium, or short duration depending on the type of strength needed.

Before discussing this topic, let's briefly clarify the terms *cyclic* and *acyclic*. *Cyclic* movements are repeated continuously, such as in running, walking, swimming, rowing, skating, cross-country skiing, cycling, and canoeing. As soon as one cycle of the motor act is learned, it can be repeated in the same sequence. *Acyclic* movements, on the other hand, constantly change and are dissimilar to most others, such as in throwing events, gymnastics, wrestling, fencing, and many technical movements in team sports.

With the exception of sprinting, cyclic sports are endurance sports. Endurance is either dominant or makes an important contribution to performance. Acyclic sports are often speed or power sports. Many sports, however, are more complex (for example, basketball, volleyball, soccer, ice hockey, wrestling, and boxing) and require speed, power, and endurance. The following analysis may refer to certain skills of a given sport and not to the sport as a whole.

Figure 1.5 analyzes various combinations of strength. The elements will be discussed in a clockwise direction starting with the F–E (force-endurance) axis. Each strength combination has an arrow pointing to a certain part of the axis between two biomotor abilities. An arrow placed closer to F indicates that strength plays a dominant role in the sport or skill. An arrow placed closer to the midpoint of the axis indicates an equal

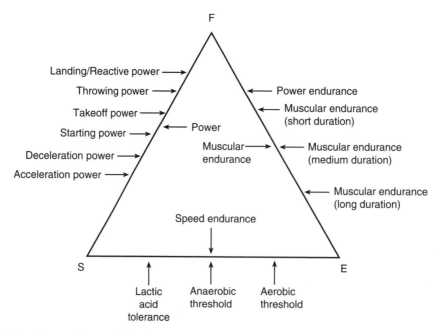

Figure 1.5 Sport-specific combinations among the dominant biomotor abilities.

or almost equal contribution of both biomotor abilities. The farther the arrow is from F, the less importance it has, suggesting that the other ability becomes more dominant. However, strength still plays a role in that sport.

The *F–E axis* refers to sports in which muscular endurance is the dominant strength combination (the inner arrow). Not all sports require equal parts of strength and endurance. For example, swimming events range from 50 to 1,500 meters. The 50-meter event is speed-endurance and power-endurance (metabolically speaking: lactic power) dominant; muscular endurance (metabolically speaking: aerobic power and capacity) becomes more important as the distance increases.

Power endurance (PE) is on top of the F–E axis because of the importance of strength in activities such as rebounding in basketball, spiking in volleyball, jumping to catch the ball in Australian football and rugby, or jumping to head the ball in soccer. All of these actions are power-dominant movements. The same is true for some skills in tennis, boxing, wrestling, and the martial arts. To perform such actions successfully throughout a game or match, athletes have to train endurance as well as power because these actions are performed 100 to 200 or more times per game or match. A basketball player must jump high to rebound a ball, but she must also duplicate such a jump 200 times per game. That is why both power and power-endurance have to be trained; however, the variables of volume and intensity are manipulated to adapt the body for repeat power performance. Nevertheless, we have to distinguish between repeated short power actions (such as in team sports) and longer lasting, continuous powerful actions (such as the 100 meters and 200 meters in track and field and the 50 meters in swimming). Both these modalities require power endurance. In intermittent sports, such as team sports, the main energy system for the powerful actions would be the alactic system but, because of short rest intervals, eventually it is the ATP production via the lactic system that predominates at certain points of the game. On the contrary, individual lactic sports rely mainly on the power of the lactic system (i.e., the ability of the lactic system to produce ATP at its maximum rate).

Muscular endurance of short duration (ME short) refers to the muscular endurance necessary for events ranging from 40 seconds to 2 minutes (a mix of lactic capacity and aerobic power). In the 100-meter swimming event, the start is a power action, as are the first 20 strokes. From the midpoint of the race to the end, muscular endurance becomes at least as important as power. In the last 30 to 40 meters, the crucial element is the ability to duplicate the force of the arms' pull to maintain velocity and increase at the finish. For events such as 100 meters in swimming, 400 meters in running, 500 to 1,000 meters in speedskating, and 500 meters in canoeing, muscular endurance strongly contributes to the final result.

Muscular endurance of medium duration (ME medium) is typical of cyclic sports two to five minutes long (aerobic power), such as 200- and 400-meter swimming, 3,000-meter speedskating, track-and-field mid-distance running, 1,000-meter canoeing, wrestling, the martial arts, figure skating, synchronized swimming, and cycling pursuit.

Muscular endurance of long duration (ME long) requires the ability to apply force against a standard resistance for a longer period (over six minutes; aerobic power to aerobic capacity) as in rowing, cross-country skiing, road cycling, long-distance running, swimming, speedskating, and canoeing.

The *speed endurance* axis (S–E) refers to the ability to maintain speed over a distance covered between 10 and 25 seconds. (50 meters in swimming, 100 and 200 meters in track and field), or repeat a high-velocity action several times per game, as in American football, baseball, basketball, rugby, soccer, and power skating in ice hockey. Athletes in these sports need to train to develop their speed-endurance.

The remaining two types of speed-endurance change in combination and proportion of speed and endurance as distance increases. For speed, sports require training velocity around the *anaerobic threshold* (4 mmol of lactate or a heart rate of approximately 170 beats per minute). For endurance, training velocity must be around the *aerobic threshold* (2 to 3 mmol of lactate or a heart rate of 125 to 140 beats per minute).

The F–S (*strength-speed*) axis refers mainly to strength-speed sports in which power is dominant.

Landing and reactive power is a major component of several sports, such as figure skating, gymnastics, and several team sports. Proper training can prevent injuries. Many athletes train only the takeoff part of a jump, with no concern for a controlled and balanced landing. The physical, or power, element plays an important role in proper landing technique, particularly for advanced athletes. Athletes must train eccentrically to be able to "stick" a landing, absorb the shock, and maintain good balance to continue the routine or perform another move immediately.

The power required to control a landing depends on the height of the jump, the athlete's body weight, and whether the landing is performed by absorbing the shock or with the joints flexed but stiff. Testing has revealed that for a shock-absorbing landing, athletes use a resistance force three to four times their body weight. Landing performed with stiff leg joints requires a force of six to eight times body weight. An athlete weighing 132 pounds (60kg) requires 180 to 528 pounds (82 to 240 kg) to absorb the shock of landing. The same athlete requires 792 to 1,056 pounds (360 to 480 kg) to land with the leg joints stiff. When an athlete lands on one leg, as in figure skating, the force at the instant of landing is three to four times body weight for a shock-absorbing landing and five to seven times for landing with stiff leg joints.

Specific power training for landing can be planned in a such a way as to gradually reach much higher tension in the muscles of the legs than specific skill training can. Through periodization of strength we can train landing power better, faster, and much more consistently, too. Higher tension means improvements in landing power. In addition, through specific power training for landing, especially eccentric training, athletes can build a power reserve that is a force greater than the power required for a correct and controlled landing. The higher the power reserve, the easier it is for the athlete to control the landing, and the safer the landing will be.

Reactive power is the ability to generate the force of jumping immediately following a landing (hence the word *reactive*; scientifically speaking this is the reduction of the coupling time—i.e., the passage from the eccentric to the concentric action). This kind of power is necessary in the martial arts, wrestling, and boxing and for quick changes in direction, as in American football, soccer, basketball, lacrosse, and tennis. The force needed for a reactive jump depends on the height of the jump and the athlete's body weight. Reactive jumps require a force equal to six to eight times body weight. Reactive jumps from a 3-foot (1 m) platform require a reactive force of eight to ten times body weight.

Throwing power refers to force applied against an implement, such as throwing a football, pitching a baseball, or throwing the javelin. The release speed is determined by the amount of muscular force exerted at the instant of release. First, athletes have to defeat the inertia of the implement, which is proportional to its mass (important only in throwing events). Then they must continuously accelerate through the range of motion so that they achieve maximum velocity at the instant of release. The force and acceleration of release depend directly on the force and speed of contraction applied against the implement.

Takeoff power is crucial in events in which athletes attempt to project the body to the highest point, either to jump over a bar as in the high jump or to reach the best height to catch a ball or spike it. The height of a jump depends directly on the vertical force applied against the ground to defeat the pull of gravity. In most cases, the vertical force performed at takeoff is at least twice the athlete's weight. The higher the jump, the more powerful the legs should be. Leg power is developed through periodized strength training, as explained in chapters 6 to 10.

Starting power is necessary for sports that require high acceleration capability to cover the space of one or two steps in the shortest time possible. Athletes must be able to generate maximum force at the beginning of a muscular contraction to create a high initial acceleration. Physiologically speaking, such ability is certainly dependent on voluntary motor unit recruitment and rate of force development (RFD). The ability to quickly overcome the inertia of the athlete's body weight depends on the athlete's relative strength (maximum strength relative to body weight) and power. Consequently, a fast start—either from a low position as in sprinting or from a tackling position in American football—depends on the power the athlete can exert at that instant and, of course, on reaction time.

Acceleration power refers to the capacity to increase speed rapidly, reaching maximum speed, usually within 6 seconds. Sprinting acceleration, just like speed, depends on the power and quickness of muscle contractions to drive the arms and legs to the highest stride frequency, the shortest contact phase when the leg reaches the ground, and the highest propulsion when the leg pushes against the ground for a powerful forward drive. Studies show that this latter characteristic (i.e., the ground reaction force during the drive phase) is the most important variable in reaching high speed (Weyand et al. 2000; Kyröläinen et al. 2001; Belli et al. 2002; Kyröläinen et al. 2005; Nummela et al. 2007; Brughelli et al. 2011; Morin 2011; Morin et al. 2012; Kawamori et al. 2013). In other words, the capacity of athletes to accelerate depends on both arm and leg force. Specific strength training for high acceleration will benefit most team sport athletes from wide receivers in American football to wingers in rugby or strikers in soccer (table 1.3).

Table 1.3   Sport-Specific Strength Development

Sport or event	Type of strength required
Athletics	
Short sprint	Reactive P, starting P, acceleration P, PE
Long sprint	Acceleration P, ME short
Middle-distance running	Acceleration P, ME medium
Distance running	ME long
Long jump	Acceleration P, takeoff P, reactive P
Triple jump	Acceleration P, reactive P, takeoff P
High jump	Takeoff P, reactive P
Throws	Throwing P, reactive P
Baseball	Throwing P, acceleration P
Basketball	Takeoff P, PE, acceleration P, deceleration P
Biathlon	ME long
Boxing	PE, reactive P, ME medium and long
Canoeing and kayaking	
500 m	ME short, acceleration P, starting P
1,000 m	ME medium, acceleration P, starting P
10,000 m	ME long

(continued)

17

Table 1.3   (continued)

Sport or event	Type of strength required
Cricket	Throwing P, acceleration P
Cycling	
Track, 200 m	Acceleration P, reactive P
4,000 m pursuit	ME medium, acceleration P
Road racing	ME long
Diving	Takeoff P, reactive P
Equestrian	ME medium
Fencing	Reactive P, PE
Field hockey	Acceleration P, deceleration P, ME medium
Figure skating	Takeoff P, landing P, PE
Football (American)	
Linemen	Starting P, reactive P
Linebackers, quarterbacks, running backs, inside receivers	Starting P, acceleration P, reactive P
Wide receivers, defensive backs, tailbacks	Acceleration P, reactive P, starting P
Football (Australian)	Acceleration P, takeoff P, landing P, ME short and medium
Gymnastics	Reactive P, takeoff P, landing P
Handball (European)	Throwing P, acceleration P, deceleration P
Ice hockey	Acceleration P, deceleration P, PE
Martial arts	Starting P, reactive P, PE
Rhythmic sportive gymnastics	Reactive P, takeoff P, ME short
Rowing	ME medium and long, starting P
Rugby	Acceleration P, starting P, ME medium
Sailing	ME long, PE
Shooting	ME long, PE
Skiing	
Alpine	Reactive P, ME short
Nordic	ME long, PE
Soccer	
Sweepers, fullbacks	Reactive P, acceleration P, deceleration P
Midfielders	Acceleration P, deceleration P, ME medium
Forwards	Acceleration P, deceleration P, reactive P
Speedskating	
Sprinting	Starting P, acceleration P, ME short
Mid-distance	ME medium, PE
Long-distance	ME long
Squash and handball	Reactive P, PE

Sport or event	Type of strength required
Swimming	
Sprinting	Starting P, acceleration P, ME short
Mid-distance	ME medium, PE
Long-distance	ME long
Synchronized swimming	ME medium, PE
Tennis	PE, reactive P, acceleration P, deceleration P
Volleyball	Reactive P, PE, throwing P
Water polo	ME medium, acceleration P, throwing P
Wrestling	PE, reactive P, ME medium

Key: ME = muscular endurance, P = power, PE = power endurance

Deceleration power is important in sports such as soccer, basketball, American football, and ice and field hockey. In these sports athletes run fast and constantly and quickly change direction. Such athletes are exploders and accelerators as well as decelerators. The dynamics of these games change abruptly: Players running fast in one direction suddenly have to change direction with the least loss of speed, and then accelerate quickly in another direction.

Acceleration and deceleration both require a great deal of leg and shoulder power. The same muscles used for acceleration (quadriceps, hamstrings, and calves) are used for deceleration, except that they *contract eccentrically*. To enhance the ability to decelerate and move in another direction quickly, athletes must train decelerating power.

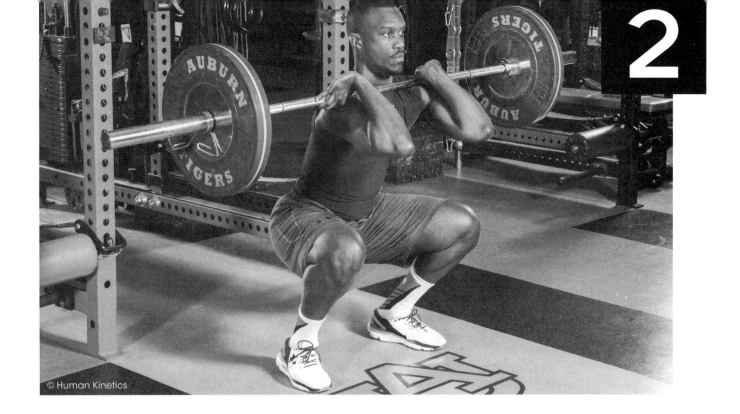
© Human Kinetics

Neuromuscular Response to Strength Training

To enhance an athlete's strength performance, coaches must understand the science behind strength training and how anatomy and physiology relate to human movement. More specifically, they need to understand muscle contraction and the sliding filament theory (discussed in this chapter) and know how the speed of contraction relates to load and why more force is exerted at the beginning of a contraction than at the end. Similarly, if they understand muscle fiber types and recognize the role played by genetic inheritance, they realize why some athletes are better than others at certain types of sporting activity (for example, speed, power, or endurance). Unfortunately, despite the value of such knowledge for effective training, many coaches (and athletes) don't read academic physiology texts or other books filled with scientific terminology. This book explains the scientific basis of strength training clearly and simply.

Understanding muscle adaptation and its dependence on load and training method makes it easier to grasp why certain types of load, exercise, or training method are preferred for some sports and not for others. Success in strength training depends on knowing the types of strength applied in athletics and how to develop them, as well as knowing the training methods best suited for a given sport. This knowledge helps both coaches and athletes understand the concept of periodization of strength faster and more easily, and improvement soon follows.

Body Structure

The human body is constructed around a skeleton. The junction of two or more bones forms a joint held together by tough bands of connective tissue called ligaments. This skeletal frame is covered by 656 muscles, which account for approximately 40% of total body weight. Both ends of the muscle are attached to the bone by dense connective tissues called tendons. Tendons direct the tension in muscles to bones: the greater the tension, the stronger the pull on the tendons and bone, and, consequently, the more powerful the limb movement.

The strength training proposed in this book consistently challenges the neuromuscular system as the load and type of training elicits physiological adaptations that generate more strength and power for sport performance. Our bodies are very pliable; they adapt to the stimuli to which they are exposed. If the proper stimulation is applied, the result is optimal physiological performance.

Muscle Structure

A muscle is a complex structure that allows movement to occur. Muscles are composed of sarcomeres, which contain a specific arrangement of contractile proteins—myosin (thick filaments) and actin (thin filaments)—whose actions are important in muscle contraction. A sarcomere is a unit of contraction in muscle fiber and is composed of the myosin and actin protein filaments.

Beyond these basics, a muscle's ability to contract and exert force depends specifically on its design, the cross-sectional area, and the length and number of fibers within the muscle. The number of fibers is genetically determined and is not affected by training; the other variables, however, can be. For example, the number and thickness of myosin filaments and the number of cross-bridges is increased by dedicated training with maximum strength (MxS) loads. Increasing the thickness of muscle filaments directly increases both the muscle's size and the force of contraction, which ultimately increase an athlete's quickness and power.

Our bodies include different types of grouped muscle fibers, with each group reporting to a single motor unit. Altogether, we have thousands of motor units, which house tens of thousands of muscle fibers. Each motor unit contains hundreds or thousands of muscle fibers that sit dormant until they are called into action. The motor unit rules over its family of fibers and directs their action by implementing the all-or-none law. This law means that when the motor unit is stimulated, the impulse sent to its muscle fibers either spreads completely—thus eliciting action by all fibers in the family—or does not spread at all.

Different motor units respond to different loads and methods in training. For instance, performing a bench press with 60% of one repetition maximum (1RM) calls up a certain family of motor units (type I and type IIA), whereas larger motor units (type IIX) are recruited with the same load only if the implement or barbell is voluntarily moved with the intention to maximally accelerate it, or if the set is taken to failure. In the latter case, fast-twitch motor units are recruited to sustain the force output, but that happens at lower discharge frequencies, in a strongly glycolytic environment, and at low angular velocities. All these characteristics of recruiting fast-twitch muscle fibers with sets taken to failure, such as for hypertrophy methods, justify the physiological conversion of the myosin heavy chain from IIX to IIA; this is the basis of the idea that strength training slows athletes down. It does so when athletes are trained like bodybuilders. When a higher load is used, such as for the MxS method, most fast-twitch muscle fibers are recruited at the start of the set. Because motor unit recruitment depends on load and methods, programs should be designed specifically to achieve activation and adaptation of the prime movers, the main muscles contracted to perform a move, and muscle fibers that dominate the chosen sport. For instance, training for short sprints and for field events (such as the shot put) should use heavy loads to facilitate the force development required to optimize speed and explosive performance.

Muscle fibers have different biochemical (metabolic) functions; specifically, some are physiologically better suited to work under anaerobic conditions whereas others work better under aerobic conditions. The fibers that rely on and use oxygen to produce energy are called aerobic, Type I, red, or slow-twitch fibers. The fibers that do not require oxygen are called anaerobic, Type II, white, or fast-twitch fibers. Fast-twitch muscle fibers are further divided into IIA and IIX (sometimes referred to as IIB, though the IIB phenotype is practically nonexistent in humans [Harrison et al. 2011]). Slow-twitch and fast-twitch fibers exist in relatively equal proportion. Depending on their function, however, certain muscle groups (e.g., hamstrings, biceps) seem to have a higher proportion of fast-twitch fibers, whereas others (e.g., the soleus) have a higher proportion of slow-twitch fibers. The characteristics of slow-twitch and fast-twitch fibers are compared in table 2.1.

These characteristics can be affected by training. Studies by the Danish researchers Andersen (2010) and Aagaard (2011) show that IIX fibers develop the characteristics of IIA fibers when subjected to a great deal of training or to training that is lactic in nature. That is, the myosin heavy chain of these fibers gets slower and more efficient at dealing with the lactic work. The change can be reversed by reducing training volume (tapering), whereupon the IIX fibers revert to their original character as the fastest-contracting fibers (Andersen and Aagaard 2000). Strength training also increases fiber size, which generates greater force production.

A fast-twitch motor unit's contraction is faster and more powerful than that of a slow-twitch motor unit. As a result, a higher proportion of fast-twitch fibers is usually found in successful athletes in speed and power sport, but they also fatigue faster. In contrast,

Table 2.1   Comparison of Fast-Twitch and Slow-Twitch Fibers

SLOW-TWITCH	FAST-TWITCH
Red, Type I, aerobic	White, Type II, anaerobic
• Slow to fatigue • Smaller nerve cell—innervates 10 to 180 muscle fibers • Develops long, continuous contractions • Used for endurance • Recruited during low- and the early part of high-intensity work	• Fast to fatigue • Large nerve cell—innervates 300 to 500 (or more) muscle fibers • Develops short, forceful contractions • Used for speed and power • Recruited only during high-intensity work

athletes with more slow-twitch fibers are more successful in endurance sports because they are able to perform work of lower intensity for a longer time.

Recruitment of muscle fibers follows the size principle, also known as *Henneman's size principle*, which states that motor units and muscle fibers are recruited in order from smallest to largest, beginning always with slow-twitch muscle fibers. If the load is of low or moderate intensity, slow-twitch muscle fibers are recruited and exercised as workhorses. If a heavy load is used, slow-twitch fibers start the contraction, but it is quickly taken over by fast-twitch fibers.

Furthermore, the recruitment of the fast and slow-twitch muscle fibers also depends on the load used in training (figure 2.1): the heavier the loads the more white muscle fibers (fast-twitch) are recruited (involved in the action) to overcome resistance.

Differences can be observed in the distribution of muscle fiber types in athletes involved in different sports. To illustrate the point, figures 2.2 and 2.3 provide a

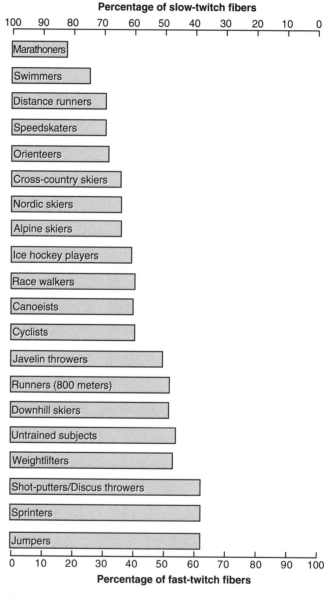

Figure 2.2 Fiber type distribution for male athletes. Note the dominance in slow-twitch fibers for athletes from aerobic-dominant sports and in fast-twitch fibers for athletes from speed- and power-dominant sports.

Data from D.L. Costill, J. Daniels, W. Evans, W. Fink, G. Krahenbuhl, and B. Saltin, "Skeletal Muscle Enzymes and Fiber Composition in Male and Female Track Athletes," *Journal of Applied Physiology* 40, no. 2 (1976): 149-154, and P.D. Gollnick, R.B. Armstrong, C.W. Saubert, K. Piehl, and B. Saltin, "Enzyme Activity and Fiber Composition in Skeletal Muscle of Untrained and Trained Men," *Journal of Applied Physiology* 33, no. 3 (1972): 312-319.

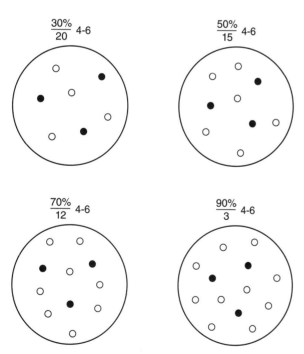

Figure 2.1 An illustration of recruitment pattern of the red and white muscle fibers for four training loads.

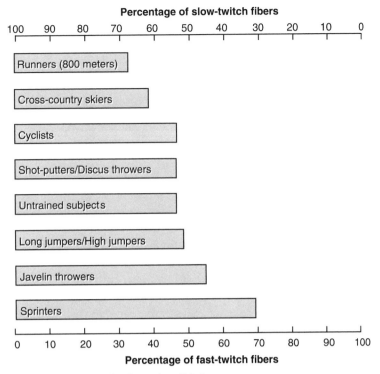

Figure 2.3 Fiber type distribution for female athletes.

Data from D.L. Costill, J. Daniels, W. Evans, W. Fink, G. Krahenbuhl, and B. Saltin, "Skeletal Muscle Enzymes and Fiber Composition in Male and Female Track Athletes," *Journal of Applied Physiology* 40, no. 2 (1976): 149-154, and P.D. Gollnick, R.B. Armstrong, C.W. Saubert, K. Piehl, and B. Saltin, "Enzyme Activity and Fiber Composition in Skeletal Muscle of Untrained and Trained Men," *Journal of Applied Physiology* 33, no. 3 (1972): 312-319.

general profile of fast- and slow-twitch fiber percentages for athletes in selected sports. For example, the drastic differences between sprinters and marathon runners clearly suggest that success in some sports is determined at least partly by an athlete's genetically established makeup of muscle fiber.

The peak power generated by athletes is also related to fiber type distribution—the higher the percentage of fast-twitch fibers, the greater the power generated by the athlete. The percentage of fast-twitch fibers also relates to speed—the greater the speed displayed by an athlete, the higher his or her percentage of fast-twitch fibers. Individuals with this natural talent should be channeled into speed-power-dominant sports such as athletics, team sport, racquet, and combat sport. Attempting to make them, say, distance runners, would be a waste of talent; they would be only moderately successful, whereas they could excel in the sports just named.

Mechanism of Muscular Contraction

Muscular contraction results from a series of events involving the protein filaments known as myosin (the thick filament) and actin (the thin filament). As illustrated by figure 2.4a, myosin filaments contain cross-bridges—tiny extensions that reach toward actin filaments. When the myosin heads reach the actins, activation of contraction begins, and the myosins and actins start binding together, initiating the muscle contraction. Activation to contract stimulates the entire fiber, creating chemical changes that allow the actin filaments to join

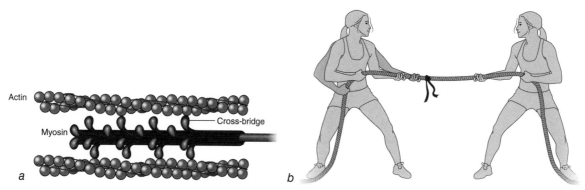

Figure 2.4 The cross-bridge theory of muscle contraction. Contractile elements of muscle. (*a*) The actin and myosin filaments and their cross-bridges. (*b*) Two athletes pulling against a rope; the athlete on the left has been exposed to MxS and as a result has a higher number of cross-bridges ("more arms" to pull).

with the myosin cross-bridges. Binding myosin to actin by way of cross-bridges releases energy, causing the cross-bridges to swivel, thus pulling or sliding the myosin filament over the actin filament. This sliding motion causes the muscle to shorten (contract), which produces force.

> The thicker the myosin filament and the higher the number of cross-bridges, the stronger the binding force (the pull). Only MxS increases the thickness of myosin and the number of cross-bridges. A stronger athlete is always more powerful, more agile, and faster.

To best visualize the cross-bridge (sliding filaments) theory and the benefits that MxS has on the increase of the number of cross-bridges, refer to figure 2.4*b*: as opposed to the athlete on the right, the athlete on the left has followed an MxS, and as a result has more cross-bridges against the rope. It is quite easy to predict the winner.

The sliding filament theory described earlier provides an overview of how muscles work to produce force. The theory involves a number of mechanisms that promote effective muscle contraction. For instance, the release of stored elastic energy and reflex adaptation are vital to optimizing athletic performance, but these adaptations occur only when the proper stimulus is applied in training. For instance, an athlete's ability to use stored elastic energy to jump higher or put the shot farther is optimized through explosive movements, such as those used in power training (medicine ball throws, plyometric).

> As an essential element to produce force, muscle contraction occurs
>
> - when there is a neural stimulation (electrical impulse),
> - when the muscle fibers are stimulated and calcium (Ca) is released into the muscle cell, allowing myosins and actins to bind (the myosin cross-bridges pull against the actin to initiate the contraction), and
> - when energy (ATP) is available to sustain work (the contraction itself).

However, the contractile part of the muscle (muscle fibers) is unable to effectively transfer energy to the movement unless the athlete strengthens the collagen structures, too, such as ligaments and tendons. For this reason, if the body is to withstand the forces and impacts that the athlete must undergo in order to optimize the muscles' elastic properties, anatomical adaptation must precede power training.

A reflex is an involuntary muscle contraction brought about by an external stimulus (Latash 1998). Two main components of reflex control are the muscle spindles and the Golgi tendon organ. Muscle spindles (stretch receptors that detect changes in the length of the muscle, such as during a contraction) respond to the magnitude and rapidity of a muscle stretch (Brooks, Fahey, and White 1996) whereas the Golgi tendon organ (stretch receptors that detect changes in the muscle found within the muscle–tendon junction [Latash 1998]) responds to muscle tension. When a high degree of tension or stretch develops in the muscles, the muscle spindles and the Golgi tendon organ involuntarily relax (inhibitory action) the muscle to protect it from harm and injury.

When these inhibitory responses are curtailed, athletic performance is increased. The only way to do so is to adapt the body to withstand greater degrees of tension, which increases the threshold for the activation of the reflexes. This adaptation can be achieved through maximum strength training that uses progressively heavier loads (up to 90% of 1RM or even more), thus causing the neuromuscular system to withstand higher tensions by consistently recruiting a greater number of fast-twitch muscle fibers. The fast-twitch muscle fibers become equipped with more protein, which aids in cross-bridge cycling and force production for the athlete's needs.

All sporting movements follow a motor pattern known as the

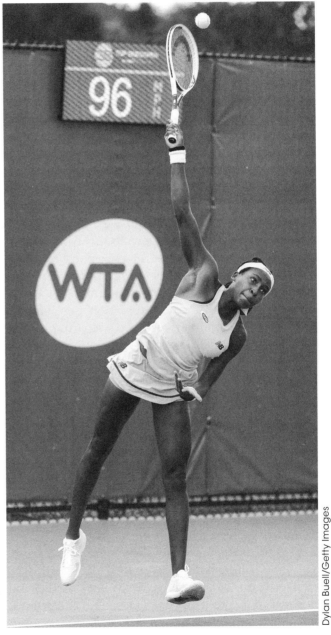

Dylan Buell/Getty Images

The peak of power generated by an athlete depends also on her muscle fibers' makeup: the more fast-twitch fibers, the more power.

stretch–shortening cycle, which is characterized by three main types of contraction: eccentric (lengthening), isometric (static), and concentric (shortening). For example, a volleyball player who quickly squats only to jump and block a spike has completed a stretch–shortening cycle. The same is true for an athlete who lowers the barbell to the chest and rapidly explodes by extending the arms. To fully use the physiological assets of a stretch–shortening cycle, the muscle must change quickly from a lengthening to a shortening contraction (Schmidtbleicher 1992).

Muscular potential is optimized when all the intricate factors that affect the stretch–shortening cycle are called into action. Their influence can be used to enhance performance only when the neuromuscular system is strategically stimulated in the appropriate sequence. Toward this end, periodization of strength builds the planning of phases on the ergogenesis (physiological makeup of the chosen sport, such as the proportion of the energy system's contribution to final performance). Once the ergogenesis is outlined, the phases of training are planned in a sequential, stepwise approach to transfer positive neuromuscular adaptations to practical hands-on human performance. Understanding applied human physiology, and a snapshot goal for each phase, helps coaches and athletes integrate physiological principles into sport-specific training.

To reiterate, the musculoskeletal frame of the body is an arrangement of bones attached to one another by ligaments at the joints. The muscles crossing these joints provide the force for body movements. Skeletal muscles do not, however, contract independently of one another. Rather, several muscles, each of which plays a different role, as discussed in the following paragraphs, produce the movements performed around a joint. Agonists, or synergists, are muscles that cooperate to perform a movement. During movement, antagonists act in opposition to agonists. In most cases, especially in skilled and experienced athletes, antagonists relax, allowing easy motion. Because athletic movements are directly influenced by the interaction between agonist and antagonist muscle groups, improper interaction between the two groups may result in motion that is jerky or rigid. The smoothness of a muscular contraction can be improved by focusing on relaxing the antagonists. Use technical training to teach athletes how and when to relax or contract a given muscle group to perform a smooth technical skill.

For this reason, co-contraction (the simultaneous activation of agonist and antagonist muscle to stabilize a joint) is advisable only during the early phases of rehabilitation from an injury. A healthy athlete, on the other hand, especially one in a power sport, should not perform exercises (such as those on unstable surfaces, balance boards, etc.) to elicit co-contractions. For instance, one distinct characteristic of elite sprinters is very low myoelectrical activity of the antagonist muscles in each phase of the stride cycle (Wysotchin 1976; Wiemann and Tidow 1995).

Prime movers are muscles primarily responsible for producing a joint action that is part of a comprehensive strength movement or a technical skill. For example, during an elbow flexion (biceps curl), the prime mover is the biceps muscle, whereas the triceps acts as an antagonist and should be relaxed to facilitate smoother action. In addition, stabilizers, or fixators, which are usually smaller muscles, contract isometrically to anchor a bone so that the prime movers have a firm base from which to pull. The muscles of other limbs may come into play as well, acting as stabilizers so that the prime movers can perform their motion. For instance, when a judoka pulls the opponent toward himself and is holding him, the back, legs, and abdomen muscles are contracted isometrically to provide a stable base for the action of the elbow flexors (biceps), shoulder extensors (rear deltoids), and scapular adductors and depressors (trapezius and latissimus dorsi).

Types of Strength and Their Training Significance

Training can involve various types of strength, each of which is significant for certain sports and athletes. We can distinguish types of strength in terms of the qualities of strength, the force–time curve, the type of muscle action, the athlete's body weight, and the degree of specificity.

Strength: Its Qualities

The desired effect of a strength training method always falls into one of the following three categories or qualities: maximum strength, power, and muscular endurance.

Maximum Strength

Maximum strength (MxS) is the highest force that can be exerted by the neuromuscular system during a contraction. This quality is increased through a combination of structural adaptation (hypertrophy) and, mostly, neural adaptation (mainly in the form of improved intermuscular and intramuscular coordination). Maximum strength refers to the heaviest load that an athlete can lift in one attempt and is expressed as 100% of maximum or one repetition maximum (1RM). For training purposes, athletes must know their maximum strength for the most important (fundamental) exercises (prime movers) because it provides the basis for calculating loads for almost every strength phase.

Power

Power is the rate of doing work, or force $\times$ velocity ($P = F \times V$); it is measured in watts. In sport training, power is the product of two abilities—strength and speed—and is itself the ability to apply the highest force in the shortest time. Although the scientific term is power, some authors incorrectly use the term speed-strength. Unlike powerlifting, in which the athlete expresses (maximum) strength without time limitation, athletes in all other sports face time constraints in applying as much force as possible. Examples include foot strikes (the force applied against the ground to overcome the force of gravity) by running athletes in individual and team sport, punches and kicks in combat sport, and bat swings and ball throws in baseball. Power is trained by using methods that enhance quick expression of force, thus improving either by recruiting more motor units or the firing rate of the active motor units. Power can be maximized only by using its specific methods following a maximum strength phase of training.

Muscular Endurance

Muscular endurance is a muscle's ability to sustain work for a prolonged period. Most sports involve an endurance component, and muscular endurance methods train both the neural and the metabolic aspects specific to a sport. We distinguish four types of sport-specific muscle endurance methods:

1. power-endurance (glycolytic power): 10 to 15 seconds
2. muscle-endurance short, or glycolytic capacity: 30 seconds to 2 minutes, often with incomplete rest
3. muscle-endurance medium, or aerobic power: 2 to 8 minutes
4. muscle-endurance long: 8 to 60 minutes, or longer

Strength: Force-Time Curve

If we analyze a force–time curve (figure 2.5), we can distinguish the following types of strength: starting strength, explosive strength (rate of force development), power (starting strength plus explosive strength), and maximum strength.

Starting Strength

Starting strength is expressed at the start of a concentric action and is usually measured at 50 milliseconds. Its level depends on the ability to voluntarily recruit as many motor units as possible (i.e., intramuscular coordination) at the beginning of the movement.

Explosive Strength or Rate of Force Development

Explosive strength is the rate at which force increases at the beginning of the concentric action. Its level depends on the ability to either recruit more motor units or increase the firing rate of the active units to increase force output.

Power

Taken together, starting strength and explosive strength represent power, or, according to other authors, "speed-strength." A high level of power is usually needed to excel in sports due to the limited time available for force application in sport actions.

Maximum Strength

Maximum strength is the maximum amount of force that an athlete can produce in a movement.

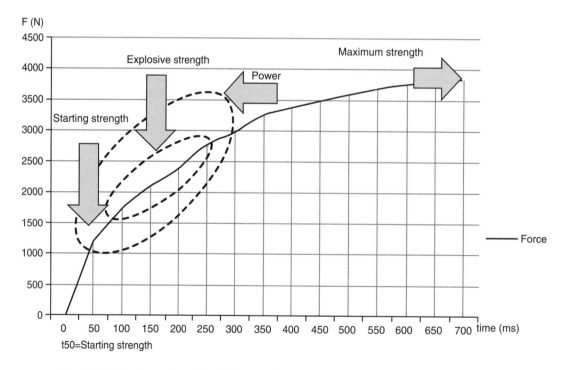

(f2-f1)/(t2-t1)=Explosive strength (or RFD, rate of force development) in N/ms

Figure 2.5 Force–time curve.

Strength: Muscle Action

We can distinguish three types of strength according to muscle action: concentric, isometric, and eccentric.

Concentric Strength

In a concentric action, the muscle creates tension while it shortens, thus creating movement in a joint. Maximum strength is normally measured as the highest load that can be lifted concentrically in one attempt (one repetition maximum, or 1RM), either preceded or followed by an eccentric action. For concentric force, 1RM represent 100% of once-maximum capacity.

Isometric Strength

In an isometric action, a muscle creates tension without shortening or lengthening; this happens either when the force generated equals the external resistance or when the external resistance is immovable. A high incidence of isometric actions by the prime movers is required in many motor sports, as well as in BMX, sailing, and combat sport. The need for such actions must be reflected in the athlete's strength training program. Isometric strength can be up to 20% higher than concentric strength. Unlike other strength-related actions, isometric contraction is assessed as time under tension, or the duration in seconds and minutes of isometric contractions.

Eccentric Strength

In an eccentric action, a muscle creates less tension than the external resistance, and so the muscle lengthens. A high level of eccentric strength is advisable for sports that require jumping, sprinting, and changing direction. Eccentric strength can be up to 40% higher than concentric strength (figure 2.6). For instance, if 1RM for a concentric contraction is 220 lb (100 kg), the same athlete can use up to 140% (310 lb [140 kg]) for an eccentric contraction.

Type of strength	Power									
		Cyclic		Acyclic						
		Muscle endurance								
			Cyclic		Acyclic					
Load	Low					Medium		Heavy	Max-imum	Super-maximum
Type of contraction	Concentric									Eccentric
% of Load	10　20	30　40	50　60	70	80	90　100	110	>120	130	
Number of repetitions	100-150	80-100　40-50	20-25　12-15	8-10	4-6	3-4	2-3	1		

Figure 2.6 Eccentric strength, which is advisable in sports that require jumping, sprinting, and changing direction, can be up to 40% higher than concentric strength.

Strength: Relation to Body Weight

Maximum strength training methods elicit both neural and muscular adaptations. As described in the following chapters, the loading parameters can be manipulated in such a way as to increase either the athlete's body weight and strength or only the athlete's strength while maintaining body weight. For this reason, we distinguish two types of strength: absolute and relative.

Absolute Strength

Absolute strength is an athlete's capacity to exert maximum force regardless of body weight. A high level of absolute strength is required in order to excel in some sports—for example, linemen in American football and rugby, most throwing events in track and field, and the heaviest weight categories in weightlifting and wrestling. Increases in strength parallel gains in body weight for those athletes who follow a training program aimed at increasing absolute strength.

Relative Strength

Relative strength is the ratio between maximum strength and body weight. A high level of relative strength is important in gymnastics, combat sport in which athletes are divided into weight categories (such as wrestling, boxing, judo, Brazilian jiu-jitsu, and mixed martial arts), team sport that requires frequent changes of direction, and track-and-field sprints and jumps. For instance, a gymnast may be unable to perform the iron cross on the rings unless the relative strength of the muscles involved is at least one to one; in other words, the absolute strength must be at least sufficient to offset the athlete's body weight. Of course, the ratio is changed by a gain in body weight—as body weight increases, relative strength decreases, unless strength increases accordingly. For this reason, the training programs aimed at increasing relative strength do so by eliciting the neural adaptations to strength training rather than by increasing muscle size and overall body weight.

Strength: Degree of Specificity

We distinguish two types of strength according to the degree of sport-specific biomechanical and physiological similarity of the training means and methods employed in a program: general strength and specific strength.

General Strength

General strength is the foundation of the entire strength training program and should be the main focus in the first years of sport training. Low general strength may limit the athlete's overall progress. It leaves the body susceptible to injury and potentially even asymmetrical shape or decreased ability to build muscle strength, as well as lower capacity for developing sport-specific skills.

Contributors to the development of an athlete's general strength include anatomical adaptation, hypertrophy, and maximum strength macrocycles. Anatomical adaptation is devoted to development of overall core strength, along with muscle balance and injury prevention through tendon reinforcement. As the name implies, anatomical adaptation prepares the body for the more difficult phases that follow. General strength is further increased through the structural changes elicited by hypertrophy macrocycles and the neural adaptations that result from maximum strength macrocycles.

Specific Strength

Specific strength training takes into account the characteristics of the sport, such as the ergogenesis (energy systems contributions), the planes of movement, the prime movers, the joints' range of motion, and the muscles' actions. As the term suggests, this type of strength is specific to each sport and requires a good deal of analysis. Therefore, it is incorrect to compare the strength levels of athletes involved in different sports. Specific strength training should be incorporated progressively, starting at the end of the preparatory phase, for all advanced athletes.

Strength Reserve

Strength reserve is the difference between maximum strength and the strength required to perform a skill under competitive conditions. For example, one study using strength-gauged techniques measured rowers' mean force per stroke during a race, which was 123 lb (56 kg) (Bompa, Hebbelinck, and Van Gheluwe 1978). The same subjects were found to have absolute strength in power-clean lifts of 198 lb (90 kg). Subtracting the mean strength per race (123 lb [56 kg]) from absolute strength (198 lb [90 kg]) indicates a strength reserve of 75 lb (34 kg). In other words, the ratio of mean strength to absolute strength is about 1:1.6.

Other subjects in the same study were found to have a higher strength reserve and a ratio of 1:1.85. Needless to say, these subjects performed better in rowing races, which supports the conclusion that an athlete with a higher strength reserve is capable of performing at a higher level. Therefore, in order to prevent a negative transfer, a strength and conditioning coach should aim to help athletes reach the highest possible level of maximum strength during the weekly time devoted to strength training in a rational ratio with more sport-specific sessions. Strength reserve is essential in sports such as throwing events and sports in which force is applied against resistance, such as swimming, canoeing, maximum velocity sports, and so on.

Strength Training and Neuromuscular Adaptations

Systematic strength training produces structural and functional changes, or adaptations, in the body. The level of adaptation is evidenced by the size and strength of the muscles. The magnitude of these adaptations is directly proportional to the demands placed on the body by the volume (quantity), intensity (load), and frequency of training, as well as to the body's capability to adapt to such demands. Training rationally adapts to the stress of increasing physical work. In other words, if the body is exposed to a demand rationally greater than it is accustomed to and enough recovery time is given to the trained physiological systems, it adapts to the stressor by becoming stronger.

Until a few years ago, we believed that strength was determined mainly by the muscles' cross-sectional area (CSA). As a result, weight training was used to increase "engine size"—that is, to produce muscular hypertrophy. However, though CSA is the single best predictor of an individual's strength (Lamb 1984), strength training research since the 1980s (and authors such as Zatsiorsky and Bompa) have shifted the focus to the neural component of strength expression. In fact, the primary role of the nervous system in strength expression was well documented by a 2001 review (Broughton).

Neural adaptations to strength training involve disinhibition of inhibitory mechanisms as well as intra- and intermuscular coordination improvements. Disinhibition affects the following mechanisms:

- Golgi tendon organ—sensory receptors, located near the myotendinous junction, that elicit a reflex inhibition of the muscle they supply when it undergoes excessive tension, either by shortening or passive stretching

- Renshaw cells—inhibitory connecting neurons (interneurons) found in the spinal cord, whose role is to dampen the rate of discharge of alpha motor neurons, thus preventing the muscular damage derived from tetanic contraction

- Supraspinal inhibitory signals—conscious or unconscious inhibitory signals that come from the brain

The components of intramuscular coordination are determinant factors for the improvement of strength, such as:

- Synchronization—the capacity to contract motor units simultaneously or with a minimum latency (that is, with a delay less than five milliseconds). Although motor units' synchronization has a minimal influence on the maximum force exerted by muscles, it is important in the rapid expression of force (RFD, rate of force development).

- Recruitment—the capacity to recruit motor units simultaneously is important in speed-power sports and can be induced or improved only via MxS. Therefore, MxS is the determinant ingredient in the achievement of the neuromuscular potential and, ultimately, to reach peak performance.

- Rate coding—or discharge rate, refers to the capacity to increase firing rate (motor unit discharge rate) in order to express more strength. Force produced by a muscle depends on the rate at which motor neurons are discharged. Discharge rate ranges from a minimal of 5 to 8 pulses per second (pps) to a maximal of 20 to 60 pps or higher (Enoka 2015). Higher force capabilities result in higher rates.

Adaptations in intramuscular coordination transfer well from one exercise to another, as long as the specific motor pattern is established (intermuscular coordination). For instance, the maximum voluntary recruitment of motor units developed through maximum strength training can be transferred to a sport-specific exercise skill as long as the athlete knows its technique. The objective of maximum strength macrocycles is to improve motor unit recruitment of the prime movers, whereas power macrocycles work mainly on quickness of discharge, or rate coding. Contrary to popular belief, these two aspects of intramuscular coordination—recruitment and rate coding—play greater determinant roles than synchronization does in muscular force production.

Intermuscular coordination, the capacity of the muscles to learn to work together, on the other hand, is the capacity of the nervous system to coordinate the links of the kinetic chain, thus making the action more efficient. With time, as the nervous system learns the action, fewer motor units get activated by the same weight, which leaves more motor units available for activation by higher weights (see figure 2.7). Therefore, to increase the weight lifted in a given exercise over the long term, intermuscular coordination training (technique training) is key.

Despite the fact that the hypertrophic response to training is immediate (Ploutz et al. 1994), the accretion (growth) of muscular protein becomes evident only after six weeks or more (Moritani and deVries 1979; Rasmussen and Phillips 2003). These proteins, which represent the specific adaptive response to the imposed training, stabilize the achieved neural adaptations. This is the way to read the famous study by Sale (1986) because the neural adaptations, once they take place, are neither at their full potential nor absolutely stable. Therefore, to increase strength over time, one must keep training the factors discussed here (figure 2.8). This is particularly true of intermuscular coordination, which

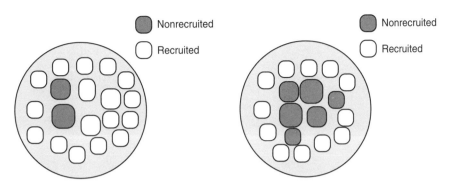

Figure 2.7 Over time, strength training for intermuscular coordination reduces the motor unit activation necessary to lift the same load, leaving more motor units available for higher loads.

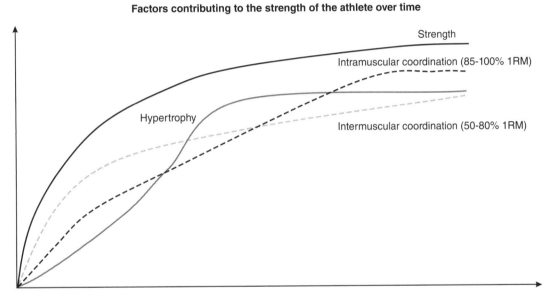

Figure 2.8 Factors contributing to the strength of the athlete over time.

allows load increase in the midterm and the long term on the basis of ever-increasing system efficiency, as well as specific hypertrophy.

When it comes to designing a maximum strength training program, the information related to weightlifting and powerlifting should be analyzed and applied with some caution. For instance, while weightlifters train daily, often several times per day, some 6,000 to 9,000 hours per year, athletes from other sports may dedicate only 15% to 20% of the time to train for MxS. Different sports have different goals and different methods of training. During this time, athletes from various sports have to improve MxS in a progressive manner, mostly using intensities 3, 2, and 1, in that order. Most athletes have to improve MxS in a much shorter time and number of sessions, which might call for a higher average work intensity. This is why you should be circumspect in applying training methods from weightlifting and powerlifting.

The field has shown us that the majority of adaptations of the neuromuscular system necessary to increase maximum strength involve loads of 80% to 95% of 1RM, and the time of exposure to loads of 90% or higher (necessary in order to elicit adaptations specific to that intensity range) should be very short.

Table 2.2   Neural Adaptations According to Strength Training Zones

Adaptations	INTENSITY ZONES (% OF 1RM)				
	5	4	3	2	1
Intramuscular coordination:	40-60	60-70	70-80	80-90	90-100
• Synchronization	****	***	***	***	****
• Recruitment	**	***	****	****	****
• Rate coding	****	***	***	***	****
Intermuscular coordination	****	***	***	**	*
Disinhibition of inhibitory mechanisms	*	**	***	****	****
Specific hypertrophy	*	**	****	***	**

Adaptation stimulus: **** = very high; *** = high; ** = medium; * = low

All loads are supposed to be moved with the most explosive (and technically correct) concentric action that the load allows.

Table 2.2 summarizes the neuromuscular adaptations for each intensity range. From this table, we learn that

- the majority of intramuscular coordination gains involve loads over 80%,
- the majority of intermuscular coordination gains involve loads under 80%, and
- we need to use the full spectrum of intensities to maximize neuromuscular adaptations and, consequently, maximum strength.

Taking into consideration the training methodology, we can infer the following points from this table.

- In a preparation phase with limited time for development of maximum strength, the average intensities used in the maximum strength macrocycles will be higher (80%-85% of 1RM). This approach is usually taken in team sports.
- In the preparation phase for an individual sport with ample time for development of maximum strength—and especially when a multiyear perspective projects continuous progression in the midterm and long term—the periodized strength plan will focus mostly on intermuscular coordination. Thus, the average, not the peak, intensities used in maximum strength macrocycles will be lower (70%-80% of 1RM).
- Nevertheless, for the development of maximum strength, every periodized plan starts with lower intensities, higher times under tension per set (which favor the anatomical adaptations), and a focus on technique so that higher intensities will elicit high muscular tension later on.

Neuromuscular Strategy to Improve Athletic Performance

The human body—in our context, the neuromuscular system—for speed-power sports, is trained, modeled to behave, and to react in a certain way, according to the training program planned by the coach. The agents that make the neuromuscular system react in a desired way is the training method used by a coach and the planning of these methods as per the specific requirements of the training phase of the annual plan. The entire training program of an annual plan is created with the scope of reaching maximum per-

Table 2.3 The Neuromuscular Strategy for Speed-Power Sports

Training phase	Preparatory			Competitive	Transition
Neuromuscular strategy	Adaptation	Increase recruitment of FT fibers	Increase discharge rate of FT fibers	Maintain the ability to recruit or discharge FT fibers	Recovery or regeneration Balance development
Training methods	AA	MxS	P/A	Maintain MxS	AA

Key: AA = anatomical adaptation, FT = fast-twitch, MxS = maximum strength, P/A = power and agility

formance at the time of the main competitions of the year, or, in the case of team sport, during the league games or international championships (table 2.3). In order to achieve this goal, periodization of strength for speed-power sports has to be composed of two physiological phases:

1. increasing the recruitment of fast-twitch muscle fibers via a maximum strength (MxS), and

2. increasing the discharge rate prior to the start of the main competitions by using the best methods to induce the development of power, maximum speed, agility, and quickness.

In the first phase, the goal can be achieved via a minimum, preferably six or more weeks of MxS training. As already discussed, MxS using loads of 80% to 90% of 1RM results in increasing the recruitment capabilities of the prime movers to involve the highest number of fast-twitch muscle fibers in action. These capabilities will translate into exerting the highest force possible to overcome resistance or to defeat the resistance of an opponent, water resistance, or the weight of an implement. Increased capabilities of recruiting a high number of fast-twitch muscle fibers facilitate the success of the second phase.

The transformation of muscle activation into muscle force is known as excitation-contraction coupling (Enoka 2015), where the interaction of actin and myosin muscle filaments and the work done by cross-bridges are determinant. A high discharge rate is quite impossible without first increasing the recruitment of fast-twitch fibers via MxS. This is why the periodization plans discussed in this book follow this physiological sequence: MxS, followed by power, speed, agility, and quickness.

In the second phase, power training, maximum velocity drills, and agility training (exercises and courses) train the neuromuscular system to increase the discharge rate, the ability to display fast and powerful or explosive actions that results in peak physiological capabilities at the time of the main competitions of the year.

The neuromuscular strategy is an essential part of the periodization of strength, the determinant two phases for achieving peak performance. Without the use of the neuromuscular strategy it is impossible to reach high performance.

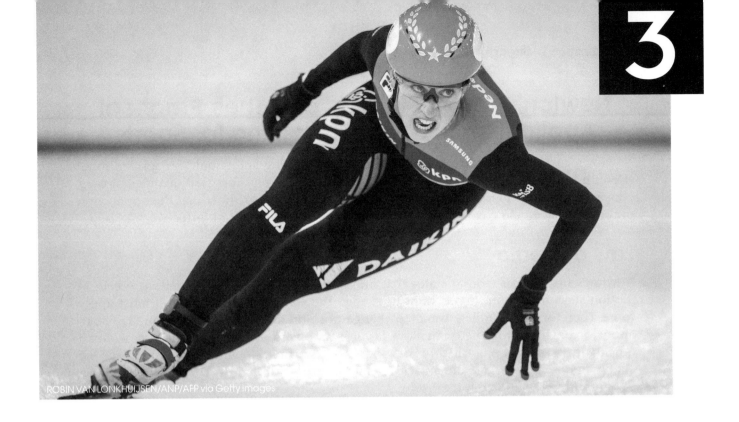

Laws and Principles of Strength Training for Sports

Proper application of scientific training laws and methodological principles can ensure superior organization of training with the fewest possible errors. The following laws and principles of strength training form the proper foundation for all strength training programs. These laws and principles are based on the laws of physics and how they are applied in sports training, whereas the methodological principles outline the practical application in strength training programs. A house is only as strong as its foundation. Both laws and principles can be applied together to produce a strong, flexible, and stable athlete who can sustain the vigor required in athletic competitions. The principles of training can ensure a steady and specific increase in strength and other abilities by specifically adapting the program to the needs of the athletes and the sport and, most important, to the physical capacity of the individual athlete.

Newton's Laws of Motion and Their Practical Application in Strength Training for Sports

Newton's laws of motion are essential to strength training and should be applied in all strength training programs for athletes, regardless of the physiological qualities of their chosen sport. We will discuss each law in a practical sense to show that the application of these laws can effectively help the athlete become stronger and faster.

Law of Inertia

Newton's first law of motion states that an object at rest stays at rest and an object in motion stays in motion. If you want to change the status of the object you must apply force. Therefore, if an athlete wants to change position from rest or in motion, he has to apply force. The same athlete can move faster by applying concentric force or slow down quickly by applying eccentric force. In both cases, starting, slowing down into a stop, or changing direction (accelerate and deceleration) are possible if force is applied against the ground (gravitational force).

More importantly, increasing acceleration or its tempo is possible only when the athlete can apply additional force. Gains in strength will always result in the capacity to increase or decrease velocity. An athlete's mass (weight) dictates the amount of force necessary to change his status: lower force for lighter athletes and higher force for heavier athletes.

Some coaches and athletes (e.g., in swimming or Nordic skiing) think strength is not needed for their sport. We strongly challenge that view. Uneducated opinions cannot stand or oppose the laws of physics.

- If you want to be faster, apply superior force against the ground.
- If you want to throw an object farther, improve your throwing force.
- If you want to defeat an opponent in combat sport, improve your strength.

Law of Acceleration

Newton's second law of motion relates to the rate of changing velocity known as *acceleration*. A constant force always produces a constant acceleration. To increase acceleration, the athlete has to increase the propulsion force exerted against the ground.

$$F = m \times a$$

Force is equal to the product of mass (m) and acceleration (a). An athlete can accelerate proportionally to the force applied against resistance. Gravity, air resistance (friction), the opponent, and the environment—such as water or terrain profile (in Nordic skiing, mountain biking, or BMX)—are some of the forces that must be overcome in order to achieve high velocity. An athlete can accelerate his mass proportional to his force, that is, to how much force he can apply against resistance. Consider the following conditions (Burkett 2018).

- If two sprinters apply same propulsion force (push-off against the ground) for the same duration, the lighter athlete can accelerate more.
- If two sprinters have the same mass, the athlete who applies more force within the same period will accelerate more.

Acceleration is measured in meters per second squared (m/s²). But when mass is also part of the equation, the final product is measured in N (Newtons). Therefore, for a sprinter with a mass of 100 kg who accelerates at 10 m/s² (i.e., gravity):

$$100 \text{ kg} \times 10 \text{ m/s}^2 = 1,000 \text{ N}$$

To overcome the resistance an athlete always encounters, he has to increase his own force and, ultimately, be able to increase acceleration.

Remember: The ability to accelerate is always proportional to the force the athlete applies against resistance. If you want to be faster, you must increase your force. There is no other way. Listen to science, not to modern gurus. Coaches cannot expect improvement of speed, acceleration, or change of direction without first improving strength, especially MxS.

Impulse, a concept derived from Newton's second law of motion, refers to a sudden transmission of force in the shortest period upon an athletic implement, such as a tennis or soccer ball, or against an opponent in contact sport. The impulse can change the state of an object (i.e., batting in baseball or serving in tennis), depending on the athlete's strength. The force of an impulse is proportional to the force of the athlete delivering it. Once again, the strength of an athlete depends directly on the quality of his training, particularly upon his MxS and power. If athletes involved in a racquet, contact, or team sport desire to improve their quality of game or match, they need to improve their strength and power. The stronger the impulse, the higher the speed achieved or the distance covered by the ball.

Law of Action-Reaction

Newton's third law of motion can be described this way: For an athlete to start a race, he has to apply force against starting blocks and gravity. The greater the athlete's force, the easier it is to overcome resistance (gravity). When force is applied against starting blocks there is a reaction of equal force but in the opposite direction.

For sports performed in or on water—such as swimming, synchronized swimming, water polo, rowing, cycling, kayaking, and canoeing—the body or the boat moves forward as a result of force. As force is applied against the water, the water exerts an equal and opposite force on the body or the boat; this is known as *drag*. As the boat or the swimmer moves through the water, the drag slows the forward motion or glide. To overcome drag, athletes must produce equal force to maintain speed and superior force to increase speed.

The equation

$$D \sim V^2$$

means that drag (D) is proportional to the square of velocity (V²). This equation is not only easier to understand but also easier to apply.

In water sports, velocity increases when an athlete applies force against the water. As force increases, the body moves faster, but as velocity increases, drag increases proportionally to the square of velocity. For example, assume that an athlete swims or rows at 2 meters (about 6.5 feet) per second:

$$D \sim V^2 = 2^2 = 4 \text{ kilograms (8.8 lb)}$$

In other words, the athlete pulls with a force of 4 kg (8.8 lb) per stroke. To be more competitive, the athlete has to swim or row faster—say, at 3 m (9.8 ft) per second:

$$D \sim V^2 = 3^2 = 9 \text{ kilograms (19.8 lb)}$$

For an even higher velocity, an athlete has to increase force by another 4 kg (8.8 lb) while drag increases to 16 kilograms (35 lb).

In order to pull with increased force, of course, one must increase MxS, because a body cannot generate increased velocity without increasing the force per stroke unit. The training implications are obvious: Not only must the athlete increase maximum strength, but the coach must also make sure that the athlete exerts almost the same force on all strokes for the duration of the race, because all water sports have a strong endurance component. This means that training must include both a phase addressing maximum strength and a phase addressing adequate muscular endurance.

Selected Principles of Strength Training for Sports

A successful strength training program should start by applying specific principles that maximize an athlete's own abilities and talent in an environment that aims to produce a superior athlete, free of injuries. The following principles are important for both young and advanced athletes.

Develop Joint Mobility

In order to increase strength and mobility (flexibility) concurrently, most strength training exercises should be used for the entire range of motion, especially for ankles, knees, hips, and shoulders. Good joint mobility can prevent strain, pain, and stress injuries. Ankle mobility, in particular dorsal and plantar flexion (bringing the toes toward and then away from the calf), should be a major concern for beginners but also for soccer, tennis, the martial arts, contact sports, and so on.

The best time for most athletes to begin mobility training is during prepubescence to make sure that at later stages of athletic development they just need to maintain it. When doing deep squats, an athlete may have evident strains and even mechanical stress if there is ankle, hip, and particularly knee mobility deficiency. Soccer is one of the sports in which ankle, knee, and hip flexibility are inadequately trained. Some exercises used in soccer are far from the range of motion needed during the game, and flexibility training is far from developing the needs of these joints. Remember that good range of motion can help prevent leg injuries.

Many exercises for improving flexibility are partner-assisted stretching and proprioceptive neuromuscular facilitation (PNF), a technique that combines passive (isometric) with active stretching. Myofascial release (in the cervical and TMJ region) increases muscle flexibility and joint mobility without negatively affecting performance (Sullivan et al. 2013; Healey et al. 2014). In fact, for peak performance, myofascial release should be planned before a competition, especially in speed and power sports.

The maximum range of motion (ROM) required during the game should be the minimum level during daily practice.

Develop Ligament and Tendon Strength

Muscle strength improves faster than tendon and ligament strength. Many training specialists and coaches overlook the strengthening of ligaments and tendons because they misuse the principle of specificity or lack long-term vision. Yet most injuries occur not at the muscle but at the myotendinous junction. The reason is that without proper anatomical adaptation, vigorous strength training can injure the tendons and ligaments. With anatomical adaptation, however, tendons and ligaments grow strong. More specifically, training tendons and ligaments causes them to enlarge in diameter, increasing their ability to withstand tension and tearing.

Ligaments, which are made up of the fibrous protein collagen, play the important role of attaching articulated bones to each other across a joint. The collagen fibrils are arranged in varying degrees of folds to help resist an increase in load. The strength of a ligament depends directly on its cross-sectional area. A ligament may rupture when excessive force is directed at a joint. During regular exercise or activity, ligaments are easily elongated to allow movement in the joint to occur naturally. However, when a high load is applied, as in competition or training, ligament stiffness increases in order to restrict excessive motion in the joint. If the load is too great, the ligament is not able to withstand the stress, and an injury can occur.

The best way to prevent such an injury is to condition the body properly to handle mechanical stress. To adapt ligaments to handle the stress, and provide adequate time for regeneration, athletes can condition them through a cycle of loading and unloading, as in the anatomical adaptation phase of training. Progressively increasing the training load improves the viscoelastic properties of ligaments and allows them to better accommodate high tensile loads such as those used in dynamic movements, maximum strength training, and plyometrics.

Tendons, on the other hand, connect muscle to bone and transmit force from muscle to bone to allow movement to occur. Tendons also store elastic energy, which is crucial to any ballistic movement, such as those used in plyometrics and other forms of jumps (stretch–shortening cycle). The stronger the tendon, the greater its capacity to store elastic energy. That is why powerful tendons are characteristic of sprinters and jumpers. Without strong tendons, they would not be able to apply such great force against their bones to overcome the force of gravity.

Ligaments and tendons are both trainable. Their material and structural properties change as a result of training, leading to increased thickness, strength, and stiffness by up to 20% (Frank 1996). Ligaments and tendons are also capable of healing, although more slowly than muscles, given the lower vascularization, and they might not recover to their preinjury capability.

With all this in mind, exercise—especially the type performed during the anatomical adaptation phase—can be considered an injury prevention method. If the strengthening of tendons and ligaments is disrupted, the athlete may experience a decline in the tendons' ability to transmit force and in the ligaments' ability to secure the anatomical integrity of the joints. The abuse of steroids increases the muscle force at the expense of the ligaments' and tendons' material properties (Woo et al. 1994). More generally, increasing force without correspondingly strengthening the ligaments and tendons results in the ligament and tendon injuries experienced by some athletes, including professional American football players.

Develop Core Strength

The arms and legs are only as strong as the trunk. Put another way, a poorly developed trunk provides only weak support for hard-working limbs. Therefore, strength training programs should strengthen the core muscles before focusing on the arms and legs.

Core muscles activate highly during jumps, rebounds, and plyometric exercises. They stabilize the body and serve as a link, or transmitter of force, between the legs and the arms. Weak core muscles fail in these essential roles, limiting the athlete's ability to perform. Most of these muscles are dominated by slow-twitch fibers because of their supporting role in the body's posture and their continuous activation during arm and leg actions. They contract constantly, but not necessarily dynamically, to create a solid base of support for the actions of other muscle groups.

Many people complain of low-back problems yet do little to correct them. The best protection against low-back problems is to have well-developed back and abdominal muscles. Coaches and athletes should not neglect this area of the body. At the same time, although core strength training is currently touted as a new theory with concomitant new exercises, some of these are in fact useless and even dangerous. This section provides our point of view regarding core training. We believe that excessively focusing on the core does nothing to promote an increase in performance but serves only as a means of distracting the athlete from performing a host of exercises that are integral to sport performance—those that work the prime movers of the sport.

The abdominal and back muscles surround the core area of the body with a tight and powerful support structure of muscle bundles running in different directions. If the abdominal muscles are poorly developed, the pelvis tilts forward, and lordosis (sway-back) develops at the lumbar area of the spine. The rectus abdominis, for example, runs vertically and keeps the spine from extending when the legs are fixed, as in sit-ups, to maintain good posture. The internal and external obliques help the rectus abdominis bend the trunk forward (spine flexion) and perform all twisting, lateral-bending, and trunk-rotating motions. They help an athlete recover from a fall in many sports and perform many actions in boxing, wrestling, and the martial arts. The anterior and lateral abdominal muscles perform delicate, precise trunk movements. These large muscles run vertically, diagonally, and horizontally.

Because many athletes have weak abdominal muscles compared to their back muscles, general and specific abdominal muscle training is recommended. Isolating the abdominal muscles requires an exercise that flexes the spine but not the hips. Exercises that flex the hips are performed by the iliopsoas (a powerful hip flexor) and to a lesser extent by the abdominal muscles (which then work mostly isometrically to prevent spine extension in the sagittal plane). The most popular abdominal exercise is the sit-up. The sit-up can be considered a basic core strengthening exercise because it strengthens the hip flexors (iliopsoas) and the abdominal muscles simultaneously. The hip flexors have been overlooked as core muscles in the last two decades, supposedly because of their negative influence on posture (short hip flexors induce an anterior pelvic tilt and lumbar spine hyperlordosis). Nevertheless, strong hip flexors are paramount to avoid neural inhibition and promote strength development of the antagonist hip extensors, which is fundamental for the running and jumping athletes. Furthermore, the hip flexors are actively involved in the first acceleration steps, where there is a lesser elastic–reactive component compared to max velocity. Finally, the hip flexors are prime movers in combat sport, where there are grappling actions, in which the opponent's body is driven not only with the strength of the upper body's pulling muscles but also and mainly via hip flexion. These important muscles can also be trained through exercises such as leg and knee lifts against resistance.

IRRADIATION

When an athlete performs a strength exercise, many core muscles are activated and contract synergistically to stabilize the body and act as a support so that a limb can perform the exercise. This synergistic contraction is called *activation overflow* or *irradiation* (Enoka 2002; Zijdewind and Kernell 2001). The process is illustrated in the following examples.

Upright Rowing

The motion of upright rowing involves standing with the feet hip width apart while the arms, holding a barbell, are lowered in front of the thighs. As the arms flex to lift the weight to and from the chest, the abdominal and back muscles, including the erector spinae (core muscles), contract to stabilize the trunk so that the arms can perform the action smoothly (an anti-flexion action in the sagittal plane). Without support from the core muscles to stabilize the trunk, the prime movers would not be effective in performing the task.

While the exercise is performed, all the core muscles (especially those of the back) are activated and contracted (activation overflow), and, as a result, are strengthened. In fact, the level of muscle contraction can be higher during this exercise than during many body weight exercises for core strength. Therefore, using it can better develop the core muscles (Hamlyn et al. 2007; Nuzzo 2008; Colado et al. 2011; Martuscello et al. 2012).

Squatting and Deadlifting

During any leg action performed against resistance in the upright position, all core muscles are strongly activated to stabilize the trunk and use it as a support (Martuscello et al. 2012). This activation also strengthens the muscles involved. In particular, heavy quarter squats (performed by elite athletes with a load three to four times body weight), for instance, elicit particularly strong contractions of the core muscles. The deadlift, on the other hand, is a great builder of back muscle strength. (The deadlift has been used to strengthen leg extensors and back muscles since the Bronze Age. It is not a weightlifting novelty. Not at all. Remember the Aeneas rowers? They used the deadlift.)

Spiking

One of the most dynamic athletic skills, volleyball spiking, could not be properly performed without the direct support of the core muscles. During spiking, the core muscles contract to stabilize the trunk so that the legs can perform an explosive takeoff and the arms can hit the ball. The core muscles also fixate and stabilize the trunk in other situations where the arms and legs need to perform an athletic task; examples include running, jumping, throwing, medicine ball exercises, and various quick or agile foot movements. Indeed, the core is engaged by any strength or sport-specific exercise in which the core must contract in order to resist flexion or extension of the spine. As a result, the overall volume of specific core strengthening exercises can be reduced to a few sets of essential exercises per session.

The back muscles, including the deep back muscles along the vertebral column, are responsible for many movements, such as back extension and trunk extension and rotation. The trunk, in turn, acts as the transmitter and supporter of most arm and leg actions. The vertebral column also plays an essential role as a shock absorber during landing and takeoff.

STABILITY BALL TRAINING

Like everything in sport-specific training, the stability ball (also known as the Swiss ball or balance ball) is not new. It first hit the scene in the 1960s and has become very popular, especially in rehabilitative settings. Since the 1990s, it has also become popular in sport and fitness. Its popularity in the fitness field is understandable, given that the field is all about variety and excitement.

Many exercises performed on the stability ball provide good upper- and lower-body strength, flexibility, and of course core strength. The benefit of these exercises for athletes is overemphasized, however, by some members of the sporting world, who claim that improvements in proprioception and balance translate to improvements in athletic performance. In reality, balance is not a limiting factor for performance; therefore, it is not in the same category as speed, strength, and endurance. The body will adapt to the unstable environment of sport through the stimulus of participating in the sport itself, as well as through the practice of technical and tactical drills related to the sport. Selected exercises can be performed on the ball, but they should be limited to the anatomical adaptation or transition phases of training, when general adaptation takes precedence over specific physiological adaptation.

Beyond these caveats, athletes and coaches should be aware that performing at maximum strength on a stability ball can be detrimental to athletic performance. The ball limits the amount of weight that the athlete can lift because more neural drive is used to stabilize the body as a whole, as well as the specific joints involved, thus reducing the activation of the fast-twitch muscle fibers of the prime movers. The only stability ball exercises we recommend are those intended for training the abdominal muscles, which allow the athlete to stretch the abdominals fully before the concentric part of the exercise. Other muscle groups can be trained more effectively through other means.

Stability balls do have a time and place in training. Activation overflow explains how all muscles involved in a movement essentially communicate with each other and offer their help. Our bodies are extremely pliable and adapt wonderfully to traditional methods of training. And, most important in sports, an athlete's body performs better when it adapts better, thereby creating stability naturally.

Back problems can result from excessive, uneven stress on the spine or from sudden movement in an unfavorable position. For athletes, back problems may result from wear and tear caused by improper positioning or forward tilting of the body. More specifically, disc pressure varies according to body position relative to external stress. For example, stress increases on the spine while lifting in seated positions or standing when the upper body swings, such as in upright rowing or elbow flexion. Sitting produces greater disc pressure than standing, and the least stress occurs when the body is supine or prone (as in bench presses or prone bench pulls). In many exercises that use the back muscles, abdominal muscles contract isometrically, stabilizing the body.

Develop the Stabilizers

Prime movers work more efficiently with strong stabilizer, or fixator, muscles. Stabilizers contract, primarily isometrically, to stabilize a joint so that another part of the body can act. For example, the shoulders are immobilized during elbow flexion, and the abdominal muscles serve as stabilizers when the arms throw a ball. In rowing, when the trunk muscles act as stabilizers, the trunk transmits leg power to the arms, which then drive the blade through the water. A weak stabilizer, therefore, inhibits the contracting capacity of the prime movers.

Improperly developed stabilizers can also hamper the activity of major muscles. When placed under chronic stress, the stabilizers spasm, restraining the prime movers and reducing athletic effectiveness. This condition is often seen in volleyball players who suffer injury as a result of inadequate muscle strength and balance in the shoulder muscles (Kugler et al. 1996). At the shoulders, supra- and infraspinatus muscles rotate the arm. The simplest, most effective exercise to strengthen these two muscles is to rotate the arm while holding a dumbbell. The resistance provided stimulates the two muscles stabilizing the shoulder. At the hips, the piriformis and gluteus medius muscles perform external (outward) rotation. To strengthen these muscles, the athlete should stand with the knees locked and lift the leg to the side with a strap connected to a cable machine.

Stabilizers also contract isometrically, immobilizing one part of the limb and allowing the other to move. In addition, they can monitor the state of the long bones' interactions in joints and sense potential injury resulting from improper technique, inappropriate strength, or spasms produced by poor stress management. If one of these conditions occurs, the stabilizers restrain the activity of the prime movers, thus avoiding strain and injury.

Stabilizers play important roles in athletic performance. However, some strength and conditioning coaches have exaggerated the training of the stabilizer muscles, especially through the use of proprioception training (also known as balance training). In fact, unstable surface training elicits high motor units activation due to co-contraction (simultaneous contraction of agonists and antagonists to stabilize a joint), which is not conducive to the neuromuscular adaptations required by speed and power athletes, who need "silent" (i.e., inactive) antagonists during powerful actions.

On the other hand, a number of studies have shown that proprioception training with balance boards does help provide stability to a previously injured or unstable ankle (Caraffa et al. 1996; Wester et al. 1996; Willems et al. 2002). The theory is that if balance board training helps promote greater stability by increasing the proprioception and strength of the stabilizer muscles of an unstable structure, it will further strengthen and prevent injury to an already stable structure. This has yet to be proven, however, and in any case the real question is how much time should be devoted to exercises intended to strengthen the stabilizer muscles.

Certain studies show that proprioception training can decrease injury to the knee (Caraffa et al. 1996), whereas other studies disprove the benefits of proprioception training for injury prevention (Söderman et al. 2000). One review study in particular challenged flaws in the design and implementation of proprioception studies (Thacker et al. 2003). Furthermore, in the last 10 years, strength and conditioning coaches who have refrained

Be selective regarding the time and energy you spend on a large variety of exercises and methods.

- Athletes are usually pressed for time; for top athletes, spending hours on balance training and the stability ball can be a waste of valuable time.
- Too much time is often spent on drills for agility and not enough on MxS/power.
- Coaches and instructors should review their training philosophy by creating a neuromuscular strategy to improve athletic performance.

from using balance boards or proprioception training for team sports (soccer and volleyball) have reported no increase in ankle or knee injuries.

That said, balance board or Swiss ball training can be helpful during the early part of the preparatory phase (the anatomical adaptation phase). Unilateral exercises are certainly the best choice for improving joint stability while training the prime movers. Nevertheless, if proprioceptive strength is trained during the anatomical adaptation phase, the board or Swiss ball should be put away in the next phase to allow time for training with methods that directly enhance the athlete's physical stature and promote sport-specific strength, speed, and stamina. After all, even if exercises worked to improve an athlete's proprioception, the slow to intermediate nature of these exercises would never protect the joint from the fast and powerful movements performed in sport (Ashton-Miller et al. 2001). Preparing the stabilizers for movement is important; specifically, training for the movements of the sport with ideal sport-specific speed and power or endurance is vital to the athlete's performance and physical state.

Train Movements, Not Individual Muscles

The purpose of strength training in sports is to load the joints' movements specifically used in performing the skills of a given sport. Athletes should resist training muscles in isolation, as is done in bodybuilding. From the start, bodybuilding has promoted the concept of working muscles in isolation, a concept that has served this activity very well for generations. However, isolation exercises do not apply to sports because athletic skills are multijoint movements performed in a certain order, forming what is called a kinetic (movement) chain.

For instance, a takeoff to catch a ball uses the following kinetic chain: hip extensions, then knee extensions, and finally ankle extensions (push-off), in which the feet apply force against the ground to lift the body. This powerful sequence, typical of so many sport actions, is called triple extensions.

According to the principle of specificity, especially during the conversion (to specific strength) phase, body position and limb angles should resemble those needed for the specific skills to be performed. When athletes train for a movement, the muscles are integrated and strengthened to perform the action with more power. Therefore, athletes should not resort to weight training alone but should broaden their training routines by incorporating medicine balls, power training with strength training machines, throwing with heavier implements, and plyometric equipment. Exercises performed with these instruments allow athletes to potentiate their athletic skills.

Multijoint exercises, such as the squat, deadlift, bench press, military press, chin-up, and weightlift, as well as throws and jumps, in sport training have been used since track-and-field athletes introduced them in the early 1930s, prior to the 1936 Olympic Games. Most athletes still follow this tradition. Such exercises are key to strength training efficiency and efficacy. A few isolation exercises (referred to as accessory exercises) can still be used to support hypertrophy of lacking muscles or to increase blood flow (necessary for tendon health) and to support the muscle protein content of the prime movers during periods of low reps and very high loads in training.

Identify the prime movers in your sport first, and then train them as per the principles of periodization of strength.

48

Focus Not on What Is New But on What Is Necessary

Over the years, the North American sport and fitness market has been deluged by many products that supposedly improve athletic performance. Often, however, they do not. In fact, an understanding of biomechanics and exercise physiology reveals that many products that claim to improve strength, speed, and power may actually inhibit them. Two methods that have captured the minds of athletes, coaches, and trainers are balance training and overspeed training. Balance training is safe but also widely overused despite the fact that it is not effective. Overspeed training—along with many training devices used in an effort to enhance speed and power—jeopardizes an athlete's running technique and decreases the rate of force development.

It is important to have a good selection of exercises, but an exercise is essential only if it targets the prime movers or the main muscle groups used in performing an athletic skill—no more, no less. It is immaterial, for example, whether the athlete uses a simple bench or a stability ball to perform bench presses. The essential goal is to perform the exercise with continuous acceleration through the range of motion. At the beginning of a bench press, fast-twitch muscle fibers are recruited to defeat inertia and the heavy load of the barbell. As the athlete continues to press the barbell upward, he or she should attempt to generate the highest possible acceleration. Under these conditions, the discharge rate is increased in the same fast-twitch muscle fibers. Maximum velocity, therefore, must be achieved toward the end of the action to coincide with the instant of releasing a ball or other athletic implement during sport performance.

Similarly, if a high level of strength adaptation is required in the leg muscles, the athlete should squat, squat, squat to develop the greatest possible levels of strength and adaptation—in other words, do what is necessary. Adding variety by implementing different exercises is fine as long as they target the same muscle group in the most specific way.

Principles of Strength Training

The purpose of any strength training program is to produce a continual increase in the athlete's physical capacity. Strength training principles offer methods for adapting the body to the various loads used in training; they also provide guidelines for individualizing the program to the specific needs of the athlete and the sport.

Progressive Increase of Load

The principle of progressive increase of load is best illustrated by the Greek myth about Milo of Croton. To become the world's strongest man, Milo lifted and carried a calf every day, beginning in his teenage years. As the calf grew heavier, Milo grew stronger. By the time the calf was a full-grown bull, Milo was the world's strongest man, thanks to long-term progression.

In more specific terms, training progressively elicits adaptations in the structure and functions of the athlete's body, increasing his or her motor potential and ultimately resulting in improved performance. Of course, the body reacts both physiologically and psychologically to the increased training load (that is, to the sum of the volume and intensity of all the training stimuli). Therefore, training also produces gradual changes in nervous reaction and functions, neuromuscular coordination, and psychological capacity to cope with stress. The entire process requires time and competent technical leadership.

Some coaches employ a consistent training load, called a standard load, throughout the year. This approach may cause decreased performance during the late competitive phase because the physiological basis of performance has decreased and prevents consistent improvements (figure 3.1). Superior adaptation and performance are produced only by steadily applying training load increments.

Another traditional strength training approach uses the overload principle. Early proponents of this principle claimed that strength and hypertrophy increase only if muscles work at their maximum strength capacity against workloads greater than those normally encountered (Hellebrand and Houtz 1956; Lange 1919). Contemporary advocates suggest that the load to exhaustion in strength training should be increased throughout the program (Fox, Bowes, and Foss 1989). Therefore, the curve of load increment can rise constantly (figure 3.2).

Proponents of overloading suggest two ways to increase strength: (1) maximum loads to exhaustion, inducing strength gains, and (2) submaximal loads to exhaustion, inducing hypertrophy (a popular approach among bodybuilders). However, athletes cannot be expected to lift to exhaustion every time they work out. This is especially true from the specific preparation onward, when most of their energy must be directed to sport-specific activities and their bodies must be well recovered in order to perform sport-specific skills optimally.

In fact, such physiological and psychological strain leads to muscle tightness, impaired sport-specific technical proficiency, fatigue, exhaustion, injury, or overtraining. To be

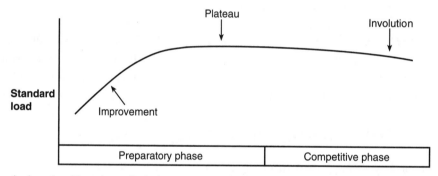

Figure 3.1 A standard load results in improvements only in the early part of the annual plan.

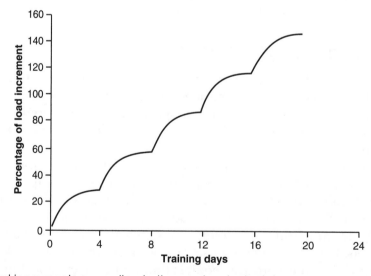

Figure 3.2 Load increments according to the overload principle.

Adapted from *Phys Ther Rev* 1956; 36(6): 371-383, with permission of the American Physical Therapy Association. Copyright © 1956 American Physical Therapy Association. APTA is not responsible for the translation from English.

effective, a strength training program must follow the concept of periodization of strength, in which specific goals for each phase lead up to either peak performance at the year's major competitions or the best possible performance throughout a championship.

To achieve these goals, a more effective approach is step-type loading (figure 3.3). The athlete's ability to tolerate heavy loads improves as the result of adaptation to stressors applied in strength training (Councilman 1968; Harre 1982). The step-type method requires a training load increase followed by an unloading phase during which the body adapts, regenerates, and prepares for a new increase.

The frequency of such unloading microcycles is determined by each athlete's needs, the rate of adaptation, and the competitive calendar. Training load increases are determined by the rate of the athlete's performance improvement; the intensity increase between steps (weeks) in a macrocycle commonly falls between 2% and 5%. An abrupt increase in training load may exceed the athlete's capacity to adapt and therefore affect his or her physiological balance.

The step-type approach does not necessarily mean increasing the load in each training session in a linear fashion. Furthermore, a single training session is insufficient to cause appreciable body adaptations. To achieve adaptation, the same exercise must be repeated several times a week but at different intensities, followed by an increase in the following week.

In figure 3.3, let's say that each horizontal line represents a week, or microcycle, of training and that the load is applied on Monday. This load fatigues the body but is still within the capability of the athlete. The body adjusts by Wednesday and adapts to the load over the next two days, and by Friday the athlete feels stronger and capable of lifting heavier loads. Thus, fatigue is followed by adaptation and then a physiological rebound or improvement. This new level can be called a new ceiling of adaptation. By the next Monday, the athlete is physiologically and psychologically comfortable. This process is the reason why it is possible either to increase the strength training load linearly throughout the microcycle (if the loading parameters at the beginning of the macrocycle were well within the athlete's capacity) or to vary it (heavy on Monday, light on Wednesday, and medium-heavy on Friday).

The third step in figure 3.3 is followed by a lower step or unloading microcycle. A reduction in overall demand allows the body to regenerate and fully adapt. During the unloading week, the athlete recovers almost completely from the fatigue accumulated in the first three steps, replenishes energy stores, and relaxes psychologically. The body accumulates new reserves in anticipation of further increases in training load. Training performance usually improves following the unloading microcycle. Testing can be planned at the end of the unloading microcycle.

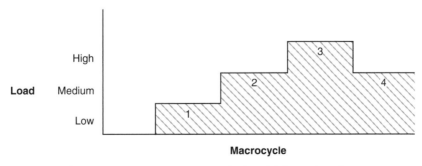

Figure 3.3 Illustration of step loading in a macrocycle, in which each column represents the weekly load, increasing in a step-like fashion (Bompa 1965a, 1965b, and 1983).

The shorter the macrocycle (for instance, a 2+1 structure, which entails two weeks of loading followed by an unloading week), the lower the increase from the beginning load. Thus, a longer macrocycle may permit a larger increase but generally starts at a lower intensity. Longer macrocycles (3+1 or even 4+1 weeks) are used during general preparation when the intensity at the beginning of the macrocycle is low, whereas shorter macrocycles are used from the specific preparation onward, as the training intensifies. It is, in fact, harder to sustain a prolonged increase of intensity when the intensity at the beginning of the macrocycle was already high. Although training load increases in steps, the load curve in the annual plan has a wavy shape that represents the ongoing increases and decreases of loading to stimulate and realize adaptations (see figure 3.4).

Although the step-loading method is applicable to every sport and athlete, two variations are possible—reverse step loading and flat loading—and they must be applied carefully and with discretion. In reverse step loading (figure 3.5), the load decreases rather than increases from step to step. Some Eastern European weightlifters maintain that this form of loading (planning the heaviest loads immediately following a microcycle of low-intensity training) is more specific to their physiological needs. Reverse step loading has been used in weightlifting since the late 1960s but has not been accepted in any other sport. The reason is simple: The goal of strength training for sport is progressive adaptation—gradually increasing the athlete's training capabilities—and performance improvements are possible only when training capabilities have increased. Reverse loading should be used only during the peaking cycle prior to competition as a tapering method. Endurance improvements are much better achieved by step loading because volume is the main factor, and it is better increased in a step-loading fashion throughout the year.

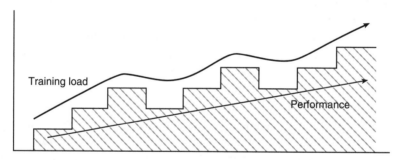

Figure 3.4 The curve of training load undulates (wavy arrow) whereas performance improves continuously (straight arrow). Some authors have claimed the undulatory concept as their own without quoting the original source (Bompa 1965a, 1965b, and 1983). Not only that, but some authors have gone so far as suggesting undulatory periodization. Undulatory periodization? How can you undulate the main training phases of the annual plan?

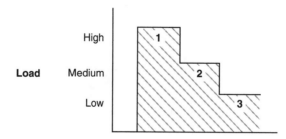

Figure 3.5 Reverse step loading as it used by some weightlifting schools. It may also be used during the unloading phase in sports training to facilitate peaking.

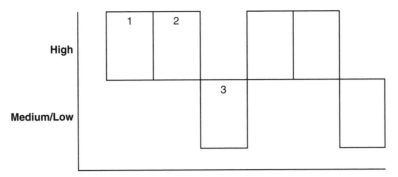

Figure 3.6 The flat loading pattern is usually employed during the specific preparation and early competitive phases for power sports (Bompa 1993).

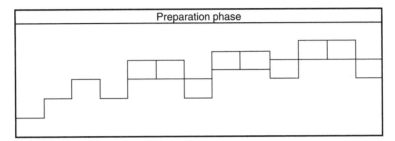

Figure 3.7 Suggested loading patterns for the preparation phase. Step loading is used at the beginning of the program since the load is increased progressively. After the first five weeks of progressive adaptation, flat step loading is used to ensure that training is very demanding and results in the specific adaptation necessary for performance improvement (Bompa 1993).

The flat loading pattern (figure 3.6) is appropriate for advanced athletes with a good strength training background, for athletes who can tolerate prolonged exposure to high-intensity training, and, generally, for power sport during the specific preparation phase. High-demand training is performed at the same level for 2 to 3 microcycles, followed by a low-load recovery week. The 2 to 3 microcycles must involve high demand for either one or all elements—technical, tactical, speed, and endurance training. When planning the lower-intensity microcycle, all the elements must be of lower demand in order to facilitate relaxation and recovery.

The dynamics of the loading pattern for a well-trained athlete are a function of the training phase and the type of desired training adaptation. During the early part of the preparatory phase for all sports, the step loading pattern prevails, ensuring better progression (figure 3.7). The flat loading pattern is better suited for the late preparatory phase, especially for power sports and for athletes competing at or beyond the national level.

Variety

Contemporary training requires the athlete to perform many hours of work. The volume and intensity of training sometimes increase yearly, and exercises are repeated numerous times. To reach high performance, an athlete who is serious about training must dedicate two to four hours each week to strength training, in addition to performing technical, tactical, and energy systems training.

Under these conditions, boredom and monotony can become obstacles to motivation and improvement. The best way to overcome these obstacles is to incorporate variety

DEFINING AND UNDERSTANDING STRENGTH TRAINING

Step loading is the favorite modality for eliciting morpho-functional adaptations through a progressive increase of muscular, metabolic, or neural stress over time. There are many ways to progress the load rationally, thereby eliciting the desired adaptations, such as higher levels of hypertrophy, muscular endurance, maximum strength, or power. In order to understand these options, we must analyze the loading variables and how they influence the final training effect. Throughout a macrocycle, we can progress one or more of these parameters according to the training effects (adaptations) we want to elicit. The parameters are described in detail in the following sections.

Repetitions

The number of repetitions per set is closely linked to the percentage of one repetition maximum (1RM). Throughout a macrocycle, we can either increase repetitions in order to increase endurance (more volume), keep repetitions the same while manipulating other parameters, or decrease repetitions to increase intensity (percentage of 1RM) or to unload or peak while maintaining or slightly reducing intensity.

Sets

Throughout a macrocycle, we can increase the number of sets in order to increase work capacity and endurance (more volume). We can also keep the same number of sets to increase one of the other parameters or to decrease the number of sets to unload or peak. The number of sets (volume) is the single most influential variable on the training's residual fatigue effect.

Rest Interval

The rest interval directly influences the final training effect. We can increase the rest interval if the macrocycle moves toward a decrease in reps and an increase in intensity (percentage of 1RM). We can decrease the rest interval in order to increase endurance (more density). Or, we can keep the rest interval the same while changing one or more of the other variables. When performing a series of sets for power endurance and muscle endurance, reducing the rest interval between sets (while maintaining their power output) allows a densification that later translates into a higher mean power output for a longer duration.

---

into the training routines. Variety improves training response and positively affects an athlete's psychological well-being. In order to implement variety effectively, however, instructors and coaches must be well versed in strength training. They should not use variety for variety's sake. You should never forget, however, that specificity is the key to physiological adaptation and performance improvements. Periodization of strength naturally includes rational variations of means and methods throughout the annual plan to elicit the best neuromuscular adaptations. The following guidelines will help you design strength training programs with sensible variations over the course of the annual plan.

- Progress from full range of motion (ROM) in the general preparation phase to sport-specific ROM in the late specific preparation phase and the competitive phase. Be mindful of the fact that full-ROM exercises cause more muscular tension than their partial counterparts; therefore, a low volume of such exercises should always be used for maintaining maximum strength (Bloomquist et al. 2013; Hartmann et al. 2012; Bazyler et al. 2014).

- Vary exercise selection, especially for children, by using more unilateral and dumbbell exercises during anatomical adaptation and compensation macrocycles.
- Vary loading by using the principle of progressive increase of load in training.
- Vary the type and speed or tempo of muscle contractions. The usual pattern goes from slow eccentrics (3 to 5 seconds) and controlled concentrics (1 or 2 seconds) in anatomical adaptation to slow eccentrics and fast concentrics (1 second or less) in the maximum strength macrocycles and then to fast eccentrics and explosive concentrics in macrocycles for power, power endurance, or muscle endurance short. This pattern is represented by a trio of numbers (King 1998); the first number is the duration in seconds of the eccentric phase, the second number is the length of the pause between the eccentric and concentric phases, and the third number is the duration of the concentric phase (an "X" means explosive).
- Vary the method. Move from body weight, dumbbells, and machines during macrocycles for anatomical adaptation and hypertrophy to mainly barbells or strength training machines in macrocycles for maximum strength, conversion to specific strength, and maintenance.

Variety in exercise selection keeps the athlete motivated and the adaptation fresh. Problems can arise, however, when coaches and athletes substitute an exercise or change a method solely for the sake of doing something new. The principle of variety should be used only if the change or substitution keeps the athlete on the path of adaptation.

When athletes reach a high level of competition and fitness, certain exercises should always be included in their regimen. Coaches can alter the load or method used in training but should always stick to the movements that best work the kinetic chain prime movers used in the sport or best elicit the threshold of stimulation needed for maximum gains.

Coaches and athletes should also remember that sport training is different from fitness training and that fitness ideals rarely work in sport training. For example, many strength training instructors preach that exercises should be altered every other week. Although this approach may be beneficial when training personal clients who require constant variety and excitement, it is not appropriate for athletes. Alternating strength exercises for a given sport can be done only if the new exercise addresses the prime movers in that sport.

Because adaptation is a physiological requirement for athletic improvement, the same type of training and muscle groups must be targeted repeatedly in order to produce the highest degree of adaptation. Without constant increase in the adaptation of bodily systems, athletes see no observable improvement in their performance. Yes, repeating the same type of exercise day in and day out is very boring. But so is constantly repeating the technical skills of running, swimming, cycling, and rowing, to name a few. Yet nobody suggests to runners, swimmers, cyclists, and rowers that they alter their primary skill training because it is boring. Coaches should choose a number of exercises that have the same functional purpose but add variety to training. In this way, they can spice up the training program but keep in mind the main focus: the athlete's level of physiological adaptation.

Individualization

Contemporary training requires individualization. Each athlete must be treated according to his or her ability, potential, and strength training background. Sometimes coaches are tempted to follow the training programs of successful athletes, disregarding their particular athlete's needs, experience, and abilities. Even worse, they sometimes insert such programs into the training schedules of junior athletes, who are not ready, either physiologically or psychologically, for such high loads.

Before designing a training program, the coach should assess the athlete. Even athletes who are equal in performance do not necessarily have the same work capacity. Individual work abilities are determined by several biological and psychological factors and must be considered in specifying the amount of work (volume), the load (intensity), and the type of strength training an athlete performs. Work capacity is also affected by training background. Work demand should be based on experience. Even when an athlete exhibits great improvement, the coach must still be cautious in estimating training load (volume plus intensity). When assigning athletes of different backgrounds and experiences to the same training group, the coach should consider individual characteristics and potential.

Another factor to consider when planning a training program is the athlete's rate of recovery. When planning and evaluating the content and stress of training, coaches should remember to assess demanding factors outside of training. They should be aware of the athlete's lifestyle and emotional involvements. Rate of recovery can also be affected by schoolwork and other activities. For help in monitoring the rate of recovery, coaches can use a heart rate variability monitoring device.

Sex-based differences also require consideration. Generally speaking, the total body strength of women is 63.5% of that of men. More specifically, the upper-body strength of women is, on average, 55.8% of that of men; the lower-body strength of women, however,

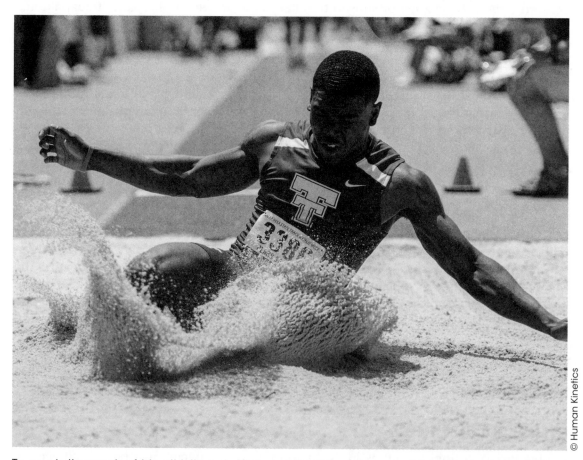

To reach the peak of his athletic potential, an athlete needs an individualized and periodized training plan.

is much closer to that of men, at an average of 71.9% (Laubach 1976). Women tend to have lower hypertrophy levels and lower work capacity than men do, mostly because their testosterone level is as much as 20 times lower (Wright 1980). Female athletes can follow the same training programs as male athletes without worrying about excessive bulky muscles. They can apply the same loading pattern and use the same training methods as men without concern, except when monitoring their recovery ability.

Strength training for women should be rigorously continuous, without long interruptions. Plyometric training should progress carefully over a long period to allow for adaptation. Because women generally tend to be physically weaker than men, improved and increased strength training can produce more visible gains in performance (Lephart et al. 2002). Further increases in strength from plyometric training promote greater power capabilities. As for training the energy systems, women can use the same training methods as men.

One major issue involving sex difference is injury in sport. Female athletes often report a higher incidence of lower-body injuries, in particular to the knee joint. Studies have been conducted in an effort to explain this fact both physiologically and anatomically. For instance, when performing the kinematics and electromyographic activity of the one-leg squat, intercollegiate female athletes, as compared with their male counterparts, demonstrated less lateral trunk flexion and more ankle dorsiflexion, ankle pronation, hip adduction, hip flexion, and external rotation (Zeller et al. 2003). Furthermore, female athletes who participate in jumping and agility exercises tend to exhibit less muscular-stiffness protection of the knee than males do (Wojtys et al. 2003). Involuntarily, females allow their knees to drift inward (knock knees), which places more stress on the knee joint and can aggravate or strain the anterior cruciate ligament.

Although sex-specific planning is not entirely required, these differences indicate that time should be dedicated to improving maximum strength, in particular the strength of the lower body, in female athletes. In particular, increased strengthening of the quadriceps and hamstrings at the end of the early preparatory phase can physiologically prepare the athlete for game-specific drills and power training, which place more stress on the knee joint and can lead to injury.

Specificity

To be effective and achieve greater adaptation, training must be designed to develop sport-specific strength. Toward this end, a coach must make a simple performance model analysis of the sport for which the strength training program is being created. The analysis should take into account the ergogenesis (i.e., the energy contribution to the sporting event of each of the three energy systems), the specific joints' range of motion, the planes of movement, and the prime movers and their actions (eccentric, isometric, concentric). Training specificity is the most important mechanism for sport-specific neuromuscular adaptations.

Specificity and the Dominant Energy System

The coach should carefully consider the dominant energy system in the chosen sport. For instance, muscular endurance training is most appropriate for endurance sports such as rowing, long-distance swimming, canoeing, and speedskating. The coach must also consider the specific muscle groups involved (the prime movers) and the movement patterns characteristic of the sport. Exercises should use the sport's key movement patterns. They must also improve the power of the prime movers. Normally, gains in power transfer to skill improvement.

Specificity Versus a Methodical Approach

The principle of specificity sprang from the idea that the optimal strength training program must be specific. According to this principle, an exercise or type of training that is specific to the skills of a sport results in faster adaptation and yields faster performance improvement. However, specificity should be applied only to advanced athletes during the competitive phase. These athletes devote a large portion of their annual strength training plan to train the dominant strength in their selected sport.

The misuse of specificity results in asymmetrical and inharmonious body development and neglects the antagonist and stabilizer muscles. Misuse can also hamper the

---

THE FALLACY OF FUNCTIONAL TRAINING

Occasionally, certain authors advance a new term intended to sound like a scientific novelty: *functional training*. This refers to exercises performed on different types of equipment, such as balls, ABS (plastic) pipes with foam, and proprioceptive platforms, all of which are designed to create a more difficult environment in order to increase participation by small and deep stabilizing muscles (Staley 2005). But is it possible that Olympic and world championship events have been won, and world records set, without the athletes having worked on specific strength, or having done so in an optimal manner, until the year 2000?

Specific strength and *functional strength* are not synonymous. Training for the specific strength needed in a given sport involves replicating the specific modality of force expression needed in the chosen event, both neurally and metabolically. This training is achieved by using specific exercises that mimic the action of the kinetic chains in the specific motor skills (including specific joints' range of motion and force vector). Particular emphasis is placed on the prime movers, without disturbing the motor patterns required for the sport's technique.

In contrast, rather than referring to the physiological and biomechanical parameters of the specific event or motor skill, the term functional strength is more commonly used to describe how strength is trained—that is, its training means free weights or cables, unilateral training, and possibly standing and moving through more than one plane of motion. (Exceptions to this definition are found in propaedeutic exercises and some core stability exercises.) In other words, in order to talk about specific strength training, the essential starting points are the biomechanical—and in particular the physiological—parameters of the event. Functional training, in contrast, is simply defined by the use of exercises with the characteristics just listed.

To state that the exercise selection fully defines the degree of functionality of a strength training program is, obviously, methodologically wrong, but it is also true that the best functionalists apply the concept of periodization of strength to their planning. In addition, not only do they consider biomechanics when selecting exercises, but they also consider physiology when choosing load parameters, even if they prefer certain exercises and methods. We should, however, ask ourselves to what extent certain functional training methods are appropriate to reach the levels of maximum strength development needed in certain power sport (e.g., one-leg squat grabbing a suspension training belt). At this point, it should be clear that periodization of strength is a more comprehensive concept than functional training, and specific strength is grounded on biomechanics and physiology rather than on exercise novelty, variation, or simple skill.

To be effective, training must address and adapt to the main functions of the body. In other words, training is functional and physiological.

development of the prime movers and result in injury. Overemphasizing specificity can result in narrow development of the muscles and one-sided, specialized muscle function. Therefore, compensation strength exercises should always be used in training, especially during the early preparatory phase and the transition phases of the annual plan. These exercises balance the strength of agonist and antagonist muscles.

Specificity of Exercises for Strength Training

When it comes to strength exercise selection for a sport, especially in the late preparatory phase, coaches must try to imitate the dynamic structure of the skill, as well as the spatial orientation or body position in relation to the surrounding environment. In other words, coaches should select exercises that place the body and limbs in positions similar to those used when performing the skill.

The angle between limbs or other body parts influences how a muscle contracts and which parts of it contract. Therefore, familiarity with these aspects (the specific joints' ROM and prime movers' muscle actions) is necessary for effective training.

To achieve maximum training specificity, exercises must

- increase the activation of the prime movers,
- imitate the angle of the skill performed, and
- be specific in the intended direction of athletic skills (neural pathway).

The order of muscles targeted by the strength training exercise (muscle chain) has to be similar to the order of muscles when performing an athletic skill.

Exercises used in strength training are often selected based on gimmicks promoted by the producers of training equipment and touted as modern training methods. But an exercise is not modern just because these manufacturers say so. Are these exercises efficient and beneficial for the athlete? Efficiency, not modernism, is essential. Exercises must aim at a specific part of the human anatomy (muscles) and must have a physiological effect. Just say no to gadgets promoted by the sports equipment industry and try to discriminate between its financial interest and your interest as a coach.

Training methods must also be specific to the speed of contraction, particularly for power and agility training, and must result in neural adaptation, called nervous system training (Enoka 2015). Neural adaptation also results in increasing the number of active motor units; maximum strength and power are the only training methods that increase the fast-twitch muscle fibers' recruitment and firing rate.

Selected Comments Regarding the Biomechanical Efficiency of Strength Training

In our many years of involvement in sport training, we have concluded that some coaches have a minimal understanding of the role and benefits strength training can have in improving athletic performance. The same can be said about the selection of exercises. Here is a compendium of methods and exercises.

- Elastic cords were first used in training in 1954 in Romania. At that time, the cords were used to develop muscle endurance in rowing, kayaking, and canoeing. From the late 1980s on, the cords also started to be used on the North American continent, at first in fitness training and a few years later for sport training. Once again, the producers of these cords misunderstood their role and benefits. It was proposed that the cords also be used for the development of power. This is an error in understanding exercise equipment and its benefit in training. Elastic cords are not conducive to the development of power for the simple reason that as the cord is stretched, resistance increases. Every time you apply force against a resistance, the movement is slowed down and you cannot accelerate through the range of motion or perform an explosive movement. That is why such an exercise does not accrue to the development of power. In addition, at least in the case of exercises that are performed in the shoulder region, you generate a strain in the shoulder's ligaments that may result in injury.

- Medicine balls (MB) are among the most effective implements for developing power. For the best adaptation to MB training you at first progressively increase the weight of the balls. Then you should progressively *decrease* the weight of the balls as you approach the competitive phase. Lowering the weight facilitates a quicker force application against the ball, which results in a forceful and powerful throw and, ultimately, in increased distance. Do you know why these balls are called medicine balls? Because in mid-1800 they were used in medical clinics in Central Europe for rehabilitation purposes.

- A takeoff is initiated first by flexing the ankles and the knees, followed by leg and arm upward actions to elevate the center of gravity, and followed by an actual jump.

- Strength training for increased takeoff in figure skating tends to be incorrectly done. If skaters increase the power of the takeoff they will be able to jump slightly higher and, as a result, have longer time to do the rotations they want.

- Strength training in Nordic skiing is more important for those who use skating technique. If you look at the leg and arm actions (legs and arms push-offs), you will see the need for better strength training programs.

- Power skating in ice hockey requires a lower position of the trunk. In this position the vertical projection of the center of gravity will be well ahead of the feet and, consequently, be able to generate higher velocity. However, this low position of the trunk cannot be properly maintained unless your low back (lumbar) and intervertebral muscle are stronger. Use trunk extensions or rotations against resistance to improve the strength of these muscles.

- During the turn in a slalom race in skiing, a centrifugal force is generated. This force may take the athlete out of the race unless he or she is able to load the downhill ski to apply centripetal force against the slope. Strong legs, via MxS, will help the skier be competitive.

- MxS does assist the athlete during many types of jumps, to overcome gravitational force but also to absorb the shock of landing. In freestyle snowboarding, ski jumping, spiking in volleyball, basketball, and so on, eccentric strength must also be trained. Unfortunately, most athletes rarely train eccentric strength.

- MxS is essential for explosive, powerful starting in most sports. The force applied against the starting block varies according to the maximum force of the athlete, which is often between 285 and 375 pounds (130 and 170 kg), measured on a force plate. This is valid also for the start in other sports, such as speedskating, bobsled, and the like.

- MxS is equally important for post-start acceleration in many sports. Why? Because during the acceleration an athlete has to apply high force to overcome the force of gravity and to move the body forward.

- The speed of a punch in boxing depends on the force of the athlete. Fear of gaining additional weight makes MxS seem to be an undesirable athletic activity. But exercises with a load of 50% to 70%, performed very fast, make the boxer faster without gaining body weight.

- Do you remember Aeneas and his rowers? If you want to increase speed in rowing, kayaking, canoeing, and swimming, you must train MxS. On the other hand, if you want to increase the capacity to apply force repetitively, you must use the muscle-endurance training method.

- There is a continuous debate whether 1-leg squats are better than 2-leg squats. People tend to forget the most important element for improving MxS: the capacity to recruit the fast-twitch (FT) muscle fibers in action. The higher the load, the higher the capacity to recruit more FT fibers. As per the data collected by the author in electromyography testing, the highest electrical activity was recorded in 2-leg squats (the level of electrical activity demonstrates the level of stimulation on the action of specific muscles). At the same time, the 2-leg squat ensures a better equilibrium, and as a result, the athlete is able to lift heavier loads.

- Some physiologists promote the idea that what is essential for the development of strength is time under tension, or how long a contraction lasts. While this is a good method to increase muscle size for bodybuilders, it is not recommended for strength training for sports. Remember what is determinant in strength training for sport: speed, explosiveness, and quick changes of direction. Time under tension is not conducive to speed and power development.

- Have you ever asked yourself why many figure skaters fall when landing from a jump? The answer is simple: they do not have good leg strength to begin with, not to mention that landing requires a good eccentric force to absorb the shock of landing. After a figure skater reaches the highest point of a jump, the body accelerates downward, toward the ice. This acceleration poses a real problem for the poorly trained athlete, especially if a jump has to be followed by another jump. To be able to jump again, the skater also needs to train reactive power, or the capacity to land and immediately jump again.

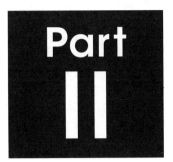

Part II

Planning, Periodization, and Program Design

In training, nothing happens by accident but rather by design. Do you want to be successful? Plan for it!

Introduction to Part II

Planning takes place during the thousands of hours you spend behind your desk and in the field, in the gym, or at the pool alongside your hardworking, perspiring athletes. Nothing is possible in athletics unless you use your time diligently to plan and periodize your athletes' work to reach peak performance.

The terms *periodization, planning,* and *programming* are often used as if they were synonymous, but they are not. *Planning-periodization* incorporates two basic concepts: periodization of biomotor abilities and short- and long-term planning, both of which are determinants for success.

Periodization of biomotor abilities, strength, speed, and endurance facilitates the development of the sport-specific combination of motor abilities to the highest level in order to reach peak performance for the time of the main competitions of the year. *Periodization of biomotor abilities* is based on the following premises.

- Improvement in sport performance is based on your ability to increase your athletes' physiological potential to the highest level without sacrificing the refinement of sport-specific skills.

- Morpho-functional adaptations, the positive changes in body structure and functions, require time to manifest themselves.

- The development of biomotor abilities and the improvement of technical and tactical factors require a progressive approach in which the intensity and volume of training should result in improving athletes' potential beyond the previous level of adaptation.

- Manipulation of training variables and the use of an appropriate planning methodology facilitates peak performance.

- An athlete cannot maintain peak performance for a prolonged period of time.

Periodization of annual plan, as the foundation of comprehending planning methodology, refers to dividing the training program into shorter, easier-to-manage training phases. Periodization of annual plan is beneficial for the following reasons.

- The scope of planning specific training phases is to reach superior adaptation that facilitates peak performance.

- It helps the coach to design a rational structure of training.

- It enhances coaches' awareness of the time available for each training phase.

- It integrates, at appropriate times, technical, tactical, physical, and nutrition plans and psychological techniques to lead to the improvement of athletes' performance.

- It facilitates the management of fatigue to help the coach plan a rational alternation of loading with unloading periods (alternating training with recovery), thus maximizing adaptation. This rational plan helps the coach avoid the accumulation of residual fatigue and consequently helps prevent overtraining.

While *planning* refers to the creation of a structure for the training process via certain planning tools such as the long-term plan, the annual plan, the macrocycles, and the microcycles, *programming* is the process of filling those tools with the details of the actual training, such as the training methods and training means to be used. Therefore, as a coach, you are not just a psychologist and a nutritionist, but also a periodizer, a planner, and a training programmer. Despite the many missions you have with your athletes, we are certain you love what you are doing and the challenges you are faced with, but you also enjoy the rewards the profession offers you. There is nothing else you would rather do!

Planning-Periodization: A Clarification of Terminologies

As examined in more detail in *Periodization: Theory and Methodology of Training* (Bompa and Buzzichelli, 2018) sports planning is not a novel creation. In simple forms it has existed since the Greek Olympic Games (776 BC–393 AD), but the sophistication of sports planning culminated with the German planning for the 1936 Berlin Olympics, the work of Leonid Matveyev and other East European specialists. While Matveyev's book (*The Problem of Periodization of Sport Training*, 1965), analyzed the training plans and diaries of Russian athletes who competed in the 1952 Olympics, Tudor Bompa was already applying periodization of training during the same period with Mihaela Penes (gold medalist in javelin throw at the 1964 Tokyo Olympic Games). His work in the early 1960s resulted in what would become his concept of the periodization of strength. The popularity of periodization has increased dramatically, especially in North America, after the first edition of Bompa's popular work (Bompa 1983).

The terminology Tudor Bompa uses is based on the original work of the Greek author Flavius Philostratus (AD 170–245), the Roman physician Claudius Galenus (Galen, AD 129–217), and the German specialists who designed the German athletes' training plans for the Berlin Olympic Games (1936):

- quadrennial, a four-year or Olympic training plan,
- annual plan, a training plan for a year, divided into smaller training phases,
- macrocycles (approximately 4 weeks),
- microcycles, a training phase of 4-7 days, usually one full week, and
- training unit, or training session.

Figure II.1 illustrates the types of plans and periodization of biomotor abilities used in training.

To the list of plans described in figure II.1, we also have to add the long-term training plan, briefly discussed in chapter 7. Part III of this book explains how to create such plans, as well as illustrating various practical examples.

The intention to critically analyze the semantics used lately in the terminology of theory and methodology of training has never concerned us. However, as each science has a terminology that defines specific concepts in its body of knowledge, the invasion of hybrid terminologies proposed by some authors requires some clarification.

The introduction of spurious terms into the theory and methodology of training since the 1990s is not justified because no new information has been added to the body of knowledge in that theory. In fact, some terms proposed lately are mostly semantics, fake terms without scientific substance. A brief analysis of contemporaneous terminologies might shed additional light on the subject.

Periodization	Periodization of the annual plan	Monocycles
		Bi-cycles
		Tri-cycles
		Multi-cycles
	Periodization of biomotor abilities	Sequential
		Simultaneous

Figure II.1   The structure of periodization of annual plan and periodization of biomotor abilities.

- *Periodization.* When Leonid Matveyev borrowed this term from history, he was referring to something new that was not yet part of the vocabulary of that period. Nor was there much written information on the subject. For better time management, the annual plan is divided into periods of training phase; he called this planning concept *periodization.* Some authors see Matveyev's periodization model as the *classical periodization.* But the true classical plans should be considered to be those actually proposed first by Flavius Philostratus (AD 170–245) and then by the German specialists who devised the training plans used for the 1936 Berlin Olympics.

- The *annual plan* has existed since the ancient Olympic Games (the *Olympic Year,* referred to by Galen). Yet the best coaches of the late 1800s to early 1900s knew about it and used simple annual planning and the breakdown of the annual plan into smaller training phases. In other words, Matveyev's work does not bring much new information about this subject. He was, however, the first author to use the term *periodization.*

- Matveyev proposed the term *macrocycle* to define an annual plan. But the German specialists used a four-week plan (*grosser,* or large, plan) to define what we call a macrocycle.

- The *microcycle* (the term proposed by Matveyev for a weekly training plan) has existed since the ancient Olympics as the *tetra system,* a four-day cycle mentioned by Philostratus.

Selected fallacies of training terminologies include

- *Block training.* Instead of using the traditional term *training phase,* some authors have adopted the term *block training* as if it brought something new. What is the difference between *training phase* and *block training*? Furthermore, the term *block* is often used incorrectly to indicate a phase of training or a macrocycle.

- *Linear periodization.* Some authors have introduced this term to refer to *traditional periodization,* which is a series of training phases intended to lead to and facilitate peak performance during the competitive phase. But why is it necessary to call something *linear* that is already recognized as being *traditional*? Besides, an annual plan has a linear format!

- *Undulatory periodization* is a hybrid term that has been proposed by some authors without logic, without any base on the way the periodization process is constructed. In fact, this term has been copied from Bompa's concept of the curve of rating training load (Bompa 1993) and is a faulty interpretation of the load alternation between training units within a microcycle. Someone unfamiliar with sport training and with the intent of being original has presumably fabricated this term in order to enlarge the terminology of periodization-planning.

- *Pendular development* and *complex development* of biomotor abilities are terms incorrectly taken from their original source (Bompa 1993). The original term for *pendular development* was *alternation of strength training* (maximum strength alternated with power training) that resulted in better power development. In fact, pendular is exactly that: an alternation of the various types of strength training. *Complex development* refers to complex training, which represents a strength-training phase in which both maximum strength and power are trained simultaneously, mostly during the precompetitive phase. Originally (Bompa 1993 and 1999), this method was called *maxex training,* or maximum explosiveness training.

- *Sequential integration* and *simultaneous integration* within periodization of training also create confusion among many authors and practitioners. Both of these planning tools are presented, totally inaccurately, as if they are mutually exclusive, but this is not the case.

- *Sequential periodization* proposes that certain biomotor abilities are developed in a specific sequence, which is true. Take, for example, periodization of strength of an annual plan (figure II.2), where anatomical adaptation (AA), maximum strength (MxS), and power (P) follow in a specific, physiologically justified sequence (neuromuscular strategy). Yet all sports, for logical and physiological reasons, also follow the simultaneous periodization model.
- *Simultaneous periodization.* In designing the periodization of dominant abilities for the majority of other sports, for physiological adaptation reasons and the methodology of developing the dominant abilities in the selected sport, coaches should follow the simultaneous periodization model (figure II.3), or the simultaneous integration of the dominant biomotor abilities of the selected sport.

If you take each ability separately, horizontally, particularly periodization of strength, this is similar to sequential periodization. However, for the vast majority of sports, where there are two or three biomotor abilities to periodize at the same time, this process has to be performed simultaneously, not independently. The dates of simultaneous periodization are dictated by the competition calendar and the duration of a biomotor ability to reach the desired standards of adaptation.

While a small number of authors have promoted the use of sequential periodization only, this type of periodization cannot be taken seriously. Physiologically and methodically you cannot train strength in one phase, followed by endurance, and then return to strength training. It is inappropriate, a physiological and methodological error, that does not result in the best performance at the desired time of the year. What happens to the adaptation and improvement of strength, specifically the neuromuscular strategy of power training while you are training endurance? How do you retain the training effect of the previous abilities? In doing so you diminish the early adaptation syndrome of strength, its training effect, and its influence on the athlete's improvement.

That is why the vast majority of sports should use simultaneous periodization, in which you integrate the periodization of dominant abilities of the selected sport, particularly team sports, for which the preparatory phase is often much shorter than for some individual sports.

Periodization of strength	AA	MxS/P	Maintain MxS/P	Competition

Figure II.2 A simple illustration of sequential periodization of strength.

Periodization of biomotor abilities	Strength	AA	MxS	• Power • Agility • Maintain MxS
	Speed	Tempo (repetitions of 200-400m, 50%-60% of maximum speed)	Maximum accelerations Maximum speed	• Starts • Maximum speed
	Endurance	Aerobic endurance (sport-specific proportions)		• Aerobic endurance • Ergogenesis (sport-specific endurance, speed-endurance)

Figure II.3 A schematic illustration of simultaneous periodization and integration of development of biomotor abilities.

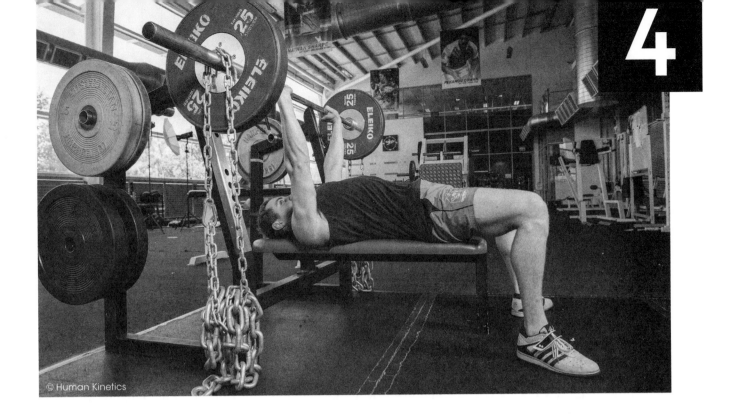

© Human Kinetics

Manipulation of Training Variables

To create successful strength training programs, coaches and athletes manipulate several training variables, mainly volume and intensity. Both the volume and the intensity of training, as well as its frequency, change according to the competition schedule and the objective of training. More specific factors within the categories of volume and intensity include load (which is generally expressed as a percentage of one repetition maximum, or 1RM), repetitions, sets, tempo or speed of execution (only for muscle endurance training), and rest intervals between sets. Manipulating these specific variables alters the volume, intensity, degree of effort, and density of training—and, consequently, the training effect.

Strength training programs must also include a mix of general and sport-specific exercises. As a rule of thumb, the early part of the yearly training program, which can include two to three months of preparatory training, should include a higher volume of training with a low proportion of sport-specific exercises. As the competitive season approaches, however, the intensity of training is stressed, the volume is decreased, and sport-specific exercises become a major part of the program.

Training Volume

Volume, or the quantity of work performed, can be measured either in terms of the weight lifted per training session, per microcycle, per macrocycle, or in terms of the total number of sets or reps performed per training session, per microcycle, per macrocycle, or per year. Instructors, coaches, and athletes should keep records of the tonnage (total weight) lifted or the sets and reps performed per session or per training phase to help them plan future training volumes.

Training volume varies based on the sport's particular physical demands, the athlete's strength training background, and the type of strength training performed. For example, athletes attempting to develop muscular endurance use a high volume of training because of the many reps they perform. Maximum strength training, on the other hand, results in lower tonnage and density, despite the high load, because of the lower number of total reps and the longer rest intervals. A medium training volume is typical for athletes in sports that require power, because the load is low to medium.

Overall training volume becomes more important as athletes approach high performance. There are no shortcuts. Athletic performance requires high weekly training frequency, which, in turn, may result in greater training volume. As athletes adapt to a higher volume of training, they experience better recovery and a higher level of structural and neural adaptation. This increase in work capacity can later translate into better handling of the intensification phases, as well as better performance overall.

Once optimal volume has been reached, the main stressor for mature athletes should be intensity. Work capacity is acquired over time; therefore, in order to increase training volume by increasing training frequency, it is necessary at first to lower the volume per training unit. This reduction is achieved by dividing the previous total volume of the microcycle by the new, higher number of training units. Increasing the number of training units while maintaining the same weekly training volume allows the work to be intensified thanks to increased recovery as the volume and duration per unit decrease. As a result, greater adaptations are possible (Bompa and Buzzichelli 2018).

Later, the volume per session can be increased, if necessary. For example, suppose that your objective is to increase strength training from three to four training units per microcycle and that your starting point is a microcycle with three strength training sessions, each with 8 tons of volume (thus 24 tons of total volume per microcycle). In this situation, here are an incorrect method and a correct method:

- *Incorrect method.* Add a training unit of 8 tons, thus abruptly increasing the total volume of the microcycle from 24 to 32 tons (an increase of 25%).

- *Correct method.* Divide the total volume of 24 tons by the new total of four training units. The total microcycle volume remains unchanged at 24 tons, but the volume of the single sessions is reduced to 6 tons each (a decrease of 25%), thus allowing a greater average intensity and better recovery. The volume per session can be increased later if need be.

Strength training volume depends on the athlete's biological makeup, the specifics of the sport, and the importance of strength in that sport. Mature athletes with a good strength training background can tolerate higher volumes, but volume should not be increased for its own sake. Rather, it should be increased if the specific situation requires it—and never at the expense of the quality of sport-specific training.

Because biomotor abilities training (increasing the athlete's motor potential) must be integrated with sport-specific training (specific performance), our starting point should be the least training volume that is effective at increasing the indexes of a certain biomotor ability. During general preparation, the volume of biomotor abilities training can be such as to temporarily affect the specific performance. During specific preparation, there should a correlation between the increase of a biomotor ability's indexes and the specific performance. And during the competitive phase, biomotor abilities training should be such as to allow maintenance, slight improvement, or peaking of the specific performance.

A dramatic or abrupt increase in volume can be detrimental, irrespective of the athlete's sport or ability, resulting in fatigue, uneconomical muscular work, and possibly injury. These pitfalls can be avoided by implementing a progressive plan with an appropriate method of monitoring load increments. Here are a few rules of thumb.

- A session dedicated to strength training should not last longer than 75 minutes unless it is a high-volume, maximum-strength session with long rest intervals, or a muscle-endurance-long session for an ultra-endurance athlete.

- The volume of an anatomical adaptation session should fall between 16 and 32 total sets; a hypertrophy session between 16 and 24 (and less than one hour in duration); a maximum strength session between 16 and 24; a power session between 10 and 16; and a power endurance or muscle-endurance-short session between 4 and 12.

- Once the sets' volume is established, it should not vary by more than 50% within a macrocycle—for example, 2 sets per exercise in the first microcycle, 3 sets per exercise in the second and third microcycles, 2 sets in the fourth (unload) microcycle.

The total volume depends on several factors, and the determinant is the importance of strength to the sport. For instance, international-class weightlifters often plan 33 short tons (30 tonnes) per training session and approximately 44,000 short tons (40,000 tonnes) per year. For other sports, the volume differs drastically (table 4.1). Power and speed sports require a much higher volume than boxing does; in sports in which muscular endurance is dominant, such as rowing and canoeing, the volume of strength per year can be three to six times higher.

Table 4.1 Suggested Guidelines for Volume (in Tonnes) of Strength Training per Year

Sport or event	VOLUME PER MICROCYCLE IN TRAINING PHASES			VOLUME PER YEAR	
	Preparatory	Competitive	Transition	Minimum	Maximum
Shot put	24-40	8-12	4-6	900	1,450
Football	30-40	10-12	6	900	1,400
Baseball, cricket	20-30	8-10	2-4	850	1,250
Downhill skiing	18-36	6-10	2-4	700	1,250
Long and triple jumps	20-30	8-10	2	800	1,200
Rowing	30-40	10-12	4	900	1,200
Kayaking, canoeing	20-40	10-12	4	900	1,200
Wrestling	20-30	10	4	800	1,200
Swimming	20	8-10	2-4	700	1,200
High jump	16-28	8-10	2-4	620	1,000
Triathlon	16-20	8-10	2-4	600	1,000
Cycling	16-22	8-10	2-4	600	950
Ice hockey	15-25	6-8	2-4	600	950

(continued)

Table 4.1 *(continued)*

| Sport or event | VOLUME PER MICROCYCLE IN TRAINING PHASES | | | VOLUME PER YEAR | |
	Preparatory	Competitive	Transition	Minimum	Maximum
Speedskating	14-26	4-6	2-4	500	930
Lacrosse	14-22	4-8	2-4	500	900
Basketball	12-24	4-6	2	450	850
Javelin	12-24	4	2	450	800
Volleyball	12-20	4	2	450	600
Sprinting	10-18	4	2	400	600
Gymnastics	10-16	4	4	380	600
Rugby	10-20	4-6	4	320	600
Squash	8-12	4	4	350	550
Figure skating	8-12	2-4	2	350	550
Tennis	8-12	2-4	2	350	550
Boxing, martial arts	8-14	3	1	380	500
Golf	4-6	2	1	250	300

Training Intensity

In strength training, intensity is expressed as a percentage of load or 1RM maximum. It is an indicator of the strength of the nervous stimuli employed in training, and it is determined by the degree to which the central nervous system (CNS) is called into action. Stimulus strength depends on load, speed of movement, and variation of rest intervals between reps. Training load, expressed as intensity percentage of 1RM, refers to the mass or weight lifted. Strength training employs the intensity zones and loads presented in table 4.2.

A *supermaximum load* exceeds one's maximum strength (1RM). In most cases, loads between 100% and 120% of 1RM can be used by applying the eccentric (yielding to the force of gravity) or isometric (maximal contraction without joint movement) method. Only

Table 4.2 Intensity Value and Load Used in Strength Training

Intensity value	Load	% of 1RM	Type of contraction	Method	Adaptations
1	Supermax	>105	Eccentric or isometric	Maximum strength	Intramuscular coordination
2	Max	90-100	Eccentric-concentric		
3	Heavy	85-90	Eccentric-concentric	Maximum strength and power (high load)	
4		80-85	Eccentric-concentric		
5	Medium	70-80	Eccentric-concentric		Intermuscular coordination
6		50-70	Eccentric-concentric	Power (low load)	
7	Low	30-50	Eccentric-concentric		

a few athletes with a robust strength training background should use supermaximum loads. Such loads should be employed for limited time periods and only for some muscle groups, in particular those muscle groups whose eccentric loading is high during the sport-specific activity (for instance, the hamstrings during sprinting or the quads during landing or changing directions). Most other athletes should be restricted to loads of no more than 100% of 1RM.

Maximum load can range from 90% to 100% of 1RM, heavy load from 80% to 90%, medium load from 60% to 80%, and low load from 30% to 60% percent. Each intensity zone elicits slightly different neuromuscular adaptations and necessitates a precise progression. Intensities above 90% percent should be used sparingly, especially to concentric failure, for their testosterone-lowering effect (Häkkinen and Pakarinen 1993; Izquierdo et al. 2006) despite their additional positive neuromuscular adaptations.

Testing the 1RM every three or four weeks at the end of a macrocycle is usually enough to reap the benefits of the 90% to 100% intensity range. Over the years, Western strength training authors have often supported the use of concentric failure as a required condition for strength gains. In reality, all of the performance-enhancing neuromuscular adaptations (except for the highest hypertrophic effect [Burd et al. 2010]) occur without the need for concentric failure.

As an athlete becomes objectively strong (thus neuromuscularly efficient), he or she can tolerate a less frequent exposure to maximum loads (figure 4.1).

Load should relate to the type of strength being developed and, more importantly, to the sport-specific combination resulting from the blending of strength with speed or of strength with endurance. For general guidelines about the load to use in developing each of these combinations, see table 4.3. The load is not the same through all training phases. Rather, periodization alters the load according to the goals of each training phase. As shown in the table, the load ranges from 30% to more than 100% of 1RM, and the corresponding intensities are shown in the second row of the table. The rows below that indicate the sport-specific combinations and the suggested load for each.

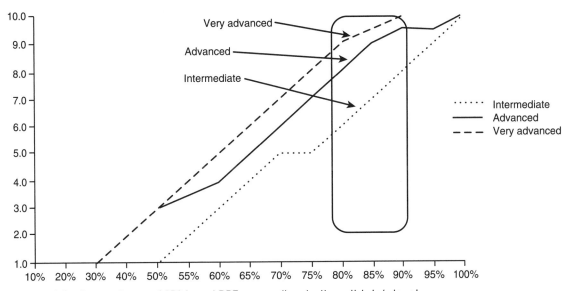

Figure 4.1 Percentage of 1RM and RPE according to the athlete's level.

Reprinted by permission from P. Evangelista, "La Programmazione Della Forza - Criteri di Scelta e Analisi Degli Schemi di Allenamento," a workshop for the Tudor Bompa Institute Italia, May 23, 2010.

Table 4.3 Relationship Between Load and Different Types and Combinations of Strength

% of 1RM	>105	100	90	80	70	60	50	40	30
Intensity	Supermax	Max	Heavy	Medium		Low			
Type of strength				Power (high load)		Power (low load)			
	Maximum strength					Muscle endurance			
Landing and reactive power	■	■	■						
Throwing power				■	■	■	■		
Takeoff power				■	■	■			
Starting power				■	■	■	■		
Deceleration power				■	■	■	■		
Acceleration power				■	■	■	■	■	
Power endurance					■	■	■	■	
Muscle endurance short					■	■	■	■	
Muscle endurance medium						■	■	■	
Muscle endurance long							■	■	■

(Left side label: Sport-specific strength combinations)

Periodization incorporates proper planning for all the performance abilities needed in the chosen sport. For instance, training for a middle-distance runner addresses training distance covered, sessions per week, and of course volume of work (e.g., sets and reps) performed in each strength training session. The more reps and sets an athlete performs in a session, the greater the volume of work. Volume and intensity are very closely related and represent the quantity and quality of work. One is not more important than the other; both should be strategically manipulated in training to produce a desired effect.

As with most body systems, a dose response exists between the total volume of work and the level of adaptation. Beginning strength trainers or athletes initially benefit from a low volume, such as one or two sets, but they eventually plateau and require greater stimulation in order to experience further adaptation. Therefore, it is not surprising to have athletes perform the squat for multiple sets (such as 6 to 8) or 50-plus reps, depending on the desired physiological effect. Keep in mind that the term *intensity*, as used in the sporting world, is strictly a representation of a percentage of load used in training. In other words, the only true way to increase intensity is to increase the load.

For instance, suppose that an athlete performs 2 reps for the first set of a lift at 90% of 1RM and then, after a four-minute rest, completes 3 reps to failure at the same load. From set 1 to set 2, the athlete has not increased the intensity. The volume has been increased, along with the stress inflicted on the muscle, but the load has remained at 90%; therefore, the intensity has not changed.

Trainers and coaches must be careful not to correlate intensity with the muscular feeling that occurs following a set. As a rule of thumb, the more sets the athlete performs, the lower the number of reps, and vice versa. For instance, during a maximum strength phase, an athlete might perform 6 sets of 3 reps with an increase load from 70% to 80% of 1RM; however, during the hypertrophy phase, the same athlete might perform only 3 sets of 10 reps with a load of 65% of 1RM.

Athletes' training programs should always be individualized, and coaches and trainers should look for signs of fatigue. One of the biggest problems in the sport training world is the sacrifice of quality for quantity. Planning should be used only as a guideline for program design. That is, it should not be carved in stone; instead, session-by-session progress and setbacks should be noted and used in revising the training program. Coaches should watch for the point at which an athlete is no longer capable of performing the suggested number of reps for a specific load or of performing the desired number of reps explosively and with sound technique. This judgment is critical, especially in the maximum strength phase of training, when the primary goal is to achieve nervous system adaptations.

Number of Exercises

The key to an effective training program is adequate exercise selection. It is difficult to establish an optimum number of exercises, and some coaches select far too many because they wish to develop more muscle groups. The resulting program is overloaded and fatiguing. Instead, the number and types of exercise must be selected according to the age and performance level of the athlete, the needs of the sport, and the phase of training.

Age and Performance Level

One of the main objectives of a training program for juniors or beginners is the development of a solid anatomical and physiological foundation. For strength training, the coach should select many exercises (9 to 12) that address the primary muscle groups (prime movers). Such a program may last one to three years, depending on the athlete's age and the expected age for achieving high performance.

On the other hand, the main training objective for advanced athletes is to reach the highest possible level of performance. Their strength programs, especially during the competitive phase, must therefore be specific, with only a few exercises (2 to 4) directed at the prime movers.

Needs of the Sport

Strength training exercises, particularly for elite athletes, should meet the specific needs of the chosen sport and address the prime movers that are dominant in that sport. For example, an elite high jumper may need to perform only three or four exercises to strengthen all prime movers adequately. A wrestler or an American football player, or athletes in a multi-planar sport in general, on the other hand, may need to perform four to six exercises to accomplish the same goal. And all sprinting athletes should do one exercise for the hip extensors with the knees straight (hamstrings), one exercise for the hip extensors with flexed knees (glutes), one exercise for the knee extensors (quads), and one exercise for the plantar flexors (calves). The more prime movers that are used in a sport the more exercises are needed. It may be possible to lower the number, however, by using well-selected multijoint exercises.

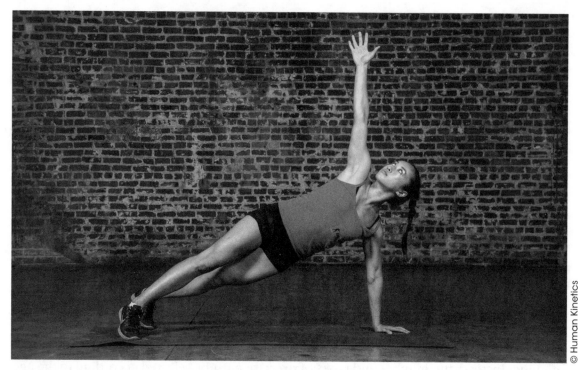

As a principle, develop core strength before limb strength.

Phase of Training

After the transition phase, a new annual plan should be used to start building the foundation for future training. In a general strength training program, anatomical adaptation is desirable early in the preparatory phase. For such a program to involve most muscle groups, the number of exercises has to be high (9 to 12), regardless of the specifics of the chosen sport.

As a program progresses, the number of exercises is reduced, culminating in the competitive phase, in which the athlete performs only two to five very specific exercises that are essential to the sport. For instance, an American football, hockey, basketball, or volleyball player will perform eight or nine exercises during the preparatory phase but only three or four during the league season. By being selective, coaches can increase training efficiency and lower the athlete's overall fatigue.

Strength training is done in addition to technical and tactical training. In short, an inverse relationship exists between the load used in training and the number of exercises per training session. A decrease in the number of exercises indicates that the athlete is training for the specifics of the sport. As the number of exercises decreases, the number of sets per exercise increases. In this way, more workload is placed on the specific prime movers of the sport in order to optimize the muscles' strength, and power for competition. Once the competitive season begins, progressive adaptation is set aside, and a low number of exercises and moderate set increments are used to maintain physiological adaptation.

Even though the upper body is only minimally involved in some sports (such as soccer, many track-and-field events, and cycling), many strength programs emphasize exercises for the upper body. In addition, many physical education instructors, still influenced by bodybuilding theories and by the commercialism and gadgets of the day, suggest far too many exercises for athletes. In reality, athletes who use a high number of exercises decrease the number of sets targeted to each prime mover. This approach leads to either very high volume per session, thus fatigue, or very low training adaptation of the prime movers and therefore very low training effect.

The desired result—high training adaptation and therefore improvement of performance—is possible only when athletes perform more sets for the chosen kinetic chain. The coach has the option of spreading all required sets for the fundamental exercises across more sessions throughout the microcycle or concentrating them in a few sessions. The first option allows the athlete to perform shorter sessions and include more accessory exercises, whereas the second option may require longer sessions and a reduction in accessory exercises.

Order of Exercises

The first determinant in exercise order is motor complexity. In fact, complex, multijoint exercises—those that normally target the prime movers in a kinetic sequence similar to the specific sport action—should always be performed first in a workout, when the nervous system is fresh. When selecting the number of exercises, strength and conditioning coaches should consider the prime movers involved in performing the skills of the sport and arrange the exercises in the order of their motor complexity.

Again, strength training for sport has been unduly influenced by the training methodologies of bodybuilding. Many strength training books and articles, for example, propose exercising the small-muscle groups first and then the large-muscle groups. But this approach results in fatiguing the small-muscle groups, which leaves athletes unable to effectively train the large-muscle groups. The large-muscle groups are the prime movers in the sport, and it is extremely important that the prime movers be trained in an unfatigued state.

Another overused training method from the world of bodybuilding is the *preexhaustion method*. Using this method, trainees exhaust the prime movers with single-joint exercises (such as seated leg extensions) before executing multijoint exercises (such as the squat). Although this theory may be useful to bodybuilders, research challenges its usefulness in sport (Augustsson et al. 2003).

For this reason, sport trainers should avoid using this method, even during the hypertrophy phase of training. Instead, the main exercises in strength training programs for sport should be multijoint exercises in which the major prime movers work together. Single-joint exercises can be used during the early preparatory phase, such as during anatomical adaptation, or to correct an assessed muscle imbalance within a kinetic chain, but should be phased out in the later stages of training. Training for sport is all about optimizing strength, power, speed, and endurance—not about improving the aesthetic appeal of the athlete.

Specific strength exercises that resemble a sport-specific motor pattern repeat similar motions, involving the chain of muscles in a pattern similar to their involvement in the sport. For instance, it makes sense for a volleyball player to perform half squats and toe raises together because spiking and blocking require the same moves. The chain of muscles involved is acting in the same sequence as in jumping. A volleyball player, then, is concerned not with whether the small-muscle groups or the large-muscle groups are involved first but only with mimicking the sport-specific motion and involving the chain of muscles in the same way as in spiking and blocking.

Two options are available for choosing the order in which to perform the exercises prescribed by the coach: horizontal and vertical (see table 4.4).

- *First option: horizontal sequence.* The athlete may perform all the sets for the first exercise, then move to the next exercise—a horizontal sequence. If the rest intervals are inadequate, this sequence may cause great local fatigue by the time all sets are performed for one exercise. As a result, it may produce hypertrophy rather than power or maximum strength, and, in the case of maximum strength sessions with lengthy rest intervals, the total duration of the sessions may become excessive.

- *Second option: vertical sequence.* The athlete may follow the order of exercises in sequence from the top down—a vertical sequence or strength circuit—as listed on the daily program sheet. This method leads to better recovery for the muscle groups involved. In fact, by the time the first exercise is performed again, the muscles have substantially recovered. To ensure better recovery, exercises should alternate either between antagonist muscle groups or between upper and lower body. If all parts of the body are exercised, the following order is suggested: lower body push, upper body push, lower body pull, upper body pull, and so on.

Table 4.4   Comparison of Sample Exercise Sequence Arrangements

Sequence	Exercise	Sets	Reps	Rest interval (min)	Sequence	Exercise	Sets	Reps	Rest interval (min)
1	Squat	4	3	3	⬇	Squat	4	3	1.5
2	Bench press	4	3	3	⬇	Bench press	4	3	1.5
3	Leg curl	4	3	3	⬇	Leg curl	4	3	1.5
4	Lat pulldown	4	3	3	⬇	Lat pulldown	4	3	1.5
5	Standing calf raise	3	6	2	⬇	Standing calf raise	3	6	1.5
6	Cable adduction	3	6	2	⬇	Cable adduction	3	6	1.5
7	Weighted sit-up	3	6	2	⬇	Weighted sit-up	3	6	2
Session duration		65 min.			Session duration		45 min.		
Rest between sets of same exercise		2-3 min.			Rest between sets of same exercise		14 min.		

Number of Reps and Speed of Execution

Although speed of execution is an important parameter of loading in strength training, it is not always properly understood. For example, in bodybuilding circles it is considered common knowledge that loads over 85% of 1RM are lifted slowly, but this is not necessarily so. Power athletes trained to lift explosively can be fast with weights up to 95% of 1RM and express high levels of power output even with such high loads.

It all comes down to training the nervous system to activate and fire all of the motor units in the shortest time. This effect can be achieved by periodizing the strength training program, going from intermuscular coordination training (moderate and heavy loads lifted explosively) to intramuscular coordination training (maximum loads lifted explosively, or at least with the intent to move them explosively) (Behm and Sale 1993). See table 4.5, and also refer back to table 2.2.

For development of maximum strength (i.e., working at 70%-100% of 1RM), the number of reps is very low (1-5). For exercises to develop power (i.e., working at 50%-80% of 1RM), the number of reps is low to moderate (1-10, performed dynamically). For muscular endurance of short duration, 10 to 30 reps will work, whereas muscular endurance of medium duration requires 30 to 60 nonstop reps, and muscular endurance of long duration requires an even higher number of reps—up to 200. Instructors who regard 20 reps as adequate for enhancing muscular endurance may find the suggested number of reps shocking. However, performing only 20 reps makes an insignificant contribution to overall performance in sports that require muscular endurance of medium or long duration, such as rowing, kayaking, canoeing, long-distance swimming, and cross-country skiing.

Speed of execution is critical in strength training. For the best training effects, the speed of execution, at least in the concentric phase, must be fast and dynamic for most types of work. The key to proper execution of speed is the way in which the athlete applies

Table 4.5 Intensities and Repetitions Used in the Maximum Strength Phases and the Power Phase

	% 1RM	MxS-II	MxS-I	Power
Intramuscular coordination	100	1		
	95	1-2		
	90	1-3		
	85	3-5		
Intermuscular coordination	80		3-5	
	75		3-5	
	70		3-5	1-2
	65			1-3
	60			3-5
	55			3-5
	50			3-5

force against resistance. For instance, when an American football player, a thrower, or a sprinter lifts a heavy load (more than 90% of 1RM), the motion may look slow, but the force against the resistance is applied as fast as possible. Otherwise, the nervous system does not recruit and fire at high frequency all the motor units necessary to defeat resistance. Only fast and vigorous application of force trains the voluntary recruitment of fast-twitch muscle fibers. In fact, one study has demonstrated that performing the concentric action of a lift at the maximal intended velocity versus half that velocity elicited a maximum strength increase over six weeks that was double that of the slow lifting, as well as an increase in velocity with all loads (Bompa 1993; González-Badillo et al. 2014).

For this reason, the speed of execution plays a very important role in strength training and should vary from phase to phase. To achieve explosive force, the athlete must concentrate on activating the muscles quickly, even when the barbell is moving slowly. Most of the time, however, the bar or training machine should in fact move fast. Only a high speed of contraction performed against a heavy load (more than 70% of 1RM) rapidly recruits the fast-twitch fibers and results in increased maximum strength and improvements of power capability. The appropriate speed of execution for each phase of the strength training program is indicated in table 4.6.

Slow to moderate speeds in the concentric phase increase the metabolic stress and the muscular force expression throughout the range of motion and can be used to increase the hypertrophic response to training. Moderate speeds can be used during the anatomical adaptation phase of training because they allow more motor control and more time under tension. The athlete can spend about three or four seconds in the eccentric portion of the lift, pause for one second for the transition from eccentric to concentric, and then spend two seconds in the concentric portion.

Fast and dynamic or explosive execution has to be applied for the rest of the annual plan; athletes should perform the concentric actions for strength exercises fast or explosively because the vast majority of sport actions require fast concentric contractions.

The intended speed of contraction should be as fast as possible during the phases focused on maximum strength, power, power endurance, and muscle endurance short. During the maximum strength phase, athletes should slowly perform a three- to four-second eccentric action followed by an explosive concentric action. The transition from the

Table 4.6   Suggested Speed of Execution per Training Phase

	SPEED OF EXECUTION	
Training objective	**Eccentric phase**	**Concentric phase**
AA	Slow	Slow or fast
Hyp	Slow	Fast
MxS	Slow	Fast
P	Fast	Fast
PE	Fast	Fast
MES	Fast	Fast
MEM	Moderate	Moderate/Fast
MEL	Moderate	Moderate

Key: AA = anatomical adaptation, Hyp. = hypertrophy, MEL = muscle endurance long, MEM = muscle endurance medium, MES = muscle endurance short, MxS = maximum strength, P = power, PE = power endurance

eccentric action to the concentric action can be manipulated during this phase. The best way to maximize concentric strength is, in fact, to remove any reflexive or elastic qualities developed during the eccentric phase of the lift by pausing for one or two seconds before performing a further concentric lift. Such a method should be used in the early part of the maximum strength phase but should not be used in the latter part of the maximum strength phase when the athlete is preparing to transition to the specific strength phase.

Let us take the bench press as an example. When performing the bench press, extending the arms forms the concentric portion of the lift, and returning the barbell to chest level and stretching the chest muscles forms the eccentric portion. Generally speaking, an athlete slowly flexes the arms to bring the bar to the chest before quickly returning the bar to the starting position and starting the cycle again. On the other hand, the eccentric portion of the lift can increase the force of the concentric lift that follows if the eccentric portion is also executed quickly, thus eliciting what is called the myotatic (stretch) reflex. This reflex is why plyometric training is so popular in sport. In essence, plyometric training improves sport performance by heightening the physiological properties of the prime movers for quick and explosive concentric actions.

As an athlete quickly lowers the bar to the chest, neural mechanisms in the muscles are heightened and elastic energy is stored in the tendons and used during the concentric or lifting portion of the exercise. Thus, a true increase in pure concentric force generation can be achieved by pausing briefly after the eccentric lift and making the upward motion of the bar a pure concentric lift without any positive influence from the eccentric action. This approach allows standardization of the range of motion for each rep by keeping the athlete from cheating or rebounding the weight. Because it encourages better technique, it improves intermuscular coordination.

This approach can also be used to help an athlete break through a strength plateau. The coach should decide whether the main focus is voluntary concentric strength maximization or imitation of the sport-specific neuromuscular pattern (usually an eccentric–concentric action). As previously stated, the focus should be switched from the former to the latter during the maximum strength phase.

Each training phase has an ideal way to perform each rep depending on the training effect pursued in that phase. This specificity applies as well to set duration, which is related to the energy system involved. The training effect for different set durations is presented in table 4.7.

Table 4.7 Set Duration and Training Effects

Set duration	Training effect
2-12 seconds	Strength improvement without hypertrophy gains (relative strength) and power
15-25 seconds	Strength improvement with hypertrophy gains (absolute strength)
30-60 seconds	Hypertrophy
15-30 seconds (sets)	Power/Power endurance
30-120 seconds (sets)	Muscle endurance short
2-8 minutes (sets)	Muscle endurance medium
More than 8 minutes	Muscle endurance long

Number of Sets

A set is the number of reps per exercise followed by a rest interval. The number of sets depends on the number of exercises and the strength combination. The number of sets per exercise decreases as the number of exercises increases because otherwise the workout would get too voluminous. There is also an inverse relationship between the number of reps per set and the number of sets per exercise. For example, for a rower, a canoeist, or a cross-country skier attempting to develop muscular endurance of long duration, the key element is the number of reps per set. Because the number of reps is high, it is difficult for these athletes to perform more than three sets.

The number of sets also depends on the athlete's ability and training capacity, the number of muscle groups to be trained, and the training phase. For instance, a high jumper or a diver in a specialized training program may use three to five exercises for 4 to 6 sets each. A higher number of exercises would require fewer sets, which would entail obvious disadvantages for the adaptation of the prime movers. Consider a hypothetical high jumper who uses eight exercises involving several muscle groups of the legs, upper body, and arms. For each exercise or muscle group, the athlete performs work of 880 lb (about 400 kg). Because the athlete can perform only 4 sets, the total amount of work per muscle group is 3,520 lb (about 1,600 kg). If the number of exercises is reduced to four, however, the athlete can perform, say, 8 total sets for a total of 7,040 lb (about 3,200 kg) per muscle group. Thus, the athlete can double the total work on the prime movers by decreasing the total number of exercises and increasing the number of sets.

The number of sets performed per training session also depends on the training phase. During the preparatory (preseason) phase—and particularly during the anatomical adaptation phase, when most muscle groups are trained—more exercises are performed with fewer sets. As the competitive phase approaches, however, training becomes more specific, and the number of exercises decreases while the number of sets increases. Finally, during the competitive phase (season), when the purpose of training is to maintain a certain level of strength or a given strength combination, everything is reduced, including the number of sets, so that the athlete's energy is spent mostly on technical and tactical work or on sport-specific training.

In team sports where the competitive season is very long, the athlete performs only a few sets per exercise (two, three, or at most four) in order to reduce residual fatigue and the chance of negative influence on recovery and specific performance. A well-trained athlete in an individual sport, on the other hand, can perform 3, 6, or even 8 sets. Certainly, it makes sense to perform a high number of sets. The more sets an athlete performs of a fundamental exercise for the prime movers, the more work that athlete can perform, ultimately leading to higher strength gains and improved performance.

Rest Interval

Energy, of course, is necessary for strength training. During training, an athlete uses mainly the fuel of a given energy system according to the load employed and the duration of the activity. During high-intensity strength training, energy stores can be greatly taxed and even completely exhausted. In order to complete the work, therefore, athletes must take a rest interval to replenish depleted fuel before performing another set.

In fact, the rest interval between sets or training sessions is as important as the training itself. The amount of time allowed between sets determines, to a great extent, how much energy can be recovered before the following set. Careful planning of the rest interval is critical in avoiding needless physiological and psychological stress during training.

The duration of the rest interval depends on several factors, including the type of strength being developed, the load employed, the set duration, the number of muscles involved, and the athlete's level of conditioning. The athlete's body weight must also be considered, because heavy athletes with larger muscles tend to recover at a slower rate than lighter athletes do.

Rest Intervals Between Sets

The rest interval is a function of the load employed in training and the type of strength being developed (table 4.8).

During a rest interval, the high-energy compounds adenosine triphosphate (ATP) and creatine phosphate (CP) are replenished proportionately to the duration of the rest interval. When the rest interval is calculated properly, CP can be restored fully or almost fully and lactic acid accumulates more slowly, thus enabling the athlete to maintain a high power output for the entire workout. If the rest interval is shorter than a minute, lactic acid concentration gets rapidly high; when the rest interval is shorter than 30 seconds, lactate levels are so high that even well-trained athletes find them difficult to tolerate. A proper rest interval, on the other hand, reduces the accumulation and facilitates the removal of lactic acid from the muscles.

Some sports require athletes to tolerate lactic acid; examples include short-distance running, swimming, rowing, canoeing, some team sports, boxing, and wrestling. Strength training for athletes in these sports should take into consideration the following factors.

- A 30-second rest restores about 50% of depleted ATP-CP.

- Using a one-minute rest interval for several sets of 15 to 20 reps is insufficient to restore the muscle's energy substrates and enable a high power output.

- Fatigue accumulated during maximum strength exercise followed by too short a rest interval results in a reduced discharge rate of motor neurons, which reduces speed. This effect does not occur following a three-minute rest interval (Bigland-Ritchie et al. 1983); in fact, a rest interval of three minutes or longer allows almost complete ATP-CP restoration.

- A longer rest interval (more than three minutes) results in greater improvement of hamstring strength (Pincivero, Lephart, and Karunakara 1997).

Table 4.8 Suggested Guidelines for Rest Intervals Between Sets

Intensity zone	Load	% of 1RM	Rest interval (minutes)
1	Supermax	>105	4-8
2	Max	90-100	3-6
3	Heavy	85-90	3-5
4		80-85	
5	Medium	70-80	2-3
6		50-70	
7	Low	30-50	0.5-2

- Sets taken to concentric failure require far more recovery time than sets not taken to concentric failure. For instance, a set of 5 reps with a 70% of 1RM load might require one to two minutes to repeat the set with the same power output, whereas the same load taken to failure with 10 to 12 reps might require more than five minutes to repeat the same mean power output, which is certainly lower than the 5 reps set (see figure 4.2). Furthermore, after an athlete works to failure, a four-minute rest interval is insufficient to eliminate lactic acid from the working muscles or to replenish all of the energy requirements, such as glycogen.

- In addition, power output and metabolic profile differ considerably between the following two options: 5 sets of 10 reps taken to concentric failure versus 10 sets of 5 reps not taken to concentric failure using the same load as a percentage of 1RM (Gorostiaga et al. 2012). Not going to failure resulted in higher mean power output, a higher ATP level after the last set (6 vs. 4.9 mmol), a higher PC level (14.5 vs. 3.1 mmol), and a lower lactate level (5.8 vs. 25 mmol); see figure 4.2 and table 4.9.

The degree to which ATP-CP is replenished between sets depends on the duration of the rest interval: the shorter the rest interval, the less ATP-CP is restored and, consequently, the less energy is available for the next set. Therefore, one consequence of an inadequate rest interval between sets is an increased reliance on the lactic acid system for energy. If the rest interval is too short, the lactic acid system provides most of the energy needed for subsequent sets. Reliance on this energy system results in lower power output and increased lactic acid accumulation in the working muscles, which leads to pain and fatigue, impairing the athlete's ability to train effectively. Unless the athlete is training for hypertrophy or lactate tolerance, a longer rest interval is required in order to maintain power output and combat excessive lactic acid accumulation.

A second consequence of an inadequate rest interval is local muscular and CNS fatigue. Most research findings point to the following possible causes and sites of fatigue.

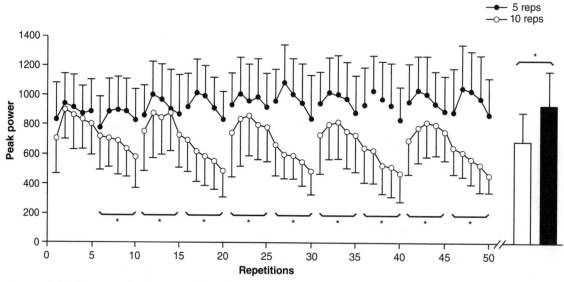

Figure 4.2 Power output comparison for each repetition of 5 sets of 10 reps taken to failure versus 10 sets of 5 reps not taken to failure.

Reprinted from E.M. Gorostiaga, I. Navarro-Amézqueta, J.A.L. Calbet, et al., "Energy Metabolism During Repeated Sets of Leg Press Exercise Leading to Failure or Not," *PLoS ONE* 7, no. 7 (2012): e40621. Distributed under the terms of the Creative Commons Attribution License.

Table 4.9   Metabolic Response to Five Sets of 10 Reps Taken to Failure Versus Ten Sets of 5 Reps Not Taken to Failure

	10 REPS			5 REPS		
	Pre	Post 1st series	Post final series	Pre	Post 1st series	Post final series
ATP	6.46 ± 0.56	6.42 ± 0.57	4.90 ± 0.39	6.58 ± 0.35	6.19 ± 0.59	6.09 ± 0.41
ADP	0.86 ± 0.03	0.91 ± 0.10	0.92 ± 0.11	0.86 ± 0.04	0.89 ± 0.08	0.87 ± 0.08
AMP	0.07 ± 0.04	0.09 ± 0.03	0.09 ± 0.04	0.08 ± 0.04	0.08 ± 0.03	0.08 ± 0.03
TAN	7.37 ± 0.59	7.42 ± 0.67	5.91 ± 0.44	7.52 ± 0.36	7.16 ± 0.66	7.04 ± 0.49
IMP	0.01 ± 0.00	0.08 ± 0.11	0.87 ± 0.69	0.01 ± 0.00	0.01 ± 0.00	0.01 ± 0.02
PCr	21.0 ± 8.86	7.75 ± 5.53	3.15 ± 2.88	19.5 ± 4.06	11.68 ± 7.82	14.47 ± 7.24
Cr	8.93 ± 4.96	25.45 ± 3.80	22.90 ± 6.89	8.40 ± 3.25	16.97 ± 6.33	15.57 ± 5.01
PCr + Cr	29.91 ± 5.19	34.55 ± 6.23	26.06 ± 8.44	27.90 ± 3.65	30.56 ± 6.19	30.15 ± 8.46
La	1.70 ± 1.18	17.20 ± 3.50	25.01 ± 8.09	2.02 ± 1.05	7.10 ± 2.54	5.80 ± 4.62
Energy change	0.933 ± 0.006	0.927 ± 0.004	0.909 ± 0.014	0.932 ± 0.007	0.927 ± 0.006	0.928 ± 0.006

Key: ATP = adenosine triphosphate; ADP = adenosine diphosphate; AMP = adenosine monophosphate; TAN = total adenine nucleotide; IMP = inosine monophosphate; PCr = phosphocreatine; Cr = creatine; La = lactate

Reprinted from E.M. Gorostiaga, I. Navarro-Amézqueta, J.A.L. Calbet, et al., "Energy Metabolism During Repeated Sets of Leg Press Exercise Leading to Failure or Not," *PLoS ONE* 7, no. 7 (2012): e40621. Distributed under the terms of the Creative Commons Attribution License.

- *Motor neuron.* The nervous system transmits impulses to muscle fibers through the motor neuron. A nerve impulse possesses a certain degree of frequency. Higher frequency of nerve impulses means stronger muscle contraction, which gives the athlete more ability to lift heavy loads or apply force rapidly for a sprint. The discharge frequency of nerve impulses is greatly affected by fatigue; specifically, as fatigue increases, the force of contraction decreases as a result of lower discharge rate (Ranieri and Di Lazzaro 2012; Taylor, Todd, and Gandevia 2006). That is why longer rest intervals (up to eight minutes) are necessary for CNS recovery during the maximum strength phase.

- *Neuromuscular junction.* The neuromuscular junction is the nerve attachment on the muscle fiber that relays nerve impulses to the working muscle. Fatigue at this site results largely from an increased release of chemical transmitters (i.e., neurotransmitters) from the nerve endings (Tesch 1980). The electrical properties of a nerve usually return to normal levels if an athlete rests for a two- to three-minute interval after performing a set. However, after performing powerful contractions, such as those typical of maximum strength training with maximal loads or speed or speed-endurance training, sufficient recovery may require a rest interval of more than five minutes.

- *Contractile mechanisms.* The muscle's contractile mechanisms (actin and myosin) can also be sites of fatigue and of performance breakdown. Specifically, the increased acidity caused by repeated muscular contraction, especially at high intensity, decreases the peak tension—or the ability of a muscle to contract maximally—and affects the muscle's ability to react to the nerve impulses (Fox, Bowes, and Foss 1989; Sahlin 1986; Enoka 2015). The contracting muscle is also fatigued by the depletion of muscle glycogen stores, which occurs during prolonged exercise (more than 30 minutes)

(Conlee 1987; Karlsson and Saltin 1971; Sahlin 1986; Stone et al. 2007). Other energy sources, including glycogen from the liver, cannot fully cover the working muscle's energy demands.

The CNS can also be affected by local muscle fatigue; in fact, this result is typical of sets taken to concentric failure. During training, chemical disturbances occur inside the muscle that affect its potential to perform work (Bigland-Ritchie et al. 1983; Hennig and Lomo 1987). When the effects of these chemical disturbances are signaled back to the CNS, the brain sends weaker nerve impulses to the working muscle, which decreases its working capacity in an attempt to protect the body. During an adequate rest interval of three to five minutes, the muscles are allowed to recover almost completely. The brain then senses the lack of danger and sends more powerful nerve impulses to the muscles, which results in better muscular performance.

Strength Training Frequency

The duration and frequency of rest intervals between strength training sessions depend on the athlete's conditioning and ability to recover, the training phase, and the energy source used in training. Well-conditioned athletes always recover faster, especially as training progresses toward the competitive phase, when they are supposed to reach their highest physical potential. Normally, strength training follows technical or tactical training, and if athletes tax the same energy system and fuel (e.g., glycogen) during technical and strength training, the next training of this type must be planned for two days later because 48 hours are required for full restoration of glycogen (Fox, Bowes, and Foss 1989; Piehl 1974; Stone et al. 2007). Even with a carbohydrate-rich diet, glycogen levels do not return to normal in less than two days.

If athletes perform only strength training, as some do on certain days during the preparatory phase, the restoration of glycogen occurs faster—55% in 5 hours and almost 100% in 24 hours. This faster restoration means that strength training can be planned more frequently. In the case of a strength training session during which multiple sets of low reps not taken to failure followed by adequate rest intervals are performed, glycogen restoration is not even a concern, because the energy system mainly involved would be the anaerobic alactic ATP-CP system.

The planning of strength training sessions should also take into account the time required for the recovery of muscle protein. Untrained subjects who take part in resistance training programs that include a combination of concentric and eccentric actions show muscle fiber breakdown (protein breakdown) that can persist as long as 48 hours after the bout of strength training (Gibala et al. 1995; Bompa and Haff 2009). The good news is that the concomitant net increase in the synthesis of muscle protein is greater than the breakdown. Protein synthesis, or the rebuilding of muscle fibers, following a strength training session can be further increased by ingesting a mix of carbohydrate and protein immediately following the session. Muscle protein recovery also likely happens faster in trained athletes.

Finally, probably the most important factor to consider in planning strength training sessions is nervous system fatigue. Scheduling high-intensity workouts on consecutive days does not allow proper time for neural recovery. For instance, many athletes perform maximum strength training on Monday followed by plyometric training on Tuesday. Because both sessions tax similar neural pathways, recovery time between the two is inadequate, and injury or signs of overtraining may appear unless the training uses a very low volume of both kinds of session.

Overall, then, scientific research overwhelmingly argues that recovery after a strength or aerobic training session must be adequate to allow time for all body systems to regenerate and adapt to the stimulus before being introduced to a similar or more aggressive training session of the same nature. In the circle of training, recovery plays as vital a role as the stimulus applied in training. Specifically, energy fuel must be restored, the nervous system must recover, and the net protein balance (synthesis minus breakdown) must remain positive in order to achieve progressive increases in muscular strength, power, endurance, or size The process can be simplified by designing training programs according to the energy systems used.

Restoration of Phosphates

Adenosine triphosphate (ATP) is the energy currency of the body, and creatine phosphate is used to form new ATP from the ADP that results from ATP metabolism. The body's energy substrates, such as the phosphates and glycogen, are lowered by the fatigue that is slowly brought on by lifting weights or performing high-level metabolic activity. The body then recovers and replenishes energy supplies to preexercise conditions (or higher) through the restoration of phosphates and glycogen.

As shown in table 4.10, phosphagen (ATP-CP) restoration reaches 50% in the first 30 seconds of recovery and 100% within three to five minutes. This pattern explains why a three- to five-minute rest is needed between sets of high-intensity resistance training, such as lifting heavy weights for four to eight reps or sprinting for 50 meters. For instance, during a sprint workout, if the rest intervals between 50-meter repetitions are insufficient (say, one or two minutes only), the workout will become progressively more lactic, thus shifting from a speed training session to a lactate tolerance session (Janssen 2001).

Beginning a set without proper phosphate recovery does not allow the athlete to maintain power output throughout the set or from one set to the next. Therefore, in the maximum strength phase of training, athletes should rest for three to five minutes before performing more sets with the same muscle group, unless they perform the set with

Table 4.10   Time Course of ATP-CP Restoration

Time (min.)	% of restoration
0.5	50
1	75
1.5	87.5
2	93.7
2.5	96.8
3	98.3
3.5	99
4	99.4
4.5	99.8
5	100

more than one repetition in reserve. For maximum recovery when exercising at very high intensity and close to failure, athletes should use the vertical method of training—moving to the next exercise after each set. In other words, they should complete one set of each suggested exercise before returning to the first exercise for the second set. This pattern allows ample time for phosphate recovery in the muscle.

Activity During the Rest Interval

When recovering between high-intensity intermittent (lactic) bouts of exercise, performance in subsequent bouts is affected more positively by engaging in aerobic activity at approximately 20% of $\dot{V}O_2$max than by than stretching or passive rest (Dorado, Sanchis-Moysi, and Calbet 2004). To facilitate faster recovery between sets, athletes could also perform relaxation exercises (such as shaking the legs, arms, and shoulders) or light massage, both of which speed up recovery. In addition, they can perform diversionary activities that involve the unfatigued muscles in light contractions, which have been reported to facilitate faster recovery of the prime movers (Asmussen and Mazin 1978).

Static stretching should *not* be performed for the muscles that are going to be trained in a strength or power session unless it is done at the beginning of a long warm-up routine that implies an escalation of intensity, because it may acutely inhibit their power output (Power et al. 2004; Cramer et al. 2005; Nelson et al. 2005; Yamaguchi et al. 2006; Samuel et al. 2008; La Torre et al. 2010). Static stretching addressing the muscles used should be planned for the end of the training session. The purpose of stretching exercises is to artificially lengthen a muscle where the myosins and actins overlap. The sooner the muscles reach their anatomical length, the faster they start their recovery and regeneration process, thus more easily eliminating the metabolites accumulated during training.

Strength Training Loading Patterns

One of the most popular strength training loading patterns is the pyramid. Its structure, shown in figure 4.3, implies that the load increases progressively to a higher intensity while the number of reps decreases proportionately. The physiological advantage of using the pyramid is that it prepares the nervous system for higher tensions in a gradual way, thus stabilizing technique and lowering inhibitory mechanisms. To facilitate the highest level of strength adaptation, athletes should avoid going to concentric failure in any set and should use a range of 10% to 15% in the loading pattern from the first set to the last set of the pyramid. Any range greater than 15% does not optimize strength gains.

Another pattern, the double pyramid, consists of two pyramids, one of which is inverted on top of the other. The number of reps decreases from the bottom up in the first pyramid, then increases again in the second pyramid. Conversely, the load gets higher as the reps decrease, then lower as the reps increase again (see figure 4.4).

Although the double pyramid has its merits, some cautions are necessary. Most proponents of this pattern suggest reaching concentric failure in all sets. In this approach, however, by the time the final sets are performed, both the CNS and the muscles involved may be exhausted, in which case these sets will not produce the expected benefits.

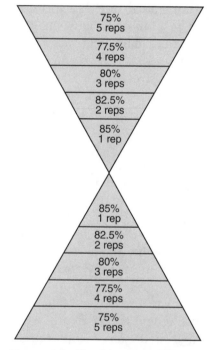

Figure 4.4 Double-pyramid loading pattern. The progression over time can involve keeping the same sets and reps scheme yet increasing the intensity by 2.5% of 1RM each microcycle to 2.5% over the entire maximum strength phase.

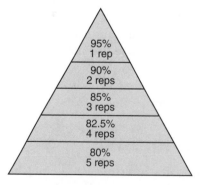

Figure 4.3 Pyramid loading pattern.

To the contrary, because the fatigue will impair the recruitment of the fast-twitch fibers, the last sets in this loading pattern result in muscle hypertrophy rather than in development of strength or power. Increases in power, in particular, can be obtained only when an athlete is in unfatigued state, which generally occurs at the beginning of a session immediately following the warm-up. However, if both maximum strength and hypertrophy training are planned in the same training session (the absolute strength method), the double pyramid may be an acceptable solution because it allows a high total time under tension for the fast-twitch muscle fibers.

For an improved variant of the double pyramid, the skewed pyramid (Bompa 1993) is suggested (see figure 4.5). In this approach, the load is constantly increased throughout the session, except during the last set, when it is lowered (e.g., 80%, 85%, 90%, 95%, and 80%). Lowering the load in that last set (i.e., the back-off set) and taking it to failure has been proven to retain muscle hypertrophy when the majority of high-intensity, low-rep sets would only stimulate relative strength (Goto et al. 2004). This method could be used during the strength maintenance phase of the annual plan.

One of the best loading patterns for maximizing strength gains is the flat pyramid (Bompa 1993) (see figure 4.6). It develops maximum strength and also elicits some hypertrophy specific to fast-twitch fibers, thanks to the higher number of total reps performed at high loads. This loading pattern starts with a warm-up set of, say, 50% of 1RM, followed by intermediary sets at 60%, 70%, and 75%, then stabilizes the load at 80% for the entire workout. The physiological advantage of the flat pyramid is that by using a load of only one intensity level, the best neuromuscular adaptation for maximum strength is achieved without imposing conflicting adaptation stimuli on the body with several intensities.

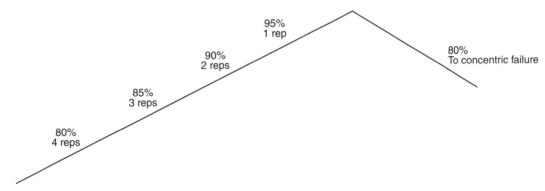

Figure 4.5 Skewed pyramid loading pattern.

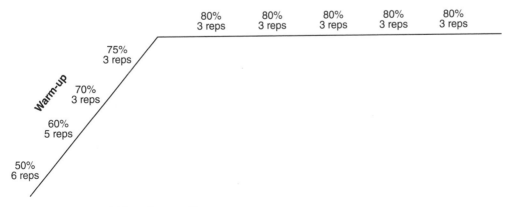

Figure 4.6 Flat pyramid loading pattern.

In traditional pyramids, the load often varies from 70% to 100%. Load variations of such magnitude cross three levels of intensity: medium, heavy, and maximum. Despite the fact that the load necessary to produce gains in maximum strength falls between 70% and 100%, each intensity zone (70%-80%, 80%-90%, and 90%-100%) elicits slightly different neuromuscular adaptations and necessitates a precise progression. The volume spent in each intensity zone determines the main neuromuscular adaptations. Thus, a traditional pyramid that uses a load of 70% to 100% may result in gains in both power and maximum strength, and, while this may be of general benefit to athletes, it does not maximize gains in either area.

Variations of intensities for the pyramid are certainly possible and necessary, as long as the load stays within the intensity range required for the desired neuromuscular adaptations in a specific macrocycle (70%-80% for intermuscular coordination, 80-90% for intramuscular coordination) from set to set.

When seeking to maximize strength gains in intermediate and advanced athletes, step (or wave) loading is an excellent pattern. Because its practical application is a bit more complex than the pyramids, we tend not to use the wave loading pattern with beginners but rather reserve it for later stages of athletic development. For a 14-week progression, see figure 4.7. Wave loading normally involves two waves, usually composed of three work sets, in which the load is increased progressively while the number of reps decreases. The same pattern of load and reps used for the first wave is repeated in the following wave.

The physiological advantage of step or wave loading hinges on the fact that a latter wave is potentiated by the higher-intensity sets of a former wave, thus increasing the power output at the same percentage of 1RM. It also leaves power athletes fresher for high-intensity sets because they do not need to do all of the more voluminous sets before the low-rep sets, as happens for other loading patterns. Some proponents of wave loading have suggested exploiting the neural potentiation of the first wave by increasing the load in the second wave. Although this approach can be used to elicit gains in both strength and hypertrophy, we prefer to progress the load from week (microcycle) to week, thus increasing strength and power and leaving more energy for sport-specific activity.

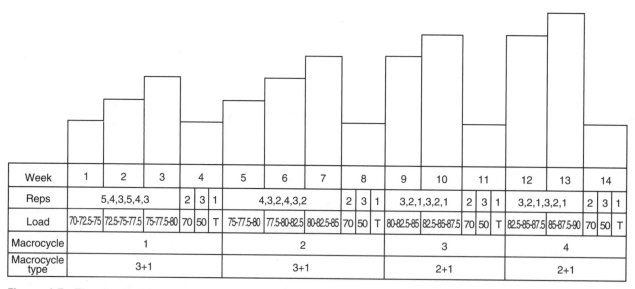

Week	1	2	3	4			5	6	7	8			9	10	11			12	13	14		
Reps	5,4,3,5,4,3			2	3	1	4,3,2,4,3,2			2	3	1	3,2,1,3,2,1		2	3	1	3,2,1,3,2,1		2	3	1
Load	70-72.5-75	72.5-75-77.5	75-77.5-80	70	50	T	75-77.5-80	77.5-80-82.5	80-82.5-85	70	50	T	80-82.5-85	82.5-85-87.5	70	50	T	82.5-85-87.5	85-87.5-90	70	50	T
Macrocycle	1						2						3					4				
Macrocycle type	3+1						3+1						2+1					2+1				

Figure 4.7 The step/wave loading pattern is particularly suited for intermediate and advanced power athletes. Here is a 14-week progression with three repetition schemes throughout the macrocycles.

Training Program Design

All training programs must be planned, designed, and measured in order to assess whether the training objective has been achieved. The following steps remove any confusion from the process of designing a program and assessing its significance to the athlete's level of development.

Analysis of the Sport's Performance Model

Analyze the contribution of each biomotor ability and determine the most specific qualities to train.

Endurance

1. Use scientific literature to determine the contribution of each energy system to the sport activity (at the competitive level of the team or athlete):
   - Anaerobic alactic (ATP-CP)
   - Anaerobic lactic (LA)
   - Aerobic (O_2)
2. Evaluate whether an activity is continuous or intermittent.
3. Determine the working intensity zones for endurance and the progression to be used throughout the training program.
4. Choose the methods to use in each macrocycle and the progression of training means.

Speed

1. Evaluate the number, intensity, and duration of sprints or quick actions.
2. Consider the differences between, and the contribution of, each of the following qualities of speed: alactic speed (acceleration, maximum speed), lactic speed short (repeated sprint ability, or RSA), and lactic speed long (speed endurance). Note that lactic speed long (speed endurance) is an expression of lactic power in which speed is maintained for more than eight seconds. In contrast, lactic speed short (repeated sprint ability or RSA) is an expression of alactic capacity in which sprints under six seconds are repeated with partial recovery until they become an expression of lactic power short, which also heavily engages aerobic power during short rest intervals to restore phosphates through aerobic phosphorylation.
3. Evaluate the type (active or passive) and duration of recovery between sprints or fast actions.
4. Evaluate whether speed is expressed linearly or nonlinearly.
5. Choose the methods to use in each macrocycle and the progression of training means.

Strength

1. Select the type of strength. Determine which of the following qualities of strength are specific to the event: power, power endurance, or muscle endurance short, medium, or long. The increase of the chosen quality or qualities will be the ultimate goal of the entire periodization of strength. Remember that for the endurance types of strength (of a more metabolic nature), the morpho-functional adaptations to training require longer exposure to the stimuli than is the case for the neural adaptations.

This factor directly affects the length of the conversion phase, and therefore the time remaining for other phases, as the program designing process works backward from the end point.

2. Determine the appropriate duration of the anatomical adaptation period based on the athlete's characteristics (including his or her athletic development stage and strength training experience) and the time available for an introductory phase.

3. Decide whether or not to implement a period devoted to hypertrophy in light of the characteristics of the athlete and of the sporting event.

4. Select the exercises to use in training. Strength and conditioning coaches should select training exercises according to the specifics of the sport, the athletes' needs, and the phase of training. Each athletic skill is performed by prime movers, which can differ from sport to sport, depending on the specific skill requirements. Coaches must first identify the prime movers and then select the strength exercises that best involve those muscles. At the same time, they must consider the athlete's needs, which depend on his or her background and individual strengths and weaknesses. Because the weakest link in a chain always breaks first, compensation exercises (also referred to as accessory exercises) should be selected to strengthen the weakest muscles. The selection of exercises is also phase specific. Normally, during the anatomical adaptation phase, most muscle groups are employed to build a better and more multilateral foundation. As the competitive phase approaches, training becomes more specific, and exercises are selected specifically to involve the prime movers. Coaches must analyze the sport movements in order to determine exercises and loading parameters. The following factors should be considered.

   • Planes on which the movements take place (sagittal, frontal, transverse)

   • Force expressed at various joint angles within the sport-specific range of motion (i.e., the zone that must be most affected by the development of the specific strength)

   • Muscle groups producing the movements (i.e., the prime movers, which also must be most affected by the development of the specific strength)

   • Muscle actions (concentric, eccentric, isometric)

5. Choose the methods to use in each macrocycle and the progression of training means.

Analysis of the Tradition of Training in a Sport

Analyze the training tradition of the chosen sport. Over the years, coaches have found solutions based more on practicality than on science. Equipped with the latest knowledge and your practical experience, you can find the ideal starting point to overcome this tradition.

Analysis of the Athlete

To determine the current state of training, you need to test the athlete's degree of development of each biomotor ability or its qualities, possibly in relation to the means that you will use in the training program. Consider test results and the athlete's competitive level in order to establish the training load progression and the performance goals for every biomotor ability in each phase of the year.

First, determine the athlete's degree of strength training. Maximum strength is the highest load that an athlete can lift in one repetition (1RM). Before designing a maximum strength or power program, a coach should know each athlete's maximum strength at least in the dominant exercises. An athlete's individual data are valid only for a certain cycle of training, usually a macrocycle, because the degree of training changes continuously. The 1RM test should be performed only by athletes with some experience in strength training and only after macrocycles involving some exposure to loads equal to or greater than 70% of 1RM. This is especially true for beginners. Coaches should also test muscle strength balance around the joints that are most important for the sport (using submaximal weights of 3RM to 8RM) and test sport-specific strength at the beginning of the year to enable monitoring of its progression and to get information about the dynamics of adaptation to your training programs.

The preceding steps give you a clear picture of the athlete's level of athletic development and degree of training in each biomotor ability. You can use this information to determine the type and number of exercises, the loading pattern, the percentage of 1RM, the number of reps, and the number of sets to prescribe for a macrocycle training program. The program cannot, however, be the same for each macrocycle. Training demand must increase progressively so that the athlete adapts to a higher workload, which translates into increased strength. Coaches should test athletes to redetermine their 1RM before each new macrocycle in order to ensure that progress is achieved in maximum strength and that the new load is related to the gains made in strength.

It is also possible to use one or more sport-specific power or conditioning tests to gain an idea of the athlete's sport-specific athletic shape throughout the whole training process.

Record the information. In order to do so effectively, one must understand the notation used in a training program chart to express load, number of reps, and number of sets.

TESTING THE ONE REPETITION MAXIMUM

Some coaches believe that testing for 1RM is dangerous—that lifting 100% can result in injury. But it is not dangerous for trained athletes to lift 100% once every three or four weeks. Most injuries occur during training and competition, not during testing. Sometimes the body of an athlete is subjected to forces up to five times his or her body weight during the sporting activity, so testing maximum strength should not constitute a safety concern. Consider, as well, that testing is performed at the end of the unloading microcycle of a macrocycle, when the athlete has recovered from the fatigue of the previous loading microcycles. A test for 1RM must follow a thorough, progressive warm-up, such as the one suggested here (in kg) for the squat (projected 1RM at 150 kg).

- 1st set: 20 kilograms × 10 reps, 30-second rest interval, 13% of 1RM
- 2nd set: 60 kilograms × 4 reps, 60-second rest interval, 40% of 1RM
- 3rd set: 80 kilograms × 2 reps, 90-second rest interval, 53% of 1RM
- 4th set: 100 kilograms × 2 reps, 2-minute rest interval, 67% of 1RM
- 5th set: 120 kilograms × 1 rep, 2-minute rest interval, 80% of 1RM
- 6th set: 130 kilograms × 1 rep, 3-minute rest interval, 87% of 1RM
- 7th set: 140 kilograms × 1 rep, 4-minute rest interval, 93% of 1RM
- 8th set: 145 kilograms × 1 rep, 5-minute rest interval, 97% of 1 RM
- 9th set: 150 kilograms × 1 rep, 6-minute rest interval, 100% of 1RM

Load is noted as a percentage of 1RM, and athletes must be tested, especially during the preparatory phase at the end of each macrocycle. Knowing an athlete's 1RM allows the coach to select the percentage to use in training according to the training goals of each phase. Notation of load, number of reps, and number of sets is expressed as follows.

$$\frac{\text{Load}}{\text{no. of reps}}\ \text{sets}$$

$$\frac{80}{10}\ 4$$

The numerator (e.g., 80) refers to the load as a percentage of 1RM, the denominator (e.g., 10) represents the number of reps, and the multiplier (e.g., 4) indicates the number of sets.

The advantage of expressing load as a percentage of 1RM is that when working with a larger group of athletes, such as a football team, the coach does not have to calculate the weight for each player; rather, each athlete uses his or her personal 1RM as the basis for calculating weight, which may vary from player to player. Thus, individualization is built into this method.

SIMPLIFIED NOTATION FOR A STRENGTH TRAINING PROGRAM

Any strength training program should be written on a sheet of paper or in the training journal or on the computer. Table 4.11 illustrates a simplified format for a strength training program, either in an equation form or in a sequence. The first column lists the exercises in sequential order. The second column specifies the load, number of reps, and number of sets. The last column indicates the rest interval to be taken following each set.

Table 4.11   Sample Strength Training Program Format

Exercise	Load/reps × sets (load as % of 1RM)	Rest interval (minutes)
1. Squat	80/4 × 4	3
2. Bench press	85/3 × 4	3
3. Deadlift	70/3 × 4	2
4. Lat pull-down	60/5 × 3	3
5. Abdominal crunch	Body weight/15 × 3	2

Exercise Prescription

The 656 muscles distributed throughout the human body are capable of performing a great variety of movements. All athletic skills and actions are performed by muscles as a result of contraction. Therefore, if an athlete wants to improve a skill or physical performance, he or she must concentrate on training the muscles that perform the action—the prime movers.

The process of prescribing exercises for a given muscle group (or groups) must be based on phase-specific considerations. During the anatomical adaptation phase, exercises must be selected that develop most muscle groups—both agonist and antagonist—to build a stronger base for the training phases to follow. As the competitive phase approaches, exercises become very specialized and are prescribed specifically for the prime movers (see table 4.12).

Exercise prescription should be based not on exercises borrowed from weightlifting or bodybuilding but on an understanding of how the muscles produce a movement. Especially from the late preparatory phase onward, an exercise is good for an athlete in a given sport if it follows the principle of specificity. This means it must involve the prime movers and the synergistic muscles used in performing the skills of that particular sport or event.

Coaches often turn to bodybuilding for exercise ideas without understanding the differences between bodybuilding and other sports. One difference lies in the method—analytic or compound—used to determine how an exercise achieves a specific training goal. Bodybuilders use the analytic method for high muscle definition. They analyze each muscle's individual action and movement, then train each muscle in isolation to achieve the best size development.

In sport, however, the compound method should be used because it involves not just an individual muscle but all muscles of the joint (or joints) necessary to produce an athletic skill. Exercises should also involve the muscles and joints in a sequence similar to that used in performing the needed skills. Use the variety of strength training machines produced by the industry to better address the prime movers. (Note: The weightlifting barbell and the rigidity of its exercises are far from meeting the specific needs of most sports regarding targeting the prime movers.)

In many cases, athletes and coaches rate the success of a strength training program according to the amount of muscle the athlete builds (hypertrophy). However, aside from exceptions such as American football linemen, shot-putters, and heavyweight boxers and wrestlers, constant increase in muscle size is not a desirable effect for most athletes.

Table 4.12 Periodization of Exercise Prescription Throughout the Annual Plan

Type of exercise	Anatomical adaptation	MxS (early prep)	MxS (late prep)	Conversion to specific strength
Unilateral	*****	***	***	**
Bilateral	***	*****	*****	*****
Full range of motion	*****	****	***	**
Specific range of motion	—	—	****	*****

The asterisks indicate the relative volume dedicated to each group of exercises.

Power and speed sports—or sports with quick, explosive action (e.g., baseball, football, hockey, most track-and-field events, volleyball)—rely on nervous system training, which includes many power exercises and moderate to high loads (greater than 70% of 1RM) that result in neural adaptation (Sale 1986; Schmidtbleicher 1992; Enoka 2015). For most sports, neural adaptation in strength training means increasing power and the speed of the contraction without increasing muscle mass—in other words, increasing relative strength and power.

Higher neural adaptation is achieved by carefully selecting training methods and exercises. Researchers and international-class coaches share similar views about what represents the specificity of strength training. These views can be summarized as follows.

- Strength training methods must be specific to the speed of contraction used in the sport (Coyle et al. 1991; Kanehisa and Miyashita 1983). This requirement means that from the second half of the preparatory phase through the competitive phase, coaches should select methods that specifically increase the speed of contraction and therefore the level of power or quickness.

- Training methods and exercises must increase the contraction force in the intended direction of movement. This requirement means selecting exercises according to the muscles used to perform the technical skills of a given sport (the prime movers). That is why bodybuilding exercises and methodology are a waste time, especially during the second part of the preparatory phase and throughout the competitive phases.

- Training methods must increase activation of the prime movers. For this reason, selected exercises must be sport-specific and primarily engage the prime movers.

- Training methods must increase the discharge rate of motor neurons (Hortobagyi et al. 1996; Enoka 2015) or stimulate the muscles to perform an athletic action with power and high speed. Motor neurons innervate, stimulate, and arouse the muscles. The more specific the training method and exercises, the better the nervous system is trained to perform quick and powerful athletic movements.

- Motor unit recruitment and firing rate increase with higher loads and faster contractions (De Luca et al. 1982). Training methods that enhance maximum strength and power are the only ones that increase fast-twitch muscle fiber recruitment and the firing rate of motor units.

- Exercise action must be performed along the neural pathway used in the sport (Häkkinen 1989). More specifically, exercises must be selected so that the muscles' contractions are performed in the same activation sequence that occurs during performance of the relevant sport skills. If an exercise does not realistically simulate, or is not specific to, a technical skill, the result is lower exercise transfer and lower performance improvement.

- Neural adaptation that results from training for specificity of strength increases the number of voluntarily activated motor units. This capability transfers from general to specific exercises. Well-selected training methods, such as maximum strength methods and power training, activate more motor units. As a result, an athlete can perform sport-specific skills with higher speed of contraction and more power.

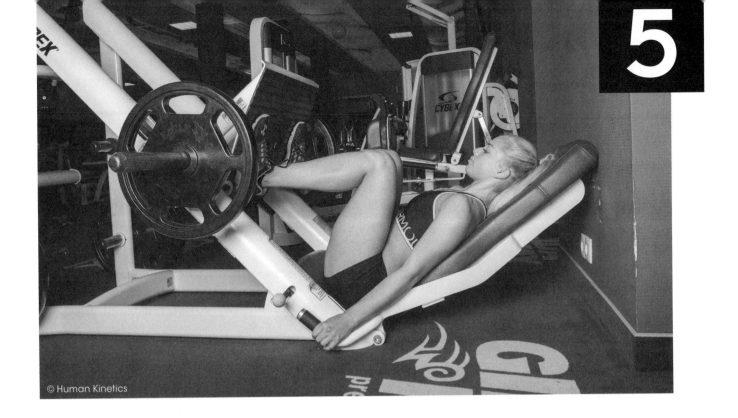

© Human Kinetics

The Microcycle Short-Term Plan

A successful strength training program should be part of a long-term training plan and not be implemented only during certain parts of the annual plan. Nor should strength training be performed just for the sake of it. If (and only if) properly implemented, strength training helps protect athletes from injury, delays the onset of fatigue, and enables the athlete to generate the high level of power output required for optimal sport performance. In order to be effective, however, strength training must meet the objectives of the particular training phase and mesh with the overall plan.

Because a training program is a methodological, scientific strategy for improving performance, it should be well organized and well designed. An effective training program incorporates the principles of periodization of strength throughout the year. Whether short-term or long-term, the training program also reflects the coach's knowledge of methodology and takes into account the performance model of the sport as well as the athlete's background and physical potential.

A good training plan is simple, objective, and flexible so that it can match the athlete's physiological adaptation and performance improvements. Planning theory, however, is very complex, and this book discusses planning only as it pertains to strength training. Further information can be found in *Periodization: Theory and Methodology of Training* (Bompa and Buzzichelli 2018). In this chapter we address the organization of the training session plan and the microcycle; in the next chapter we cover the annual plan for the periodization of strength. Refer to the periodization sections in chapter 6 for more sport-specific information.

Training Session Plan

The training session is the main tool for organizing the daily workout program. To achieve better management and organization, the training session can be structured into four main segments. The first two (introduction and warm-up) prepare the athlete for the main part, in which the concerted training takes place, and the last part (cool-down) returns the athlete to the normal physiological state.

Introduction

During the introduction to a training session, the coach or instructor shares with the athletes the training objectives for the day and how they are to be achieved. The coach also organizes the athletes into groups and gives them necessary advice regarding the daily program.

Warm-Up

The specific purpose of the warm-up is to prepare athletes for the program to follow. During the warm-up, body temperature is raised, which appears to be one of the main factors in facilitating performance. The warm-up stimulates the activity of the central ner-

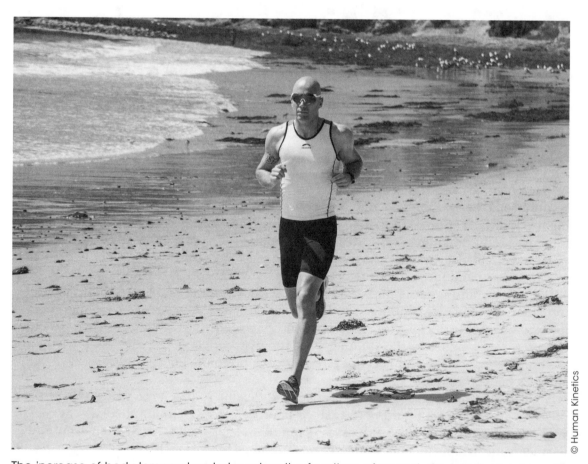

© Human Kinetics

The increase of body temperature helps prime the functions of several physiological systems for the work to come.

vous system (CNS), which coordinates all systems of the body, speeds up motor reactions through faster transmission of nerve impulses, improves the biomechanical performance of the motor system, increases the contraction speed and peak power that muscles can produce, and improves coordination (Wade et al. 2000; Enoka 2015). The elevation of body temperature also warms up and facilitates the stretching of muscles, myofascia, and tendons, thus preventing or reducing ligament sprains and tendon and muscle strains. Warmed-up muscle tissue is able to accommodate higher-velocity stretches before the tendon–bone coupling experiences damage (Enoka 2015).

The warm-up for strength training includes two parts: general and specific. The general warm-up (5-10 minutes) involves light jogging, cycling, or step-ups, followed by calisthenics and dynamic stretching exercises to increase blood flow, which raises body temperature. This activity prepares the muscles and tendons for the planned program. During the warm-up, athletes should also prepare mentally for the main part of the training session by visualizing the exercises and motivating themselves for the strain of training. The specific warm-up for strength training is much shorter than is necessary, for instance, for a speed training session (3-5 minutes); in fact it is a short transition to the working part of the session. In this portion, athletes prepare themselves for a successful workout by performing multiple sets of a few reps on the equipment to be used and employing gradually heavier loads leading to those planned for the day (which means fewer warm-up sets for high-rep sets and more warm-up sets for heavier sets of fewer reps).

Main Part

The main part of the training session is dedicated to the concerted training program, in which training objectives are accomplished, including strength training. In most sports, technical and tactical work are the main objectives of training, and strength development is a secondary priority. First-priority activities are performed immediately after the warm-up, followed by strength training. The types of training to be performed in a given day depend on the phase of training as well as the training objectives. Table 5.1 provides sample options for sequencing your training for several training sessions.

The training program must be based on scientific principles, and the fundamental guidelines are determined by the dominant energy systems in the chosen sport. When discussing certain combinations for both the training session and the microcycle, coaches and athletes should remember the following key points.

Table 5.1 Sample Sequence Options for Training Sessions

Session 1	Session 2	Session 3	Session 4
1. Warm-up 2. Phosphagen (alactic) technical skills 3. Speed 4. Maximum strength or power	1. Warm-up 2. Glycolytic (lactic) technical and tactical skills 3. Power endurance	1. Warm-up 2. Oxidative (aerobic) tactical skills 3. Muscular endurance	1. Warm-up 2. Phosphagen (alactic) tactical skills 3. Power

- In sports characterized by short-duration (less than 10-second) explosive actions, power is the most specific quality of strength. Examples include sprinting, jumping, and throwing events in track and field; sprinting in cycling; ski jumping; free-style skiing; diving; pitching and batting; American football throwing; any takeoff or quick change of direction in a team sport; and quick limb actions in boxing, wrestling, and the martial arts.

- Speed endurance (glycolytic speed, 15- to 50-second) activities characterized by fast actions interspersed with quick changes of direction, jumps, and short rest intervals tend to rely on power endurance or muscle endurance short. These actions include 50- to 100-meter swimming; 200- to 400-meter events in track and field; 500-meter speedskating; tennis; figure skating; and many game elements in team sports.

- Prolonged activities performed against any type of resistance (be it gravity, ground, water, snow, or ice) depend mainly on muscular endurance. These activities include rowing, swimming events longer than 100 meters, kayaking and canoeing, cross-country skiing, and certain elements of team, combat, and racket sports. Therefore, strength coaches must carefully analyze their sport and decide the proportions in which their athletes need to be exposed to power, power endurance, and muscular endurance.

Cool-Down

While the warm-up serves as a transition from the normal biological state of daily activities to high-intensity training, the cool-down is a transition with the opposite effect: It brings the body back to its normal functions. Therefore, athletes should not leave for the showers immediately after the last exercise. Instead, during a cool-down of 10 to 20 minutes, they can perform activities that facilitate faster regeneration and recovery from the strains of training.

As a result of training, especially intensive work, athletes build up high amounts of lactic acid, and their muscles are exhausted, tense, and rigid. To overcome this fatigue and speed up the recovery process, they should perform relaxation and stretching exercises. Specifically, at the end of the training, they should perform 5 to 10 minutes of low-intensity, continuous aerobic activity that causes the body to continue perspiring, followed by 5 to 10 minutes of stretching. Doing so improves general recovery and the removal of metabolites through their passage from the muscle cells to the circulatory system, thus reducing body temperature, heart rate, and blood pressure (Moeller et al. 1985; Hagberg et al. 1979; Bompa and Haff 2009).

The cool-down also lowers the level of cortisol, which can otherwise disturb night rest and remain at high levels up to 24 hours following training. This can delay the recovery process and the adaptations to training, and it lowers catecholamines, particularly adrenaline and noradrenaline (Jezova et al. 1985; Stone et al. 2007). Cool-down activities also reduce the athlete's emotional tension, thus favoring recovery even at a mental level. Finally, stretching in particular allows the muscles to go back to their anatomical length and restores the joint range of motion, a process that may otherwise require up to 24 hours.

Once the cool-down has begun to dissipate the results of fatigue, it is fundamental to speed up recovery and training adaptations by starting the restoration of energy substrates. In fact, we underline the fact that the rates of recovery and adaptation are determined not only by the type of training performed but also by the athlete's training level, his or her internal load at the end of the session, and his or her nutritional interventions (Bompa and Buzzichelli 2018).

Training Session Models

Many sports require technical and tactical training, as well as training for maximum speed, speed endurance, and aerobic endurance—all of which tax different energy systems. How can these components of training be combined without producing a high degree of fatigue and without letting the adaptation of one element interfere with the improvement of the others? These concerns can be addressed in one of two ways: (1) by combining training components so that the athlete taxes only one energy system per training session or (2) by alternating the energy systems in each microcycle so that the athlete trains according to the prevailing energy systems in the particular sport. The following sections describe training session models that tax the various energy systems used in sports.

Model Training Taxing the Phosphagen (Alactic) System

1. Warm-up
2. Technical training drills of short duration (3-6 seconds)
3. Maximum speed and agility training (2-6 seconds)
4. Maximum strength training
5. Power training

The order of activities in this model was established based on the physiological and mental needs of the athlete. Training must focus first on activities that require more nervous system concentration, mental focus, and thus a fresh mind—in other words, technique, speed, or both. Maximum speed should be trained before maximum strength because gains in maximum strength and power have been found to be more effective when preceded by maximum-velocity sprints (Enoka 2015).

This particular training model is applicable to team sports, including American football, soccer, baseball, softball, and cricket; sprinting, jumping, and throwing events in track and field; diving; racket sports; the martial arts; contact sports; and other sports in which the anaerobic alactic system is dominant. Although there are two strength training options, we suggest using only one type according to the phase of training. This does not exclude the possibility of using both.

The duration of a strength training session in this model depends both on the importance of strength in the sport and on the training phase. During the preparatory phase, a strength training session can last 45 to 75 minutes. In the competitive phase, it is much shorter (20-40 minutes), and the work is dedicated primarily to maintaining strength gained during the preparatory phase. Exceptions to this basic rule are made for throwers in track and field, linemen in American football, and wrestlers in the heavyweight category, who require more time for strength training (60-90 minutes).

Model Training Taxing the Glycolytic (Lactic) System

1. Warm-up
2. Technical or tactical training of medium duration (10-60 seconds)
3. Training for speed endurance and agility of longer duration (15-50 seconds) or short reps (3-10 seconds) with short rest intervals
4. Training for power endurance or muscular endurance of short duration

This model is suggested for any sport in which the anaerobic lactic system is taxed (10-60 seconds of activity burst). Thus, tactical training, especially in the form of prolonged but intensive drills, can be followed by a combination of strength training in which a certain degree of lactic endurance is used—either power endurance or muscular endurance of short duration. Applying this model once or twice a week is beneficial to athletes in most sports that use the anaerobic lactic energy system, such as in 50- to 100-meter swimming, track and cycling; 200 to 800 meters in track and field; as well as team, racket, and contact sports and the martial arts.

Model Training Taxing Both the Lactic (Glycolytic) and the Oxidative (Aerobic) System

1. Warm-up
2. Technical or tactical training of long duration (1.5-8 minutes)
3. Training for muscular endurance of medium duration

Aerobic endurance includes endurance of medium duration that involves both the anaerobic lactic acid system and the aerobic system. Aerobic system training is generally of a long duration and dedicated to training strictly the aerobic system with little adaptation of the anaerobic system. The model depicted previously combines tactical training of long duration (1.5-8 minutes) with muscular endurance of medium duration, both of which tax the anaerobic lactic system but mostly the athlete's aerobic endurance or ability to delay the onset of fatigue. This organization of the training session is good for training the power output maintenance in the last part of the game or match, for team, racket, and contact sports, and the martial arts.

Model Training Taxing the Oxidative System

1. Warm-up
2. Aerobic endurance training
3. Training for muscular endurance of long duration (>8 minutes)

The previous model is most effective for sports in which aerobic endurance is either dominant or especially important for achieving the expected athletic performance. These sports include distance running, triathlon, road cycling, cross-country skiing, rowing, canoeing, kayaking, mountain cycling, and marathon canoeing. For these sports, muscular endurance is trained at the end of the session because the resulting fatigue may affect the athlete's ability to achieve the objectives of aerobic training.

Model Training to Develop Power and Agility in Fatigue

1. Warm-up
2. Technical and tactical training taxing the aerobic system (1.5-8 minutes)
3. Power and agility training

The result of a competition is frequently decided in the final minutes. Athletes must be trained for such conditions in order to generate greater power and quickness, display a high level of agility at the end of the competition, and, as a result, perform at a higher level. The most efficient way to enhance these abilities is to train athletes under conditions of fatigue similar to those they will encounter in competition. Training sessions geared toward meeting this objective should first fatigue the athlete via metabolic conditioning (intensity zone 3 or 4), followed by 20 to 30 minutes of high-intensity power and agility drills. These drills can be both specific and nonspecific. Another option, especially for racket sports, the martial arts, boxing, and wrestling, is to use muscular endurance training for 20 to 30 minutes, followed by power and agility drills of high intensity. This model is good for specialized training sessions for team, racket, and contact sports and the martial arts, in which the scope of training is to stress the last part of the game or match.

Planning the Microcycle

The microcycle, or weekly training program, is probably the most important planning tool. Throughout the annual plan, the structure and dynamics of microcycles change according to the phase of training, the training objectives, and the physiological and psychological demands faced by the athlete. A macrocycle, on the other hand, is a training plan composed of two to six weeks or microcycles, whose structure and duration depend on the training objectives of the phase.

Load Increments

Throughout macrocycles, the load in strength training is increased depending on the type of cycle and training phase. The work within each macrocycle follows a step-type progression. From an intensity standpoint, microcycles follow the principle of progressive increase of load in training. As illustrated in table 5.2, *a* through *c*, the load is progressively increased during the first three cycles, which are followed by a regeneration cycle in which the load is decreased to facilitate recuperation and replenishment of energy. Then a maximum strength test is performed before another macrocycle begins. Based on this model, the tables provide suggested load increments using the notation system described in chapter 4, in which the numerator indicates the load as a percentage of 1RM, the denominator indicates the number of reps, and the multiplier indicates the number of sets. The following are three possible modalities of load progression.

- In table 5.2*a*, the volume stays the same, the intensity increases, the repetitions in reserve for the main working sets decrease, and a 1RM test is performed at the end of the fourth (unloading) microcycle.
- In table 5.2*b*, the volume stays the same, the intensity increases, the number of reps decreases, the repetitions in reserve stay the same, and a 1RM test is performed at the end of the fourth microcycle.
- In table 5.2*c*, the volume increases and the intensity and the repetitions in reserve stay the same.

As shown, the work, or the total load in training, is increased in steps, with the highest load occurring in microcycle 3. To increase the work from microcycle to microcycle, the coach has three options: increasing the load while decreasing the repetitions in reserve (table 5.2*a*), increasing the load while keeping the same repetitions in reserve, thus loading the reps per set (table 5.2*b*), or increasing the number of main work sets from microcycle 1 to microcycle 3 (table 5.2*c*).

Table 5.2a Macrocycle: Volume Stays the Same and the Intensity of the Main Working Sets Increases by 2.5% Each Week*

Training load	$\frac{70}{6}1\ \frac{75}{4}1\ \frac{80}{3}3$	$\frac{70}{6}1\ \frac{75}{4}1\ \frac{80}{3}3$	$\frac{70}{6}1\ \frac{75}{4}1\ \frac{85}{3}3$	Day 1 $\frac{70}{2}4$	Day 2 $\frac{50}{3}3\ \frac{80}{1}1$	Day 3 1RM test
Microcycle	1	2	3	4 (unloading)		

*The load suggested in each microcycle refers to the work per day, which can be repeated two to four times per week depending on the training goals.

Table 5.2b Macrocycle: Volume Decreases While Mean Intensity* Increases by 5% Each Week**

Training load	$\frac{70}{6}1\ \frac{75}{4}1\ \frac{80}{3}3$	$\frac{75}{5}1\ \frac{80}{3}1\ \frac{85}{2}3$	$\frac{80}{3}1\ \frac{85}{2}1\ \frac{90}{1}3$	Day 1 $\frac{70}{2}4$	Day 2 $\frac{50}{3}3\ \frac{80}{1}1$	Day 3 1RM test
Microcycle	1	2	3	4		

*Mean intensity = [(intensity1 × reps × sets) + (intensity2 × reps × sets) + (intensity3 × reps × sets)]/total reps. In this case: [(70 × 6 × 1) + (75 × 4 × 1) + (80 × 3 × 3)]/(6+4+9) = 75.8%; [(75 × 5 × 1) + (80 × 3 × 1) + (85 × 2 × 3 ×)]/(5+3+6) = 80.3%; [(80 × 3 × 1) + (85 × 2 × 1) + (90 × 1 × 3)]/(3+2+3) = 85%.

**The load suggested in each microcycle refers to the work per day, which can be repeated two to four times per week depending on the training goals.

Table 5.2c Macrocycle: Volume of the Main Working Sets Increases by One Unit Each Week*

Training load	$\frac{70}{6}1\ \frac{75}{4}1\ \frac{80}{3}3$	$\frac{70}{6}1\ \frac{75}{4}1\ \frac{80}{3}4$	$\frac{70}{6}1\ \frac{75}{4}1\ \frac{80}{3}5$	Day 1 $\frac{70}{2}4$	Day 2 $\frac{50}{3}3\ \frac{80}{1}1$	Day 3 1RM test
Microcycle	1	2	3	4 (unloading)		

*The load suggested in each microcycle refers to the work per day, which can be repeated two to four times per week depending on the training goals.

The approach can be chosen to suit the needs of different classifications of athletes. For example, young athletes have difficulty tolerating a high number of sets. It is true that they should have a high number of exercises that develop the entire muscular system and adapt the muscle attachments on the bones (i.e., the tendons) to strength training. But because it is difficult for them to tolerate a high number of exercises and a high number of sets at the same time, it is advisable to opt for a high number of exercises at the expense of the number of sets.

Microcycle 4 represents a regeneration week in which volume and is lowered and the repetitions in reserve are increased to reduce the fatigue resulting from the first three steps, to replenish the energy stores, and to promote psychological relaxation.

Again, in athletics, strength training is subordinate to technical and tactical training. Consequently, the load of strength training per week should be calculated in light of the overall volume and intensity of training.

Before discussing strength training options per microcycle, it is important to mention that the total work per week is also planned according to the principle of progressive increase and alternation of load in training. Figures 5.1 through 5.3 illustrate three micro-cycles, each of which is suggested for each of the conventional steps referred to earlier.

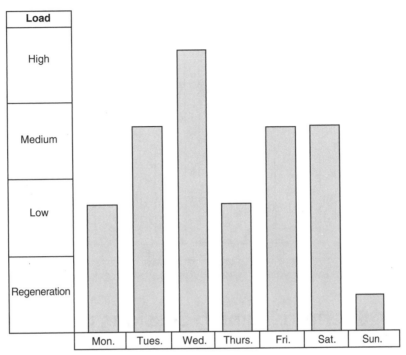

Figure 5.1 Low-workload microcycle with one high-load day and several medium- and low-load days (Sunday is a rest day).

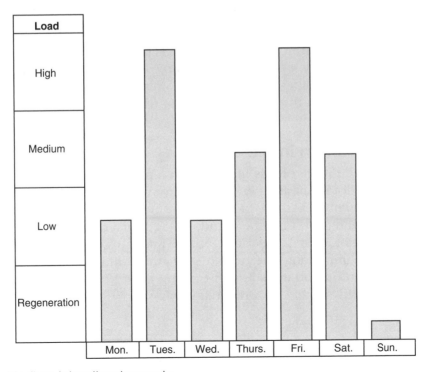

Figure 5.2 Medium-intensity microcycle.

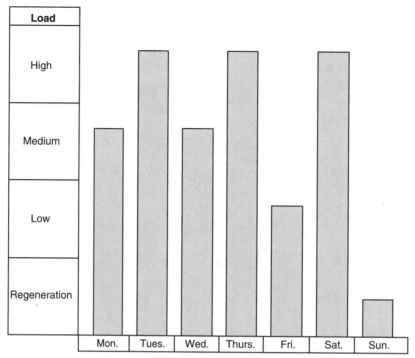

Figure 5.3 High-workload microcycle with three high-intensity training days.

Number of Strength Training Sessions per Microcycle

The number of strength training sessions per microcycle depends on the following factors: the athlete's classification, the importance of strength in the chosen sport, and the phase of training.

Athlete's Classification

Young athletes should be introduced to strength training progressively. At first, they can be exposed to one or two short strength training sessions per microcycle following technical or tactical work. Progressively, over a period of two to four years, this exposure can be increased to three or four sessions. Senior athletes competing in national or international competitions can take part in three or four strength training sessions per week, mainly during the preparatory phase.

Importance of Strength in the Sport

Strength training may be more or less important in a particular sport depending on the sport's relevant skills, dominant abilities, and energy system requirements. For example, strength is less important in a sport in which aerobic endurance is clearly dominant, such as marathon running. On the other hand, strength plays a crucial role in sports in which power is dominant, such as American football and track-and-field throwing events. When strength is less important, one or two strength training sessions per week may suffice. When it is more important, strength training must be done at least three times per microcycle, especially during the preparatory phase.

Phase of Training

The number of strength training sessions also depends on the phase of training. Depending on the sport, two to four sessions per microcycle should be performed during the preparatory phase, and one to three sessions per microcycle should be performed during the competitive phase.

Athletes who perform four strength training sessions per week will have to perform some sessions on consecutive days. In such cases, coaches have two options: (1) train the same muscle groups in every session but alternate intensities—maximum strength one day and power the next—or (2) split the exercises for upper body and for lower body to achieve faster recovery. With the first option, some form of intensity alternation is necessary because it would be impossible for the same muscle groups to recover fully if the same loading parameters were used for two sessions within 24 hours or, even worse, four sessions within 96 hours.

In sport, strength training is performed in addition to technical and tactical training. For maximum effectiveness—and for the most economical use of energy—strength training exercises must be chosen to stress mainly the prime movers. When we talk about strength training for sports, in order to increase effectiveness the number of strength training exercises in a workout should be reduced as much as possible, especially after the anatomical adaptation phase. This reduction allows the athlete to perform more sets and forces the prime movers to contract many times. The outcome is more strength and power development for the required muscles. A special concern, though, is represented by multiplanar (i.e., acting on multiple planes of movement) sports, such as team sports, contact sports, and the martial arts. For this sport, a higher number of exercises should be employed to address, for instance, the high force demands in the transverse plane.

Types of Strength and Restoration of Energy Systems

Some proponents suggest that strength training should be planned on "easy" days. This does not make much sense from a physiological standpoint. To some extent, the majority of sports require training of most, if not all, of the motor abilities of speed, strength, and endurance. Each ability uses and depends on a particular energy system, and the systems differ in their rate of recovery and restoration of fuel.

The full restoration of glycogen starts after 5 minutes of rest, but it might take up to 48 hours to be completed, depending on the sport-specific training and the type of strength training performed in a day. In fact, glycogen can be fully restored given an appropriate dietary intake of carbohydrate in 24 hours after an intermittent activity and 48 hours after a highly taxing metabolic session (Hermansen and Vaage 1977; Stone et al. 2007). It takes about 48 hours after continuous intensive work but only about 24 hours after intermittent activity, such as strength training (Fox 1989; Bompa and Haff 2009). Following high-intensity strength or speed training sessions in which the CNS is also taxed, complete nervous system recovery may take 48 hours. And after maximum-intensity efforts that highly stress the CNS, such as a 100-meter race or a powerlifting competition, the athlete may need up to seven days of lower loading in order to repeat the same level of performance, which indicates full regeneration of all the physiological systems involved.

The time course of substrate restoration is heavily influenced by the quality and timing of food intake, as well as by the extent of damage caused to the myofibrils during the training session (Bompa and Haff 2009). The rate of regeneration from low-intensity aerobic activities is much faster—approximately eight hours. Restoration of energy stores and nervous system recovery may be sped up by aerobic compensation sessions or lower-intensity tactical work. These types of training day can be considered easy and can be planned after the hardest days of the week or after competition.

The largest effect of a training session falls, of course, on the energy system that is mainly trained during the session; the other two systems are affected to a lesser extent. This means that the trained energy system requires more recovery time than the others do. For instance, whenever an anaerobic system is trained first in a given week, it is possible to train the aerobic system the next day, then the other anaerobic system (the one not trained on the first day), and finally the first anaerobic one again. When the aerobic system is trained first, it can be followed by the anaerobic alactic system. Anaerobic alactic exercises, in fact, need less support from the aerobic system than do anaerobic lactic exercises because the former induces a lower oxygen debt than the latter.

Especially in power and speed sports, a microcycle should alternate between the anaerobic and aerobic systems. Here are three options, depending on the sport and the training phase:

- Alactic-aerobic-lactic-aerobic-alactic-aerobic-rest
- Alactic-aerobic-lactic-aerobic-alactic-lactic-rest
- Alactic-lactic-aerobic-alactic-lactic-aerobic-rest

In the case of long-aerobic-endurance sports, on the other hand, the training menu is limited in terms of energy systems alternation. Therefore, the aerobic system is trained daily at various intensities (e.g., at anaerobic threshold pace, below race pace, slightly above race pace, at restoration pace, etc.).

Let us assume that a coach plans intensive training sessions on Monday, Wednesday, and Friday and easy days on Tuesday and Thursday. Because the intensive days are separated by 48 hours—and especially because an easy day is scheduled during those 48 hours—glycogen can reach full restoration and the CNS can recover before the next planned intensive day. This dynamic changes drastically, however, if the coach schedules intensive strength training sessions on the easy days. In that case, the athlete taxes the anaerobic energy systems on the easy days as well as on the intensive days, thus taxing the nervous system and the glycogen stores every day. As a result, strength training becomes an obstacle to restoration. This pattern complicates the ratio of energy expenditure to restoration and the recovery of the nervous system—a state of affairs that can bring the athlete to fatigue or even exhaustion. And it is only a short step from exhaustion to overtraining.

That is why strength training must be planned on the same days as technical and tactical training or speed and power training—that is, on the anaerobic days. In this approach, the athlete heavily taxes the glycogen stores and the nervous system, but the overall training program does not interfere with recovery and regeneration before the next high-intensity training, which is scheduled for 48 hours later. As a guideline for organizing a microcycle, table 5.3 shows activities grouped by energy system and thus possibly trained on three different days. Furthermore, this sequence has a double advantage: (1) it allows a higher load for strength training because the neuromuscular system has a full 48-hour window to recover before the next intensive specific session and (2) it allows strength training volume and intensity to be tweaked according to the subjective and objective status of the athlete during the specific session that follows.

In addition to determining the sequence of training sessions within a microcycle, we must also consider the sequence of training means within the sessions themselves. In fact, certain training objectives can be achieved only in the right circumstances—namely, when the athlete's level of residual fatigue is adequate for the development, retention, or refinement of certain biomotor abilities. Table 5.4 shows the acceptable level of residual fatigue for training certain biomotor abilities.

Table 5.3 Classification of Training Methods According to the Main Energy System Taxed (Ergogenesis)

Phosphagen (anaerobic alactic) day	Glycolytic (anaerobic lactic) day	Oxidative (aerobic) day
1. Technical skills (1-10 seconds) 2. Tactical skills (5-10 seconds) 3. Acceleration and maximum speed 4. Maximum strength and power	1. Technical skills (10-60 seconds) 2. Tactical skills (10-60 seconds) 3. Speed endurance (10-60 seconds) 4. Power endurance, muscle endurance short	1. Long-duration technical skills (>60 seconds) 2. Long- and medium-duration tactical skills (>60 seconds) 3. Aerobic endurance 4. Muscle endurance medium and long

Table 5.4 Training Objectives and Fatigue State

Athlete's residual fatigue	Training objectives*
Absent (fresh)	Technique, tactic (learning), acceleration, maximum speed, power
Low	Technique, tactic, acceleration, speed endurance, maximum strength, power, power endurance
Moderate	Sport-specific endurance, oxidative (aerobic) power, muscle endurance short and medium
High (fatigued)	Oxidative (aerobic) capacity, technical and tactical refinement under specific fatigue conditions, muscular endurance long

*Training objectives that require minimal residual fatigue should be trained after an easy day and placed first in the sequence of a training session.

The following tables provide examples of strength training programs related to other athletic activities and to the dominant energy systems. Table 5.5 suggests a microcycle for individual speed and power sports (sprints and jumps in track and field) in which energy systems are alternated. Strength training is consistently planned on days when other types of activity tax the same energy system. For instance, drills for speed training, which tax the anaerobic alactic system, are followed by training for power. In addition, each day of anaerobic activity (Monday, Wednesday, and Friday) is followed by a day when aerobic training is taxed in the form of tempo running (100-200 yards or meters at 60% of maximum speed for 8-20 reps).

Table 5.5 Alternation of Energy Systems for Speed- and Power-Dominant Sports

Monday	Tuesday	Wednesday	Thursday	Friday	Saturday	Sunday
Phosphagen (alactic) Technical training	Speed Power endurance	Tempo running Tactical training	Phosphagen (alactic) Technical training	Speed-endurance Power endurance	Tempo running Tactical training	

Table 5.6 illustrates how the energy systems and the specifics of strength can be alternated for a sport in which aerobic endurance is dominant, such as rowing, kayaking, canoeing, cycling, triathlon, cross-country skiing, or a swimming event of more than 400 meters. Each time aerobic endurance is trained, the only type of strength training proposed is muscular endurance. When anaerobic training is planned (Tuesday), it is followed by power endurance, which taxes the same system (anaerobic lactic).

Two taxing days of training (Monday and Tuesday) are followed by a lighter aerobic training day for compensation and to supercompensate the glycogen stores depleted the day before. The same approach is used again in the second part of the cycle.

For sports with high-complexity training (technical, tactical, and physical), the alternation of energy systems and strength training could follow the model presented in table 5.7. Examples include all team sports, the martial arts, and racket sports. Every day, all proposed activities tax the same energy system. Obviously, no more than three of the suggested training activities may be planned, which for strength training may mean choosing either maximum strength or power.

On Tuesday, an anaerobic lactic day can be planned (tactical and specific endurance training). To tap the same energy system, the strength training program should consist of activities aimed at developing power endurance or muscle endurance short. Wednesday is a compensation day of less demanding technical and tactical training. For the remaining three training days, the same sequence pattern is used (AL-LA-O_2).

During the competitive phase, the approach used to maintain strength training depends strictly on the competition schedule. There are three possibilities: one competition per week, two competitions per week, or one tournament per week.

Table 5.6 Alternation of Energy Systems for Aerobic-Endurance-Dominant Sports

Monday	Tuesday	Wednesday	Thursday	Friday	Saturday	Sunday
Oxidative (aerobic) endurance	Glycolytic (anaerobic) endurance Power endurance	Oxidative endurance Compensation	Mixed training Power endurance	Oxidative endurance Muscular endurance	Oxidative endurance Compensation	

Table 5.7 Alternation of Energy Systems for High-Complexity Sports

Monday	Tuesday	Wednesday	Thursday	Friday	Saturday	Sunday
Phosphagen technical training Maximum strength	Glycolytic tactical training Power endurance and muscular endurance	Oxidative technical or tactical training Compensation	Phosphagen technical or tactical training Speed Maximum strength	Glycolytic technical/tactical training Speed endurance Power endurance or muscular endurance	Technical or tactical training Oxidative Compensation	—

Table 5.8 presents types of activity to plan between two competitions that fall at the end of consecutive weeks. Because the typical days of competition vary from sport to sport, we have numbered the training sessions rather than specifying a day of the week for each session. The postcompetition day is intended for recovery and regeneration, to remove fatigue from the systems, and to ready the athlete to resume training on the next day.

As in other microcycles, the suggested training programs consider the physiological need to alternate and thus tax mostly one energy system per day. As a result, maximum strength training is planned on days when the anaerobic alactic system is taxed and has the scope of strength maintenance. Certainly, the suggested maximum strength training is short and uses selected exercises specific to the sport for which the athlete is training. The workload of training must be subdivided into low-, medium-, and high-intensity days. Planning the training sessions accordingly helps the athlete better manage the demands and stress associated with training and competition. Keep in mind the need for alternation between training, unloading, competition, and recovery before resuming training.

Table 5.9 illustrates a microcycle with three competitions over the course of a week—a situation common in team sports where the team plays championship and cup simultaneously or the championship itself requires two games a week. Under such conditions, the maintenance of strength is slightly different—one day of maximum strength and

Table 5.8 Suggested Training Program for a Microcycle Falling Between Two Competitions

Day	1	2	3	4	5	6	7	8
Type of activity	Competition	Day off for recovery and regeneration	Technical training Tactical training of longer duration	Technical or tactical training Phosphagen training Maximum strength or power	Technical or tactical training Model training	Technical or tactical training Speed or agility Power training	Model training	Competition
Loading pattern	High	Off	Low-medium	High	Medium-high	Medium	Low	High

Table 5.9 Suggested Strength Training Program for a Microcycle With Three Competitions

Day	1	2	3	4	5	6	7	8
Type of activity	Competition	Off Recovery and regeneration	Technical or tactical training	Competition	Recovery and regeneration	Technical or tactical training Speed Maximum strength	Tactical training Model training	Competition
Loading pattern	High	Off	Medium	High		High	Low	High

one for power, power endurance, or muscular endurance. On day 5, the postcompetition day, we suggest activities that can stimulate recovery and regeneration, such as massage, stretching, sauna, and low-intensity training. To accommodate these activities best, day 5 can be divided into two parts (for those athletes who can afford free time): recovery and regeneration in the morning and short, low-intensity technical and tactical training in the afternoon. On precompetition days, athletes engage in tactical training similar to the activities they will meet the next day in competition.

Table 5.10 illustrates a microcycle for sports that use weekend tournaments (such as Friday, Saturday, and Sunday). Because such tournaments can be organized either a few weeks apart or repeated for several weeks in a row (e.g., high school and university competitions), the same structure can be used for one week or more. Coaches will want to make changes in the microcycle based on their athletes' specific conditions, level of fatigue, and classification, as well as other factors, such as travel and the feasibility of organizing daily training sessions.

On Thursday, coaches should organize a tactical training to model the strategies that their athletes will use for the duration of the tournament. Coaches who have time for a short training session during the tournament can even use very low-intensity activities, say, in the morning, to mimic the strategies that their athletes will use in an afternoon or evening competition.

Table 5.10 Suggested Strength Training Program for a Microcycle for a Weekend Tournament

Day	Monday	Tuesday	Wednesday	Thursday	Friday	Saturday	Sunday
Type of activity	Recovery Regeneration	Technical Tactical Longer duration drills	Technical Tactical Phosphagen Speed and agility Maximum strength	Technical Tactical Model training	Competition	Competition	Competition
Loading pattern	Off	Medium	Medium to high	Low	High	High	High

Integration of Microcycles Into Macrocycles

A microcycle should not be an isolated entity; rather, it should be integrated thoughtfully into the larger macrocycle. This integration should always occur.

The integration of different types of microcycles into a macrocycle depends on the training phase, the athlete's classification, the athlete's strength training background, and the type of macrocycle. Two types of macrocycles are used during the preparatory phase: the step macrocycle and the flat macrocycle. Step loading is useful in developmental macrocycles. Consisting of progressive increases in load, step loading is less stressful and therefore more applicable to the early part of the preparatory phase. It is advisable to use the step macrocycle all year long for entry-level and intermediate athletes and for endurance athletes, whereas it can be limited to the early general preparation for more advanced athletes in power sports.

The flat macrocycle subjects athletes to a higher average level of training volume, intensity, or both and thereby challenges their level of adaptation even more. It is suggested for advanced athletes with extensive training backgrounds or simply for macrocycles where the training is very intense or specific, which requires more frequent unloading. In fact, it is suggested that a 2+1 structure for flat loading be used instead of the 3+1 normally used in step loading.

As illustrated in figure 5.4, the height of each block reflects the demand training. The letter L indicates a loading microcycle, and the letter U indicates an unloading microcycle, which is placed at the end of each macrocycle for recovery purposes. During the competitive phase, the integration of microcycles into macrocycles depends directly on the competition schedule. Because the schedule varies by the sport, the structure of the macrocycle does so too. As an example, let us consider the competitive phase for an individual sport. The macrocycle, shown in table 5.11, consists of a postcompetition recovery and regeneration microcycle to eliminate fatigue before resuming normal training. This microcycle is followed by two developmental microcycles, which are used to train the athlete to further improve or retain the specific biomotor abilities. Next comes a precompetition peaking microcycle, in which the volume of training is reduced dramatically (up to a 60% reduction) while the intensity is reduced only slightly, in order to peak for the competition.

Strength training can normally be performed during developmental microcycles to ensure that detraining doesn't affect the athlete's ability to reach peak performance at the end of the competitive phase, when championship competitions are scheduled.

The structure of a macrocycle differs for team sports, in which each week represents an opportunity to compete, sometimes twice. As a result, strength training must be implemented according to the microcycles exemplified in this chapter, especially in figures 5.1 through 5.3. Because team sports have such a large number of competitions, the scope

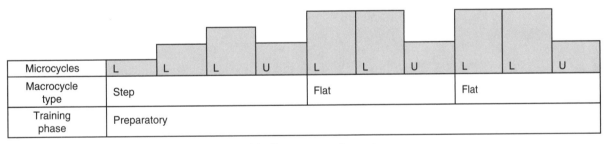

Microcycles	L	L	L	U	L	L	U	L	L	U
Macrocycle type	Step				Flat			Flat		
Training phase	Preparatory									

Figure 5.4 Step and flat macrocycles within the preparatory phase.

Table 5.11 The Structure of a Macrocycle for the Competitive Phase of an Individual Sport

Type of micro-cycle	Postcompetition recovery and regeneration	Developmental	Developmental	Precompetition peaking	Competition
Number of strength training sessions per micro-cycle	1 or 2 (toward the end of the micro-cycle)	2-4	2-4	1 (in the early days of the microcycle)	

of strength training programs must be to maintain specific strength gains made during the preparatory phase. This approach avoids detraining. Moreover, thanks to the physiological benefits from maintaining high levels of specific strength, an athlete's levels of athletic competence is maintained throughout the entire competitive season.

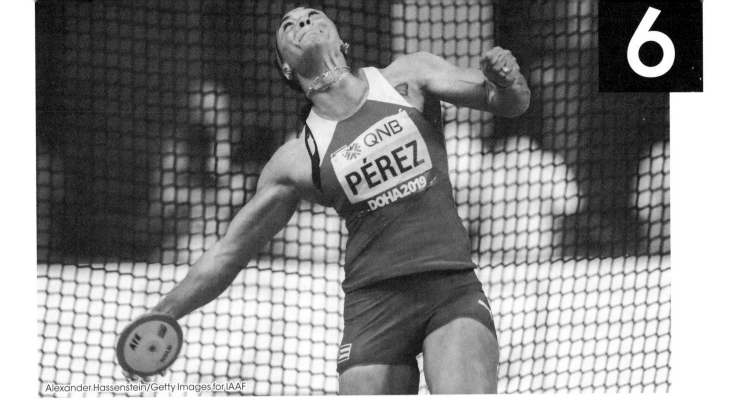

Alexander Hassenstein/Getty Images for IAAF

The Annual Plan

The annual training plan is as important a tool for achieving long-term athletic goals as the microcycle is for achieving short-term athletic goals. An organized and well-constructed annual training plan is required for maximizing the athlete's motor potential improvements. To be effective, it must be based on the concept of periodization and employ its training principles as guiding precepts. One primary objective of training is for the athlete to reach peak performance at a specific time, usually for the main competition of the year. For the athlete to achieve this high level of performance, the entire training program must be properly periodized and planned so that the development of skills and motor abilities proceeds logically and methodically throughout the year.

Periodization consists of two basic components. The first component, periodization of the annual plan, addresses the various training phases throughout the year. The second component, periodization of the biomotor abilities, addresses the development of biomotor abilities training to increase the athlete's motor potential. In particular, the periodization of strength structures strength training to maximize its effectiveness in meeting the needs of the specific sport.

Periodization of the Annual Plan

The first component of periodization consists of dividing the annual plan into shorter, more manageable training phases. Doing so enhances the organization of training and allows the coach to conduct the program systematically. In most sports, the annual training cycle is divided into three main phases of training: preparation (preseason), competitive (season), and transition (off-season). Each training phase is further subdivided into cycles.

The duration of each training phase depends heavily on the competition schedule as well as on the time needed to improve skills and develop the dominant biomotor abilities. During the preparation phase, the coach's primary objective is to develop the athlete's physiological foundations. During the competitive phase, it is to strive for perfection according to the specific demands of competition.

Figure 6.1 illustrates the periodization of the annual plan into phases and cycles of training. This particular plan has only one competitive phase, so athletes have to peak only once during the year; such a plan is called a monocycle or single-peak annual plan. Of course, not all sports have only one competitive phase. For example, track and field, swimming, and several other sports have indoor and outdoor seasons or two major competitions for which athletes must peak. This type of plan is usually called a bi-cycle or double-peak annual plan (see figure 6.2). Advanced athletes competing at the international level, on the other hand, have to peak up to three times a year. Think of most individual-sport athletes that have to peak for the winter championship, summer championship (that usually functions as national selection trials), and, finally, for the world championship or the Olympics. In that case, we speak of a tri-cyclical annual plan.

Yearly plan						
Phases of training	Preparatory			Competitive		Transition
Sub-phases	General preparation		Specific preparation	Pre-competitive	Competitive	Transition
Macro-cycles						
Micro-cycles						

Figure 6.1 Periodization of a monocycle.

Annual plan					
Preparatory (I)	Competitive (I)	Transition (I)	Preparatory (II)	Competitive (II)	Transition (II)

Figure 6.2 Periodization of a bi-cycle.

Periodization of Strength

Coaches should be more concerned with deciding what kind of physiological response or training adaptation will lead to the greatest improvement than with deciding what drills or skills to work on in a given training session or phase. Once they have made the first decision, they will have an easier time selecting the appropriate type of work to produce the desired development. Only by considering these overriding physiological factors can coaches choose an approach that results in the best training adaptation and ultimately leads to increases in physiological capacity and improved athletic performance.

Such an innovative approach is facilitated by periodization. Recall from chapter 1 that the purpose of strength training for sports is not the development of strength for its own sake. Rather, the goal is to maximize power, power endurance, or muscular endurance, according to the needs of the chosen sport. This chapter demonstrates that the best approach for achieving that goal is the periodization of strength, with its specific sequence of training phases.

As illustrated in figure 6.3, periodization of strength includes seven phases with specific strength training objectives. Training phases are conventionally divided by a vertical bar, illustrating where one phase ends and another begins. However, the type of strength training does not change from one phase to another as abruptly as the chart implies. To the contrary, a smoother transition can be made from one type of strength to another one (e.g., from maximum strength to power).

Preparation				Competitive		Transition
Anatomical adaptation	Hypertrophy if necessary	Maximum strength	Conversion to specific strength (power; power endurance; or muscular endurance short, medium, or long)	Maintenance of maximum strength and specific strength	Cessation of strength training	Compensation training

Figure 6.3 Periodization of strength for a monocycle.

Phase 1: Anatomical Adaptation

Periodization of strength has become very popular worldwide, and many training specialists and authors have discussed and written about this very efficient strength training concept. However, in their attempt to be different or to claim originality, some authors suggest a periodization of strength plan that starts with hypertrophy training. This might be acceptable in bodybuilding, but it is definitely not acceptable in strength training for sport. In fact, except for some throwers in track and field and some position players in American football, hypertrophy or muscle size is not a determining factor in high-performance athletics.

To the contrary, athletes in most sports—such as basketball, soccer, and swimming, not to mention sports divided into weight-class categories—are extremely reluctant to increase nonfunctional muscle hypertrophy. Furthermore, to maximize hypertrophy, athletes must work each set to exhaustion, which at times may result in a high level of discomfort that negatively affects the sport-specific training or even causes injury. For this reason, the original model of periodization of strength starts with an anatomical adaptation phase.

Following a transition phase, during which athletes usually do very little strength training, it is scientifically and methodologically sound to start a strength program aimed at adapting the anatomy for the heavy loads to follow. The main objectives of this phase are to involve most muscle groups and to prepare the muscles, ligaments, tendons, and joints to endure the subsequent lengthy and strenuous training phases. Strength training programs should not focus only on the legs or arms; they should also focus on strengthening the core area—the abdominal muscles, the low back, and the spinal column musculature. These sets of muscles work together to ensure that the trunk supports the legs and arms during all movements and also act as shock-absorbing devices during the performance of many skills and exercises, especially landing and falling.

Additional objectives for anatomical adaptation are to balance strength between agonist and antagonist muscles surrounding each joint; to balance the two sides of the body, especially the legs, shoulders, and arms; and to strengthen the stabilizer muscles. The volume of strength training must be balanced between muscle functions (see figure 6.4)—in other words, between agonists and antagonists around a joint. Failing to do so may result in postural imbalances and injuries.

In some cases, balanced development between agonist and antagonist muscles is impossible because some agonist muscles are larger and stronger than others. For instance, the knee extensors (quadriceps) are stronger than the knee flexors (hamstrings). The same is true for the ankle plantar flexors (gastrocnemii) and extensors (tibialis anteriori). The knee extensors and ankle plantar flexors are exposed to more training because activities such as running and jumping are used heavily in most sports. Professionals in the field, however, must be aware of the agonist-to-antagonist ratios and attempt to maintain them through training. If they neglect to do so and instead constantly train the agonists—the prime movers of given sport skills—the imbalance will likely result in impaired performance due both to neural inhibition of force expression of the prime movers and to injuries (for example, rotator cuff injuries in baseball).

The transition and anatomical adaptation phases are ideal for balanced development of antagonist muscles because they occur at a time in the training cycle when there is no pressure from competition. Little information exists about the agonist-to-antagonist ratios, especially for the high-speed limb movements typical of sports. Table 6.1 provides some information on the subject for low, isokinetic speeds. This information should be used only as a guideline for maintaining these ratios, at least during the anatomical adaptation and transition phases.

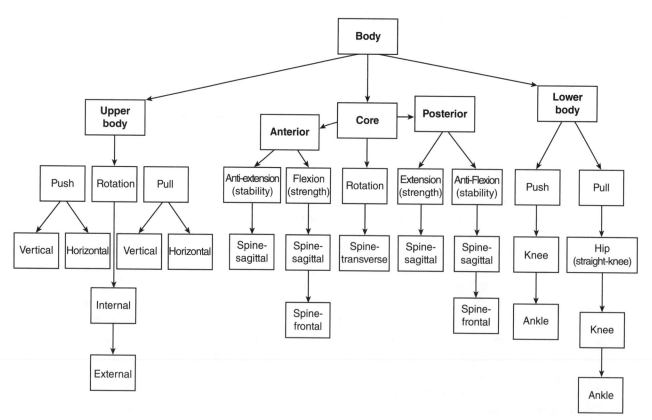

Figure 6.4 One way to achieve muscular balance is to use the same volume of work for the agonist and the antagonist muscles around a joint.

Table 6.1 Agonist-to-Antagonist Ratios for Slow Concentric Isokinetic Movements

Joint	Strength training	Ratio
Ankle	Plantar flexion (gastrocnemius, soleus) to dorsiflexion (tibialis anterior)	3:1
Ankle	Inversion (tibialis anterior) to eversion (peroneus)	1:1
Knee	Extension (quadriceps) to flexion (hamstrings)	3:2
Hip	Extension (spinal erectors, gluteus maximus, hamstrings) to flexion (iliopsoas, rectus femoris, tensor fascia latae, sartorius)	1:1
Shoulder	Flexion (anterior deltoids) to extension (trapezius, posterior deltoids)	2:3
Shoulder	Internal rotation (subscapularis, latissimus dorsi, pectoralis major, teres major) to external rotation (supraspinatus, infraspinatus, teres minor)	3:2
Elbow	Flexion (biceps) to extension (triceps)	1:1
Lumbar spine	Flexion (abdominals) to extension (spinal erectors)	1:1

Reprinted by permission from D. Wathen, "Muscle Balance." In *Essentials of Strength Training and Conditioning*, edited for the National Strength and Conditioning Association by T.R. Baechle (Champaign, IL: Human Kinetics, 1994), 425.

Throughout the anatomical adaptation phase, the goal is to involve most, if not all, muscle groups in a multilateral program. Such a program should include a high number of exercises (9-12) performed comfortably without pushing the athlete. Remember, vigorous strength training always develops the strength of the muscles faster than the strength of the muscle attachments (tendons) and joints (ligaments). Consequently, applying such programs too early often result in injuries to these tissues.

In addition, when large-muscle groups are weak, the small muscles have to take over the strain of the work. As a result, the small-muscle groups may become injured more quickly. Other injuries occur because insufficiently trained muscles lack the force to control landings, absorb shock, and balance the body quickly to be ready to perform another action (not because of a lack of landing skills). This is the reason why plyometric training is introduced gradually after two or three weeks of anatomical adaptations, using low-intensity jumps and bounds to reach the highest intensities right after the maximum strength phase when a solid base of muscular strength has been laid down.

The duration of the anatomical adaptation phase depends on the length of the preparation phase, the athlete's background in strength training, and the importance of strength in the given sport. A long preparation phase, of course, allows more time for anatomical adaptation. Logically, athletes who have a weak strength training background require a much longer anatomical adaptation phase. This phase fosters progressive adaptation to training loads and improves the ability of muscle tissue and muscle attachments to withstand the heavier loads of the phases that follow.

Young or inexperienced athletes need eight to ten weeks of anatomical adaptation training. In contrast, mature athletes with four to six years of strength training require no more than two or three weeks of this phase. Indeed, for these athletes, a longer anatomical adaptation phase likely provides no significant additional training effect.

Phase 2: Hypertrophy

In some sports, an increase in muscle size is an important asset. However, as mentioned throughout this text, hypertrophy training, which is extremely popular in bodybuilding, is overused in the sporting world. When applied to strength training for sports, hypertrophy training must extend beyond the old definition of training to exhaustion. Specifically, it can be used as a primer for the maximum strength phase to follow by adapting the body to using progressively heavier loads.

If some athletes need to increase muscle size (e.g., competitors in shot put, heavy weight categories in wrestling, boxing, and martial arts, or scrum players in rugby), they can use two different approaches: hypertrophy I, hypertrophy II, or both. Hypertrophy I is often used with athletes who require a distinct increase in muscle size and strength. It relies on using loads between 15RM (i.e., 15 reps to failure) and 10RM with little rest (60-90 seconds maximum) between sets. If bodybuilding techniques such as rest-pause and drop sets are used during this phase to increase the tension and protein synthesis within the musculature, the load used is between 8RM and 5RM, because these techniques further increase the total time under tension per set.

Hypertrophy II involves a more hybrid kind of work between hypertrophy and maximum strength that prepares the fast-twitch muscle fibers for the hard work to follow during the maximum strength training phase. Hypertrophy II increases absolute strength by eliciting both neural and structural adaptations. This phase uses loads from 8RM to 5RM with relatively long rest intervals (120-180 seconds).

For both hypertrophy I and hypertrophy II, the time devoted and the loads are determined by the athlete's age, physical development, and strength training experience. At the end of the hypertrophy phase, a maximum strength test is performed in order to plan the training percentage of the first maximum strength macrocycle.

Phase 3: Maximum Strength

The main objective of this phase is to develop the highest possible level of strength. This goal can be achieved only by using heavy loads in training: 70% to 95% of 1RM or, less often, 90% to 100%.

For a better training progression, you can divide the maximum strength phase into two distinct parts: maximum strength I and II:

- Maximum strength I works mainly on the intermuscular coordination and is composed of one or two 3+1 macrocycles, in which the load for the main strength exercises is between 70% to 80% of 1RM.

- Maximum strength II has the objective of training mainly the intramuscular coordination via a 2+1 structure with heavy loads of 80% to 90 % of 1RM (figure 6.5). This

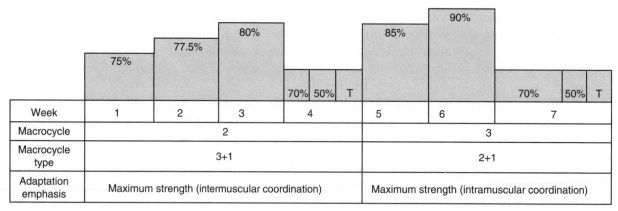

Figure 6.5 Suggested load progression for a 7-week maximum strength phase (a 3+1 and a 2+1 structure) in which the unloading phases have the scope of testing a new 1RM. The 3+1 structure is suggested for a national level athlete.

Key: T = maximum strength testing

type of strength training plan is suggested for athletes up to national level competitions. The other examples are suggested for above national, that is, international level athletes (figures 6.6-6.7).

The duration of this phase, roughly from one to three months, is a function of the chosen sport or event and the athlete's needs. A shot-putter or an American football player may need a lengthy phase of slightly more than three months, whereas many other athletes may need only one or two months to develop the necessary type of strength. The load can be increased in a three-week macrocycle, and it usually progresses by 5% per microcycle. Macrocycles for the intermuscular coordination type of maximum strength use loads up to 80% of 1RM, whereas a macrocycle for the *intra*muscular coordination type of maximum strength uses loads above 80%.

This phase is characterized by a higher number of sets with a lower number of exercises. The duration of this phase also depends on whether the athlete follows a monocycle or bi-cycle annual plan. For obvious reasons, young athletes may have a shorter maximum strength phase with lower loads.

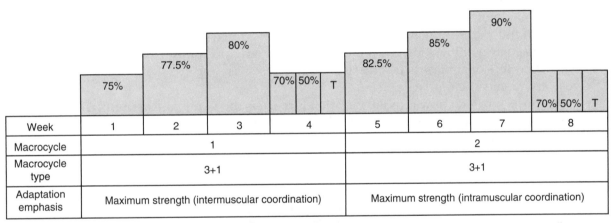

Figure 6.6 Suggested load progression for an 8-week, high-demand maximum strength phase. During the last days of the low step microcycle (step 1), a test is planned to find the new 1RM.

Key: T = maximum strength testing

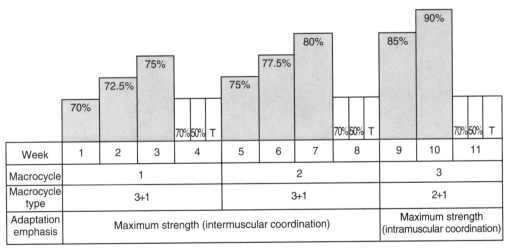

Figure 6.7 Suggested load progression for a three-macrocycle (11 weeks) maximum strength phase for a well-adapted athlete to high training demand/heavy loads.

Key: T = maximum strength testing

Most sports require either power (e.g., for jumps and throws in track and field), power endurance (e.g., for sprints in track and field), muscular endurance (e.g., for 800- to 1,500-meter swimming), or all three (e.g., for rowing, canoeing, wrestling, combat sports, the martial arts, and some team sports). Each of these types of specific strength is affected by the level of maximum strength. For instance, without a high level of maximum strength, an athlete cannot reach high levels of power. Because power is the product of force and velocity, it is logical to develop maximum strength first, then convert it to power.

Phase 4: Conversion to Specific Strength

The main purpose of this phase is to convert gains in maximum strength into competitive, sport-specific combinations of strength. Depending on the characteristics of the chosen sport or event, maximum strength must be converted into power, power endurance, or muscular endurance short, medium, or long. By applying an adequate training method for the type of strength sought and using training methods specific to the selected sport (for example, speed training), athletes gradually convert maximum strength into power.

Throughout this phase, depending on the needs of the sport and the athlete, a certain level of maximum strength must be maintained (usually employing both sport-specific range and full-range-of-motion exercises). If not, power may decline (due to detraining of neuromuscular qualities) toward the end of the competitive phase. This is certainly the case for professional players in American football, soccer, and baseball, because each of these sports has such a long season.

For sports in which power or muscular endurance is the dominant strength, the appropriate method must be dominant in training. When both power and muscular endurance are required, the training time and methods should adequately reflect the optimal ratio

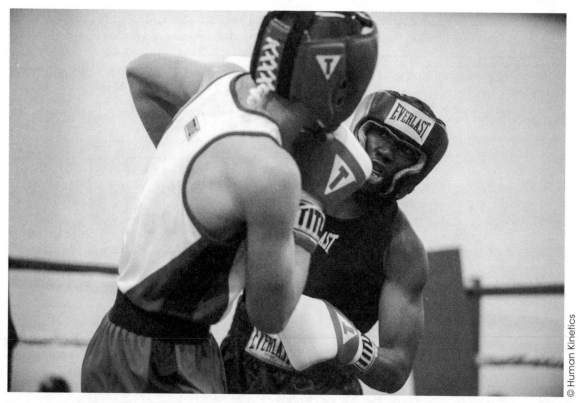

© Human Kinetics

The conversion-to-specific-strength phase helps the athlete transfer his strength gains to performance.

between these two abilities. For instance, for a wrestler, the ratio should be almost equal; for a speedskater in a 500-meter event, power endurance should dominate; and for a rower, muscular endurance should dominate. In team sports, the martial arts, wrestling, boxing, and most other power-dominant sports, coaches should combine power training with exercises that lead to the development of agility and quick reaction and movement times during the conversion phase. Only this type of approach prepares athletes for the sport-specific requirements of competition.

The duration of the conversion phase depends on the ability that needs to be developed. Conversion to power can be achieved in four to eight weeks of specific power training. On the other hand, conversion to muscular endurance requires as many as six to nine weeks because both the physiological and the anatomical adaptations to such demanding work take much longer.

Phase 5: Maintenance

The tradition in many sports is to eliminate strength training when the competitive season starts. However, athletes who do not maintain strength training during the competitive phase experience a detraining effect with the following repercussions.

- Muscle fibers decrease to their pretraining size, resulting in a strength and power loss (Thorstensson 1977; Staron, Hagerman, and Hikida 1981; McMaster et al. 2013).
- Loss of strength also results from decreases in motor unit recruitment. The athlete fails to voluntarily activate the same number of motor units as before, which causes a net decrease in the amount of force that can be generated (Edgerton 1976; Hainaut and Duchateau 1989; Houmard 1991; Kraemer and Ratamess 2005).
- Power decreases ensue because the rate of force production depends on the firing rate.
- Detraining becomes evident after four weeks, when athletes begin to be unable to perform skills requiring strength and power as proficiently as they did at the end of the conversion phase (Bompa 1993; Kraemer and Ratamess 2005).

As the term suggests, the main objective of strength training during this phase is to maintain the standards achieved during the previous phases. Once again, the program followed during this phase is a function of the specific requirements of the chosen sport. Such requirements must be reflected in the training ratio between maximum strength and the specific strength. For instance, a shot-putter may plan two sessions to train for maximum strength and two to train for power, whereas a jumper may consider one for maximum strength and two for power. Similarly, a 100-meter swimmer may plan one session to train for maximum strength, one for power, and one to train for muscular endurance short, whereas a 1,500-meter swimmer may dedicate the entire strength program to perfecting muscular endurance long.

For team sports, ratios should be calculated according to the role of strength in the particular sport; in addition, they should be position specific. For instance, a pitcher should perform maximum strength and power equally while also doing compensation work to avoid rotator cuff injury. Similarly, distinctions should be made between linemen and wide receivers in American football, and sweepers, midfielders, and forwards in soccer. Linemen and wide receivers should spend equal time on maximum strength and power but use different percentages of 1RM (linemen use a lower velocity of the application of force in their specific activity). Soccer players have to maintain both power and power endurance short—that is, the ability to repeat numerous power actions with incomplete rest.

Between one and four sessions per week must be dedicated to maintaining the required strength qualities, depending on the athlete's level of performance and the role of strength in skill performance. Studies show that at least one strength maintenance session per week is necessary to maintain most of the strength gains and the power output reached during preparation (Graves et al. 1988; Wilmore and Costill 2004; Rønnestad et al. 2011).

Compared with the preparation phases, the time allocated to the maintenance of strength in the maintenance phase is much lower. Therefore, the coach has to develop a very efficient and specific program. For instance, two to (at most) four exercises involving the prime movers will enable the athlete to maintain previously reached strength levels. As a result, the duration of each strength training session will be short—20 to 40 minutes.

Phase 6: Cessation

As the main competition of the year approaches, most of the athlete's energy must be directed to the main sport-specific biomotor ability or mix of biomotor abilities. Again, the purpose of the cessation phase is to conserve the athlete's energy for competition and peak his or her sport-specific biomotor abilities. For this reason, the strength training program should end at least three to fourteen days before the main competition. The exact timing depends on multiple factors.

- *The athlete's sex.* Female athletes, who retain strength gains less easily than males do, should usually maintain strength training until three days before competition.

- *The chosen sport.* A longer cessation phase, one to two weeks long, may result in improved alactic speed performance due to overshooting of the fast-twitch Type IIX muscle fibers. For long endurance sports for which strength is not as important as for anaerobic sports, strength training can be ended two weeks before the main competition for the year.

- *Body type.* Heavier athletes tend to retain both adaptations and residual fatigue longer and therefore should end strength training earlier than lighter athletes.

Phase 7: Compensation

Traditionally, the last phase of the annual plan has been inappropriately called the off-season; in reality, it represents a transition from one annual plan to another. The main goal of this phase is to remove fatigue acquired during the training year and replenish the exhausted energy stores by decreasing both volume (through a decrease in frequency) and intensity of training. During the months of training and competition, most athletes are exposed to numerous psychological and social stressors that drain their mental energy. During the transition phase, athletes can relax psychologically by getting involved in various physical and social activities that they enjoy.

The transition phase between two parts of the annual plan should last no longer than two weeks, and usually lasts only one week. On the other hand, the transition phase at the end of the annual plan can last between four and eight weeks, depending on the level of the athlete: Beginners must have shorter transition phases because they have not stabilized their adaptations, and their competition phase is usually shorter than that of professional athletes. A longer phase results in detraining effects, such as the loss of most training gains, especially strength gains. Professional athletes in an Olympic sport, on the other hand, can take up to eight weeks of transition at the end of the quadrennial Olympic cycle. The detraining that results from neglecting strength training in the off-season can be detrimental to an athlete's rate of performance improvement in the following year.

DETRAINING

Strength can be improved or maintained only if an adequate load or training intensity is administered continually. When strength training is decreased or ceased, as often happens during competitive or long transition phases, a disturbance occurs in the biological state of the muscle cells and the bodily organs. This disturbance results in a marked decrease in the athlete's physiological well-being and work output (Fry, Morton, and Keast 1991; Kuipers and Keizer 1988; McMaster et al. 2013).

Decreased or diminished training can leave athletes vulnerable to "detraining syndrome" (Israel 1972). The severity of strength loss depends on the elapsed time between training sessions. Many organic and cellular adaptation benefits may be degraded, including the protein content of myosin.

When training proceeds as planned, the body uses protein to build and repair damaged tissues. When the body is in a state of disuse, however, it begins to catabolize or break down protein because it is no longer needed (Edgerton 1976; Appell 1990; Mujika and Padilla 2000). As this process of protein degradation continues, some of the gains made during training are reversed. Testosterone levels, which are important for strength gains, have also been shown to decrease as a result of detraining, which may, in turn, diminish the amount of protein synthesis (Houmard 1991; Kraemer and Ratamess 2005).

Total abstinence from training is associated with a range of symptoms, including a rise in psychological disturbances, such as headache, insomnia, a feeling of exhaustion, increased tension, increased mood disturbance, lack of appetite, and psychological depression. An athlete may develop any one of these symptoms or a combination of two or more. The symptoms all have to do with lowered levels of testosterone and beta-endorphin, a neuroendocrine compound that is the main forerunner of euphoric postexercise feelings (Houmard 1991, Petibois and Deleris, 2003).

Detraining symptoms are not pathological and can be reversed if training resumes shortly. If training is discontinued for a prolonged period, however, athletes may display symptoms for some time. This pattern indicates the inability of the human body and its systems to adapt to the state of inactivity. The length of time needed for these symptoms to incubate varies from athlete to athlete, but they generally appear after two to three weeks of inactivity and vary in severity.

Coaches of athletes involved in speed- and power-dominant sports must be aware of the fact that when muscles are not stimulated with strength or power training activities, muscle fiber recruitment is disrupted. This disruption results in a deterioration of performance (Wilmore and Costill 2004). Wilmore and Costill (2004) reported that strength gained during a 12-week program decreased by 68% as a result of 12 weeks of strength training interruption; this is a substantial loss for some athletes, especially those in speed- and power-dominant sports. In contrast, subjects who kept performing at least one strength training session per week retained all of the strength they had gained in the 12 weeks of training.

The decrease in muscle fiber cross-sectional area is quite apparent after a few weeks of inactivity. The fastest rate of muscle atrophy, especially the degradation of contractile protein, takes place in the first two weeks. These changes result from lower glycogen content in the muscle, and especially from protein breakdown, as a result of inhibition of the cellular anabolic pathways (Kandarian and Jackman 2006; Zhang et al. 2007). In addition, the tendons' tensile strength diminishes as a consequence of atrophy in collagen fiber, and the ligaments' total collagen mass diminishes as well (Kannus et al. 1992).

(continued)

Slow-twitch fibers are usually the first to lose their ability to produce force. Fast-twitch fibers are generally least affected by inactivity. In fact, when exposed to lactic training, fast-twitch glycolytic muscle fibers of Type IIX (more precisely, their myosin-heavy chains) take on the characteristics of fast-twitch oxidative glycolytic fibers of Type IIA (Andersen et al. 2005). Yet they regain their faster characteristics when training volume is greatly reduced. This is not to say that atrophy does not occur in these fibers—it just takes a little longer than in slow-twitch fibers.

After an initial increase due to rebound in fast-twitch fibers, speed is affected by longer detraining because the breakdown of muscle protein and the loss of neural adaptation decrease the power capabilities of muscle contractions. The loss in power becomes more pronounced as a result of diminished motor recruitment. The reduction in nerve impulses to the muscle fibers makes muscles contract and relax at slower rates. Reduction in the strength and frequency of these impulses can also decrease the total number of motor units recruited during a series of repeated contractions (Edgerton 1976; Hainaut and Duchateau 1989; Houmard 1991; Mujika and Padilla 2000).

Detraining also affects aerobic-dominant sports. Coyle and colleagues (1991) observed that an 84-day training stoppage did not affect glycolytic enzyme activity but did decrease the activity of oxidative enzymes by 60%. This finding demonstrates that anaerobic performance can be maintained longer than aerobic performance, although both lactic capacity and aerobic power are affected by decreases in muscle glycogen of up to 40% that result from at least four weeks of detraining (Wilmore and Costill 2004).

Athletes and coaches should remember that strength is hard to gain and easy to lose. Athletes who perform no strength training at all during the transition phase may experience decreased muscle size and considerable power loss (Wilmore and Costill 2004; Mujika and Padille 2000). Because power and speed are interdependent, such athletes also lose speed. Some authors claim that the disuse of muscles also reduces the frequency of discharge rate and the pattern of muscle fiber recruitment; thus, strength and power loss may be the result of not activating as many motor units.

Although physical activity volume is reduced by 50% to 60% during the transition phase, athletes should find time to work on the maintenance of strength training. Specifically, it can be beneficial to work on the antagonists, stabilizers, and other muscles that may not necessarily be involved in the performance of the sport-specific skills. Similarly, compensation exercises should be planned for sports in which an imbalance may develop between parts or sides of the body—for example, pitching, throwing events, archery, soccer (work the upper body more), and cycling.

Variations in the Periodization of Strength Model

The periodization of strength example presented earlier in this chapter (see figure 6.3) was helpful for illustrating the basic concept, but it cannot serve as a model for every situation or every sport. Each individual or group of athletes requires specific planning and programming based on training background, sex, and the specific characteristics of the chosen sport or event. This section of the chapter explains variations of periodization of strength and offers follow-up illustrations of specific periodization models for certain sports and events.

Some sports, and some positions in team sports, require strength and heavy muscle mass. For instance, it is advantageous for throwers in track-and-field events, linemen in American football, and heavyweight wrestlers and boxers to be both heavy and powerful. These athletes should follow a unique periodization model with a long phase of training planned to develop hypertrophy. Developing hypertrophy first seems to increase force potential faster, especially if followed by maximum strength and power development phases, which are known to stimulate the activation and firing rate of fast-twitch muscle fiber.

Figure 6.8 shows a periodization model for heavy and powerful athletes. The traditional anatomical adaptation phase is followed by a hypertrophy phase of at least six weeks, which in turn is followed by maximum strength training and conversion to power. During the maintenance phase, these athletes should dedicate time to preserving maximum strength and power that will also preserve the hypertrophy gains obtained in the previous stages. The annual plan concludes with compensation training specific to the transition phase.

Because the preparation phase in power sports can be very long (e.g., in U.S. and Canadian college football), the coach may decide to build even more muscle mass. To this end, another model can be followed—see figure 6.9—in which phases of hypertrophy are alternated with phases of maximum strength. The numbers above each phase in figure 6.10 and some of the following tables indicate the duration of that phase in weeks.

Figure 6.10 illustrates a periodization with a longer preparation phase and alternation between maximum strength and power macrocycles. The longer preparation phase assumes either a summer sport or a sport played during the winter and early spring. The alternation between different abilities (H, MxS and P) consistently results in higher

Prep.				Comp.	T
AA	Hyp.	MxS	Conv. to P	Maint.: P, MxS	Compens.

Figure 6.8 Periodization model for athletes requiring hypertrophy.

Key: AA = anatomical adaptation, comp. = competitive, compens. = compensation, conv. = conversion, hyp. = hypertrophy, maint. = maintenance, MxS = maximum strength, P = power, prep. = preparation, T = transition

Prep.								Comp.	T
3 AA	7 Hyp.	6 MxS	3 Hyp.	3 MxS	3 Hyp.	3 MxS	4 Conv. to P	16 Maint.: P, MxS	4 Compens.

Figure 6.9 Variation of periodization for development of hypertrophy and maximum strength.

Key: AA = anatomical adaptation, comp. = competitive, compens. = compensation, conv. = conversion, hyp. = hypertrophy, maint. = maintenance, MxS = maximum strength, P = power, prep. = preparation, T = transition

Prep.							Comp.	T
7 AA	6 MxS	3 P	6 MxS	3 P	3 MxS	4 P	16 Maint.: P, MxS	4 Compens.

Figure 6.10 Periodization model for advanced power athletes requiring frequent alternations of strength training emphasis.

Key: AA = anatomical adaptation, comp. = competitive, compens. = compensation, maint. = maintenance, MxS = maximum strength, P = power, prep. = preparation, T = transition

improvement of power and is indicated for sports characterized by a few concentrated competitions throughout the year (e.g., racket and combat sports), which means that a longer maximum strength phase could be detrimental to sport-specific skills (Bompa 1993).

Furthermore, similar variations of power and maximum strength phases are necessary because gains in power are faster if muscles are trained at various speeds of contraction (Bührle 1985; Bührle and Schmidtbleicher 1981; Bompa 1993; McMaster et al. 2013). Both power and maximum strength training train the fast-twitch fibers. In addition, maximum strength training results in motor unit recruitment patterns that display high levels of force, and power training increases the frequency or speed at which the muscles carry out the work. Anyone who has witnessed the performance of a shot-putter, javelin thrower, or hammer thrower can appreciate the force and speed characteristics involved. Macrocycles alternating maximum strength and power can also be employed by power athletes such as sprinters and jumpers in track and field at a more advanced stage of development.

If the same methods and loading pattern are maintained for longer than two months, especially by athletes with a strong strength training background, the pattern of fiber recruitment becomes standard, eventually reaching a plateau. At that point, no drastic improvement can be expected. Thus, bodybuilding methods defeat their purpose in sports in which speed and power are dominant abilities. This explains why several of the figures in this chapter propose a sequence of maximum strength and power macrocycles.

In addition, the importance of maximum strength phases should not be underestimated because any deterioration in maximum strength affects the athlete's ability to maintain power or muscle endurance at the desired level throughout the competitive phase. In sports in which athletes must peak twice a year (e.g., swimming and track and field), a bi-cycle annual plan is optimal. Figure 6.11 presents the periodization of strength plan for a double-peak (bi-cycle) annual plan.

For sports with three competitive phases, athletes must peak three times a year. Examples include wrestling, boxing, and international-level swimming and track and field, which feature a winter season, an early summer season ending with national championships or trials, and a late summer season ending with the world championship or Olympics. The annual plan for such sports is called a tri-cycle plan; a periodization model for this plan is presented in figure 6.12.

For sports with a long preparation phase—such as softball, American football, and track cycling—figure 6.13 shows a periodization option with two peaks: an artificial peak at the end of April and a real peak (e.g., for the football season) during the fall. This model was developed at the request of a football coach who wanted to improve his players'

OCT.	NOV.	DEC.	JAN.	FEB.	MAR.	APR.	MAY	JUNE	JULY	AUG.	SEPT.
Prep. I			Comp. I			T	Prep. II		Comp. II		T
AA	MxS		Conv. to P	Maint.		AA	MxS	Conv. to P	Maint.	Compens.	

Figure 6.11 Periodization model for a bi-cycle annual plan.

Key: AA = anatomical adaptation, comp. = competitive, compens. = compensation, conv. = conversion, maint. = maintenance, MxS = maximum strength, P = power, prep. = preparation, T = transition

	OCT.	NOV.	DEC.	JAN.	FEB.	MAR.	APR.	MAY	JUNE	JULY	AUG.		SEPT.
	Prep. I				Comp. I		T	Prep. II	Comp. II			Prep. III	Comp. III	T
Periodization of strength	3	9		4	6		1	6	4	6		1	2	3	3
	AA	MxS		Conv. to P	Maint.: P and MxS		AA	MxS	Conv. to PE	Maint.: PE and MxS		AA	MxS, PE	Maint.: PE and MxS	Compens.

Figure 6.12 Periodization model for a tri-cycle annual plan.

Key: AA = anatomical adaptation, comp. = competitive, compens. = compensation, conv. = conversion, maint. = maintenance, MxS = maximum strength, P = power, PE = power endurance, prep. = preparation, T = transition

DEC.	JAN.	FEB.	MAR.	APR.	MAY	JUNE	JULY	AUG.	SEPT.	OCT.	NOV.
Prep.				T	Prep. II			Comp.		T	
AA	MxS		Conv. to P	AA	MxS		Conv. to P		Maint.: P, MxS	Compens.	

Figure 6.13 Double-peak periodization.

Key: AA = anatomical adaptation, comp. = competitive, compens. = compensation, conv. = conversion, maint. = maintenance, MxS = maximum strength, P = power, prep. = preparation, T = transition

maximum strength and power. The model was very successful, both with the football players and with cycling sprinters; all of the athletes increased their maximum strength and power to the highest levels ever. This new approach for a typical monocycle sport was based on the following reasons:

- A very long preparation phase with heavy loading and little variety was considered too stressful and therefore of dubious physiological benefit.
- A double-peak periodization offers the advantage of planning two phases for maximum strength training and two for power training. American football linemen followed a slightly different approach, in which hypertrophy training preceded the maximum strength phase. The benefits expected by the coach were realized: an increase in overall muscle mass, an increase in maximum strength, and the highest level of power ever achieved by his players.

Periodization Models for Sports

To make this book practical and readily applicable, we have included several sport-specific periodization models for strength. For each model, we include five factors that indicate the physiological characteristics for the relevant sport.

- Dominant energy systems
- Ergogenesis (percentage of each energy system's contribution to final performance)
- Main energy substrates

- Limiting factors for performance
- Objectives for strength training

Strength training should be linked to the sport-specific energy system. Doing so makes it relatively easy to decide the strength training objectives. For instance, for sports in which the anaerobic alactic system is dominant, the limiting factor for performance is power. On the other hand, sports dominated by the anaerobic lactic system or the aerobic system always require a certain component of muscular endurance.

In this way, coaches can better train their athletes physiologically and, as a result, improve their performance. Increments in power should never be expected if the training applies bodybuilding methods. The phrase "limiting factors for performance" means that the desired performance cannot be achieved unless those factors are developed at the highest possible level. More specifically, good performance is limited or hindered if the athlete possesses only a low level of the required sport-specific combination of strength.

The following examples cannot cover all possible variations for each sport. To develop such a model, one would have to know the specific competition schedule, as well as the competition level and objectives of the individual athlete. Thus, for example, for sports such as track and field and swimming, the periodization models are designed around the main competitions in winter and summer.

Sport Finder

AMERICAN FOOTBALL: LINEMEN

Linemen must be able to react explosively when the ball is put into play. They must also withstand an opponent's strength. Therefore, in order to build bulk, a hypertrophy phase is included. For a sample periodization model for college football linemen, see figure 6.14. For a sample model for elite football linemen, see figure 6.15.

- Dominant energy systems: anaerobic alactic, anaerobic lactic
- Ergogenesis: 70% alactic, 30% lactic
- Main energy substrates: creatine phosphate, glycogen
- Limiting factors: starting power, maximum strength
- Training objectives: maximum strength, hypertrophy, power

Periodization	Mar.	Apr.	May	June	July	Aug.	Sept.	Oct.	Nov.	Dec.	Jan.	Feb.
	Prep.						Comp.				T	
Strength	3 AA	6 Hyp.	9 MxS			6 Conv. to P	18 Maint.: MxS, P				6 Compens.	
Energy systems	Lactic cap., alactic P	Alactic P, lactic cap.	Alactic P, lactic P short								O_2 P, alactic P	

Figure 6.14 Periodization model for college football linemen.

Key: AA = anatomical adaptation, cap. = capacity, comp. = competitive, compens. = compensation, conv. = conversion, hyp. = hypertrophy, maint. = maintenance, MxS = maximum strength, P = power, prep. = preparation, T = transition

Periodization	Apr.	May	June	July	Aug.	Sept.	Oct.	Nov.	Dec.	Jan.	Feb.	Mar.
	Prep.				Comp.							T
Strength	2 AA	8 Hyp.		6 MxS	4 Conv. to P	22 Maint.: MxS, P						6 Compens.
Energy systems	Lactic cap., alactic P			Alactic P, lactic P short								O_2 P, alactic P

Figure 6.15 Periodization model for elite football linemen.

Key: AA = anatomical adaptation, cap. = capacity, comp. = competitive, compens. = compensation, conv. = conversion, hyp. = hypertrophy, maint. = maintenance, MxS = maximum strength, P = power, prep. = preparation, T = transition

AMERICAN FOOTBALL: WIDE RECEIVERS, DEFENSIVE BACKS, AND TAILBACKS

Unlike linemen, these players require speed and agility rather than muscular bulk. For a sample periodization model for college football wide receivers, defensive backs, and tailbacks, see figure 6.16. For a sample model for players at these positions in professional football, see figure 6.17.

- Dominant energy systems: anaerobic alactic, anaerobic lactic
- Ergogenesis: 60% alactic, 30% lactic, 10% aerobic
- Main energy substrates: creatine phosphate, glycogen
- Limiting factors: acceleration power, reactive power, starting power
- Training objectives: power, maximum strength

Periodization	Mar.	Apr.		May	June	July	Aug.	Sept.	Oct.	Nov.	Dec.	Jan.	Feb.
	Prep.							Comp.					T
Strength	4 AA	4 MxS	3 P	3 MxS	3 P	3 MxS	4 P	18 Maint.: P, MxS					6 Compens.
Energy systems	O_2 P, lactic cap., alactic P	Lactic cap., alactic P, O_2 P		Lactic P, alactic P, O_2 P			Alactic P, lactic P						O_2 P, alactic P

Figure 6.16 Periodization model for college football wide receivers, defensive backs, and tailbacks.

Key: AA = anatomical adaptation, cap. = capacity, comp. = competitive, compens. = compensation, maint. = maintenance, MxS = maximum strength, O_2 = aerobic, P = power, prep. = preparation, T = transition

Periodization	Apr.		May	June	July		Aug.	Sept.	Oct.	Nov.	Dec.	Jan.	Feb.	Mar.
	Prep.							Comp.						T
Strength	2 AA	3 MxS	3 P	3 MxS	3 P	3 MxS	3 Conv. to P	22 Maint.: P						6 Compens.
Energy systems	O_2 P, lactic cap., alactic P	Lactic cap., alactic P, O_2 P		Lactic P, alactic P, O_2 power			Alactic P, lactic P							O_2 P, alactic P

Figure 6.17 Periodization model for pro football wide receivers, defensive backs, and tailbacks.

Key: AA = anatomical adaptation, cap. = capacity, comp. = competitive, compens. = compensation, conv. = conversion, maint. = maintenance, MxS = maximum strength, O_2 = aerobic, P = power, prep. = preparation, T = transition

BASEBALL, SOFTBALL, AND CRICKET

The dominant ability in these three sports is power displayed in the specific drills of batting and pitching, reaction, and high acceleration. Any restriction placed on training during long preparation phases, especially in professional baseball, may reduce the amount of preparation time, and the long competition schedule can lead to fatigue or injury. Since power and acceleration depend greatly on the ability to recruit the highest possible number of fast-twitch muscle fibers, maximum strength is very important in these athletes' quest for success. Maintaining power and maximum strength helps players succeed throughout the season. For a sample periodization model for an elite baseball team, see figure 6.18. For a sample model for an amateur baseball, softball, or cricket team, see figure 6.19.

- Dominant energy system: anaerobic alactic
- Ergogenesis: 95% alactic, 5% lactic
- Main energy substrate: creatine phosphate
- Limiting factors: throwing power, acceleration power, reactive power
- Training objectives: maximum strength, power

Periodization	Dec.	Jan.	Feb.	Mar.	Apr.	May	June	July	Aug.	Sept.	Oct.	Nov.
	Prep.			Precomp.		Comp.						T
Strength	4 AA	9 MxS		6 Conv. to P		23 Maint.: power, MxS						6 Compens.
Energy systems	O$_2$ P, lactic cap.	Alactic P, lactic P short										O$_2$ compens.

Figure 6.18 Periodization model for an elite baseball team.

The metabolic training represents the cumulative effect of tempo training and specific tactical drills. The suggested order of energy systems training also implies the priority of training for each training phase. Since the competition phase is very long, detraining of strength may occur; therefore, players must maintain power and maximum strength.

Key: AA = anatomical adaptation, cap. = capacity, comp. = competitive, compens. = compensation, conv. = conversion, maint. = maintenance, MxS = maximum strength, O$_2$ = aerobic, P = power, prep. = preparation, T = transition

Periodization	Nov.	Dec.	Jan.	Feb.	Mar.	Apr.	May	June	July	Aug.	Sept.	Oct.
	Prep.						Comp.					T
Strength	4 AA	4 MxS	4 P	4 MxS	4 P	4 MxS	4 P	16 Maint.: P, MxS				4 Compens.
Energy systems	O$_2$ P, lactic cap.	Alactic P, lactic P short										O$_2$ compens

Figure 6.19 Periodization model for an amateur baseball or softball team.

Key: AA = anatomical adaptation, cap. = capacity, comp. = competitive, compens. = compensation, maint. = maintenance, MxS = maximum strength, O$_2$ = aerobic, P = power, prep. = preparation, T = transition

BASKETBALL

Basketball requires players to be strong, agile, and capable of quick acceleration, deceleration, and changes of direction. Proper strength and power training prepare a basketball player for the rigors of the season. For a sample periodization model for a college basketball team, see figure 6.20. For a sample model for an elite basketball team, see figure 6.21.

- Dominant energy systems: anaerobic alactic, anaerobic lactic, aerobic
- Ergogenesis: 60% alactic, 20% lactic, 20% aerobic
- Main energy substrates: creatine phosphate, glycogen
- Limiting factors: takeoff power, acceleration power, power endurance
- Training objectives: maximum strength, power, power endurance

Periodization	July	Aug.	Sept.	Oct.	Nov.	Dec.	Jan.	Feb.	Mar.	Apr.	May	June
	Prep.				Comp.							T
Strength	4 AA	8 MxS		8 Conv. to P	22 Maint.: P, MxS							6 Compens.
Energy systems	O_2 P, lactic cap., alactic P	Lactic cap., alactic P, O_2 P		Lactic P short, alactic P, O_2 P								O_2 compens.

Figure 6.20 Periodization model for a college basketball team.

Key: AA = anatomical adaptation, cap. = capacity, comp. = competitive, compens. = compensation, conv. = conversion, maint. = maintenance, MxS = maximum strength, O_2 = aerobic, P = power, prep. = preparation, T = transition

Periodization	Aug.	Sept.	Oct.	Nov.	Dec.	Jan.	Feb.	Mar.	Apr.	May	June	July
	Prep.			Comp.								T
Strength	3 AA	7 MxS	6 Conv. to P	26 Maint.: P, MxS								6 Compens.
Energy systems	O_2 P, lactic cap., alactic P	Lactic cap., alactic P, O_2 P	Lactic P short, alactic P, O_2 P									O_2 compens.

Figure 6.21 Periodization model for an elite basketball team.

Aerobic training (O_2) represents the cumulative effect of tempo running during the anatomical adaptation phase and the specific drills for O_2 training during the other training phases (two to five minutes nonstop). The suggested order of energy systems training also implies the priority of training for each training phase.

Key: AA = anatomical adaptation, cap. = capacity, comp. = competitive, compens. = compensation, conv. = conversion, maint. = maintenance, MxS = maximum strength, O_2 = aerobic, P = power, prep. = preparation, T = transition

BOXING

Boxers must be able to attack and react quickly and powerfully to an opponent's attack throughout the duration of the match. They require both aerobic and anaerobic energy. For a sample periodization model, see figure 6.22.

- Dominant energy systems: anaerobic lactic, aerobic
- Ergogenesis: 10% alactic, 40% lactic, 50% aerobic
- Main energy substrates: creatine phosphate, glycogen
- Limiting factors: power endurance, reactive power, muscular endurance medium
- Training objectives: power endurance, maximum strength, muscular endurance medium

Period-ization	Sept.	Oct.	Nov.	Dec.		Jan.	Feb.	Mar.	Apr.		May	June	July	Aug.
	Prep. I		Specific prep. I	Match	T	Prep. II	Specific prep. II	Match	T	Prep. III	Specific prep. III		Match	T
Strength	3 AA	6 MxS, P	3 Conv. to MEM	2 Maint.: MEM, MxS	2 AA	4 MxS, P	4 Conv. to MEM	4 Maint.: MEM, MxS	1 AA	3 MxS, P	4 Conv. to MEM	8 Maint.: MEM, MxS		Compens.
Energy systems	O$_2$ cap.	O$_2$ P, alactic P, lactic cap.	Lactic cap., O$_2$ P, alactic P		O$_2$ cap.	O$_2$ P, alactic P, lactic cap.	Lactic cap., O$_2$ P, alactic P		O$_2$ cap.	O$_2$ P, alactic P, lactic cap.	Lactic cap., O$_2$ P, alactic P			O$_2$ compens.

Figure 6.22 Periodization model for boxing.

Maximum strength training is performed at 70% to 80% of 1RM for two of the three phases and 80% to 90% for the third phase. For heavyweights, use loads of 80% to 90% of 1RM for the second and third phases. Aerobic (O$_2$) training should include specific boxing drills performed nonstop for two to five minutes. The suggested order of energy systems training also implies the priority of training for each training phase.

Key: AA = anatomical adaptation, cap. = capacity, compens. = compensation, conv. = conversion, maint. = maintenance, MEM = muscular endurance medium, MxS = maximum strength, O$_2$ = aerobic, P = power, prep. = preparation, T = transition

CANOEING AND KAYAKING: 500 AND 1,000 METERS

Flatwater sprints are all about speed and specific endurance. In order to move quickly to the finish line, the racer must quickly pull the paddle against the resistance of the water. For a sample periodization model, see figure 6.23.

- Dominant energy systems: aerobic, anaerobic lactic, anaerobic alactic
- Ergogenesis: 500-meter—16% alactic, 22% lactic, 62% aerobic; 1,000-meter—8% alactic, 10% lactic, 82% aerobic
- Main energy substrates: creatine phosphate, glycogen
- Limiting factors: muscular endurance, power endurance, starting power
- Training objectives: power endurance, maximum strength, muscular endurance short and medium

Periodization	Oct.	Nov.	Dec.	Jan.	Feb.	Mar.	Apr.	May	June	July	Aug.	Sept.
	Prep.							Comp.				T
Strength	4 AA	6 MxS	4 PE	6 MxS	3 MES	3 MxS	6 Conv. to MEM	12 Maint.: MEM, MxS				4 Compens.
Energy systems	O_2 cap.	O_2 cap., O_2 P, lactic cap.	O_2 P, O_2 cap., alactic P, lactic cap.	O_2 P, lactic cap., alactic P, O_2 cap.		O_2 P, lactic P, alactic P, O_2 cap.						O_2 cap.

Figure 6.23 Periodization model for canoeing and kayaking (500 and 1,000 meters).

The suggested order of energy systems training also implies the priority of training for each training phase.

Key: AA = anatomical adaptation, cap. = capacity, comp. = competitive, compens. = compensation, conv. = conversion, maint. = maintenance, MxS = maximum strength, MEM = muscular endurance medium, MES = muscular endurance short, O_2 = aerobic, P = power, prep. = preparation, T = transition

CANOEING AND KAYAKING: MARATHON

Unlike sprints, marathon races require muscular endurance of long duration. In addition, a racer must have a well-developed aerobic energy system to endure the length of the race. For a sample periodization model, see figure 6.24.

- Dominant energy system: aerobic
- Ergogenesis: 5% lactic, 95% aerobic
- Main energy substrates: glycogen, free fatty acid
- Limiting factor: muscular endurance long
- Training objectives: muscular endurance long, power endurance, maximum strength

Periodization	Nov.	Dec.	Jan.	Feb.	Mar.	Apr.	May	June	July	Aug.	Sept.	Oct.
	Prep.						Comp.					T
Strength	6 AA	6 MxS	4 MEM	4 MxS	12 Conv. to MEL				12 Maint.: MEL, MxS			4 Compens.
Energy systems	O_2 cap.	O_2 cap., O_2 P		O_2 P, O_2 cap., lactic cap.								O_2 cap.

Figure 6.24 Periodization model for canoeing and kayaking (marathon).

Key: AA = anatomical adaptation, cap. = capacity, comp. = competitive, compens. = compensation, conv. = conversion, maint. = maintenance, MEL = muscle endurance long, MEM = muscular endurance medium, MxS = maximum strength, O_2 = aerobic, P = power, prep. = preparation, T = transition

CYCLING: ROAD RACING

Road racing overwhelms the aerobic system. The only times that cyclists tax the anaerobic energy system are during steep climbing and at the finish of the race. Cyclists must be prepared to work hard over a long distance, generating constant rotations per minute to maintain speed and power against the resistance of the pedals, the environment, and the terrain. For a sample periodization model, see figure 6.25.

- Dominant energy system: aerobic
- Ergogenesis: 5% lactic, 95% aerobic
- Main energy substrates: glycogen, free fatty acid
- Limiting factors: muscular endurance long, power endurance
- Training objectives: muscular endurance long, power endurance, maximum strength

Periodization	Nov.	Dec.	Jan.	Feb.	Mar.	Apr.	May	June	July	Aug.	Sept.	Oct.
	Prep.						Comp.					T
Strength	4 AA	6 MxS		6 MEL	3 MxS	9 Conv. to MEL		14 Maint.: MEL, PE, MxS				6 Compens.
Energy systems	O_2 cap.			O_2 P, O_2 cap., lactic cap.								O_2 cap.

Figure 6.25 Periodization model for road racing.

Key: AA = anatomical adaptation, cap. = capacity, comp. = competitive, compens. = compensation, conv. = conversion, maint. = maintenance, MEL = muscular endurance long, MxS = maximum strength, O_2 = aerobic, PE = power endurance, prep. = preparation, T = transition

FIGURE SKATING

In order to complete the required jumps, figure skaters must develop powerful take-off (concentric) strength and landing (eccentric) strength. They also need strong anaerobic and aerobic energy systems, especially for long programs. For a sample periodization model, see figure 6.26.

- Dominant energy systems: anaerobic lactic, aerobic
- Ergogenesis: 40% alactic, 40% lactic, 20% aerobic
- Main energy substrates: creatine phosphate, glycogen
- Limiting factors: takeoff power, landing power, reactive power, power endurance
- Training objectives: power, power endurance, maximum strength

Periodization	May	June	July	Aug.	Sept.	Oct.	Nov.	Dec.	Jan.	Feb.	Mar.	Apr.
	Prep.							Comp.				T
Strength	8 AA		4 MxS	4 P	4 MxS	4 P	4 MxS	4 PE	10 Maint.: P, PE, MxS			6 Compens.
Energy systems	O_2 cap., O_2 P			Lactic cap., O_2 P		Lactic P, O_2 P, alactic P		Lactic P, alactic P, O_2 P				Alternative activities

Figure 6.26 Periodization model for figure skating.

The aerobic training (O_2) is achieved by performing specific drills, lines, and repetitions. The suggested order of energy systems training also implies the priority of training for each training phase.

Key: AA = anatomical adaptation, cap. = capacity, comp. = competitive, compens. = compensation, maint. = maintenance, MxS = maximum strength, O_2 = aerobic, P = power, prep. = preparation, T = transition

GOLF

The paramount factors in this popular sport are the golfer's power in hitting the ball off the tee and his or her precision in putting on the green. Good aerobic endurance helps any player cope with the fatigue of the sport and therefore improves concentration and effectiveness, especially during the last holes. For a sample periodization model, see figure 6.27.

- Dominant energy system: aerobic
- Ergogenesis: 100% aerobic
- Main energy substrates: creatine phosphate, glycogen
- Limiting factors: power, mental concentration, aerobic endurance
- Training objectives: power, maximum strength

Periodization	Oct.	Nov.	Dec.	Jan.	Feb.	Mar.	Apr.	May	June	July	Aug.	Sept.
	Prep.						Comp.					T
Strength	6 AA	5 MxS	1 T	8 MxS, P	2 T	4 Conv. to P	18 Maint.: P, MxS					4 Compens.
Energy systems	O_2 cap.			O_2 P								O_2 cap.

Figure 6.27 Periodization model for golf.

Key: AA = anatomical adaptation, cap. = capacity, comp. = competitive, compens. = compensation, conv. = conversion, maint. = maintenance, MxS = maximum strength, O_2 = aerobic, P = power, prep. = preparation, T = transition

HOCKEY

Important elements in this sport include acceleration and quick changes of direction. Training should focus on refining skills and developing power and both aerobic and anaerobic endurance. For a sample periodization model, see figure 6.28.

- Dominant energy systems: anaerobic lactic, aerobic
- Ergogenesis: 10% alactic, 40% lactic, 50% aerobic
- Main energy substrates: creatine phosphate, glycogen
- Limiting factors: acceleration power, deceleration power, power endurance
- Training objectives: maximum strength, power, power endurance

Periodization	June	July	Aug.	Sept.	Oct.	Nov.	Dec.	Jan.	Feb.	Mar.	Apr.	May
	Prep.				Comp.							T
Strength	4 AA	6 MxS	3 P	3 MxS	4 Conv. to PE	22 Maint.: P, PE, MxS					6 Com- pens.	
Energy systems	O_2 cap., O_2 P, alactic P	Lactic cap., O_2 P, alactic P		Alactic and lactic P short, O_2 P							O_2 cap.	

Figure 6.28 Periodization model for ice hockey.

Key: AA = anatomical adaptation, cap. = capacity, comp. = competitive, compens. = compensation, conv. = conversion, maint. = maintenance, MxS = maximum strength, O_2 = aerobic, P = power, PE = power endurance, prep. = preparation, T = transition

LONG-DISTANCE AND MARATHON RUNNING

High aerobic capacity is an essential physical attribute of distance runners. In fact, it is necessary to maintain a steady, fast pace throughout the long race. Glycogen and free fatty acid are the fuels used to produce energy for the race. For a sample periodization model, see figure 6.29.

- Dominant energy system: aerobic
- Ergogenesis: 10,000-meter—3% lactic, 97% aerobic; marathon—100% aerobic
- Main energy substrates: glycogen, free fatty acid
- Limiting factor: muscular endurance long
- Training objectives: muscular endurance long (all), power endurance (10,000-meter).

Periodization	Oct.	Nov.	Dec.	Jan.	Feb.	Mar.	Apr.	May	June	July	Aug.	Sept.
	Prep.							Comp.			T	
Strength	8 AA		6 MxS, P	6 MEM, MxS, PE		8 Conv. to MEL		14 Maint.: MEL, MxS, PE			6 Compens.	
Energy systems	O_2 cap.			O_2 cap., O_2 P		O_2 cap., O_2 P, lactic cap.					Alternative activities	

Figure 6.29 Periodization model for long-distance and marathon running.

MxS < 80% of 1RM

Key: AA = anatomical adaptation, cap. = capacity, comp. = competitive, compens. = compensation, conv. = conversion, maint. = maintenance, MEL = muscular endurance long, MEM = muscular endurance medium, MxS = maximum strength, O_2 = aerobic, P = power, PE = power endurance, prep. = preparation, T = transition

LONG SPRINTING AND MIDDLE-DISTANCE RUNNING

Long sprinters and middle-distance runners are fast runners who can also tolerate a large buildup of lactic acid during the race. Good performance requires the ability to respond quickly to changes in running pace. Therefore, these athletes need both good aerobic power and good lactic capacity, as well as lactic acid tolerance. A sample periodization model is presented in figure 6.30.

- Dominant energy systems: anaerobic lactic, aerobic
- Ergogenesis: 400-meter—12% alactic, 50% lactic, 38% aerobic; 800-meter—6% alactic, 33% lactic, 61% aerobic; 1,500-meter—2% alactic, 18% lactic, 80% aerobic
- Main energy substrates: creatine phosphate, glycogen
- Limiting factors: 400-meter—starting power; 400-meter—acceleration power; 400-meter, 800-meter elite level—muscle endurance short; 800-meter, 1,500-meter—muscle endurance medium
- Training objectives: 400-meter—power endurance; 400-meter, 800-meter—muscle endurance short; 800-meter, 1,500-meter—muscle endurance medium; all—maximum strength

Periodization	Oct.	Nov.	Dec.	Jan.	Feb.	Mar.	Apr.	May	June	July	Aug.	Sept.
	Prep. I			Comp. I		T	Prep. II			Comp. II			T
Strength	3 AA	6 MxS	5 Conv. to ME	6 Maint.: ME, MxS		1 A A	6 MxS	6 Conv. to ME	15 Maint.: ME, MxS			4 Compens.
Energy systems	O₂ P		Lactic cap., O₂ P, lactic P, alactic P			O₂ P		Lactic cap., O₂ P, lactic P, alactic P				O₂

Figure 6.30 Periodization model for long sprinting and middle-distance running.

The suggested order of energy systems training also implies the priority of training for each training phase.

Key: AA = anatomical adaptation, cap. = capacity, comp. = competitive, compens. = compensation, conv. = conversion, maint. = maintenance, ME = muscle endurance, MxS = maximum strength, O₂ = aerobic, P = power, prep. = preparation, T = transition

MARTIAL ARTS

Martial artists need flexibility, power, agility, and quick reflexes based on energy supplied by all three energy systems. Figure 6.31 shows a sample periodization model for the martial arts *without* a considerable endurance component. Figure 6.32 shows a sample for the martial arts *with* a considerable endurance component.

- Dominant energy systems: anaerobic alactic, anaerobic lactic, aerobic
- Ergogenesis: 50% alactic, 30% lactic, 20% aerobic
- Main energy substrates: creatine phosphate, glycogen
- Limiting factors: starting power, power endurance, reactive power, muscular endurance short
- Training objectives: power, maximum strength, power endurance, muscular endurance short

Periodization	June	July	Aug.	Sept.	Oct.	Nov.	Dec.		Jan.	Feb.	Mar.	Apr.	May
	Prep. I						Comp. I	T	Prep. II			Comp. II	T
Strength	4 AA	12 MxS			8 Conv. to P		4 Maint.: P, MxS	2 AA	6 MxS		4 Conv. to P	4 Maint.: P, MxS	4 Compens.
Energy systems	O_2 cap.	O_2 P, lactic cap., alactic P			Alactic P, lactic P, O_2 P			O_2 cap.	O_2 P, lactic cap., alactic P		Alactic P, lactic P, O_2 P		Alternative activities

Figure 6.31 Periodization model for martial arts without a considerable endurance component.

Aerobic (O_2) training can be done via specific drills. The suggested order of energy systems training also implies the priority of training for each training phase.

Key: AA = anatomical adaptation, cap. = capacity, comp. = competitive, compens. = compensation, conv. = conversion, maint. = maintenance, MxS = maximum strength, O_2 = aerobic, P = power, prep. = preparation, T = transition

Periodization	June	July	Aug.	Sept.	Oct.	Nov.	Dec.		Jan.	Feb.	Mar.	Apr.	May
	Prep. I						Comp. I	T	Prep. II			Comp. II	T
Strength	4 AA	8 MxS	4 P	3 MxS	6 Conv. to MEM	3 Maint.: MEM MxS		1 AA	7 MxS		4 Conv. to MEM	3 Maint.: MEM MxS	5 Compens.
Energy systems	O_2 cap.	O_2 P, lactic cap., alactic P		O_2 P, alactic P, lactic P			O_2 cap.		O_2 P, lactic cap., alactic P		O_2 P, alactic P, lactic P		Alternative activities

Figure 6.32 Periodization model for martial arts with a considerable endurance component.

Aerobic (O_2) training can be done via specific drills. The suggested order of energy systems training also implies the priority of training for each training phase.

Key: AA = anatomical adaptation, cap. = capacity, comp. = competitive, compens. = compensation, conv. = conversion, maint. = maintenance, MEM = muscular endurance medium, MxS = maximum strength, O_2 = aerobic, P = power, prep. = preparation, T = transition

RACKET SPORTS:
TENNIS, RACQUETBALL, SQUASH, AND BADMINTON

Racket sports involve fast and reactive play in which success is determined by reaction time and quick, precise changes of direction. For a sample periodization model for an amateur tennis player, see figure 6.33. For a sample model for a professional player, see figure 6.34. For a sample model for racquetball, squash, and badminton, see figure 6.35.

- Dominant energy systems: alactic, aerobic, anaerobic lactic
- Ergogenesis: tennis—50% alactic, 20% lactic, 30% aerobic; squash—40% alactic, 20% lactic, 40% aerobic; badminton—60% alactic, 20% lactic, 20% aerobic
- Main energy substrates: creatine phosphate, glycogen
- Limiting factors: power, reactive power, power endurance
- Training objectives: power, power endurance, maximum strength

Periodization	Oct.	Nov.	Dec.	Jan.	Feb.	Mar.	Apr.	May	June	July	Aug.	Sept.
	Prep.					Comp.					T	
Strength	6 AA	8 MxS, P		6 Conv. to PE		20 Maint.: P, PE, MxS					8 Compens.	
Energy systems	O_2 P, lactic cap.	Lactic cap., alactic P, O_2 P		Alactic P, lactic P short, O_2 P							O_2 compens.	

Figure 6.33 Periodization model for an amateur tennis player.

Key: AA = anatomical adaptation, cap. = capacity, comp. = competitive, compens. = compensation, conv. = conversion, maint. = maintenance, MxS = maximum strength, O_2 = aerobic, P = power, PE = power endurance, prep. = preparation, T = transition

Period-ization	1	2	3	4	5		6	7	8	9	10	11	12
	Prep. I		Comp. I	T	Prep. II	Comp. II	T	Prep. III	Comp. III	T	Prep. IV	Comp. IV	T
Strength	4 AA	6 MxS, PE	4 Maint.: PE, MxS	2 AA	4 MxS, PE	4 Maint.: PE, MxS	2 AA	4 MxS, PE	4 Maint.: PE, MxS	2 AA	4 MxS, PE	4 Maint.: PE, MxS	4 Compens.
Energy systems	O_2 P, lactic cap.	Lactic cap., alactic P, O_2 P	Alactic P, lactic P short, O_2 P	O_2 P, lactic cap.	Lactic cap., alactic P, O_2 P	Alactic P, lactic P short, O_2 P	O_2 P, lactic cap.	Lactic capacity, alactic P, O_2 P	Alactic P, lactic P short, O_2 P	O_2 P, lactic cap.	Lactic cap., alactic P, O_2 P	Alactic P, lactic P short, O_2 P	O_2 cap.

Figure 6.34 Periodization model for a professional tennis player.

This model assumes a program with four major tournaments. Since dates for major tournaments vary, the months of the year are numbered rather than named. Aerobic (O_2) training means specific drills of longer duration performed nonstop (three to five minutes). The suggested order of energy systems training also implies the priority of training for each training phase.

Key: AA = anatomical adaptation, cap. = capacity, comp. = competitive, compens. = compensation, maint. = maintenance, MxS = maximum strength, O_2 = aerobic, P = power, prep. = preparation, T = transition

Periodization of Strength Training for Sports

Periodization	1	2	3	4	5	6	7	8	9	10	11	12
	Prep. I				Comp. I		T	Prep. II	Comp. II		T	Prep. III		Comp. III			T
Strength	3 AA	6 MxS	3 PE	4 Maint.: P, MxS	2 AA	6 MxS	4 Maint.: PE, MxS	2 AA	3 MxS	3 PE	4 Maint.: PE, MxS	8 Compens.
Energy systems	O$_2$ P, lactic cap.	Lactic cap., alactic P, O$_2$ P	Alactic P, lactic P short, O$_2$ P		O$_2$ P, lactic cap.	Lactic cap., alactic P, O$_2$ P	Alactic P, lactic P short, O$_2$ P	O$_2$ P, lactic cap.	Lactic cap., alactic P, O$_2$ P		Alactic P, lactic P short, O$_2$ P	O$_2$ compens.

Figure 6.35 Periodization model for racquetball, squash, and badminton.

Because competition dates vary by geographical region, months are numbered rather than named. This model is a tri-cycle. The order of energy systems training also represents the priority of training in a given phase. Aerobic training (O$_2$) can be done via tempo training and by performing specific drills.

Key: AA = anatomical adaptation, cap. = capacity, comp. = competitive, compens. = compensation, maint. = maintenance, MxS = maximum strength, O$_2$ = aerobic, P = power, prep. = preparation, T = transition

ROWING

Rowing requires aerobic endurance and the ability to generate powerful strokes against water resistance. The athlete should also develop strong starting power and muscular endurance. For a sample periodization model, see figure 6.36.

- Dominant energy systems: anaerobic lactic, aerobic
- Ergogenesis: 10% alactic, 15% lactic, 75% aerobic
- Main energy substrates: creatine phosphate, glycogen
- Limiting factors: muscular endurance medium and short, starting power
- Training objectives: muscular endurance medium, muscle endurance short, maximum strength

Periodization	Sept.	Oct.	Nov.	Dec.	Jan.	Feb.	Mar.	Apr.	May	June	July	Aug.
	Prep.							Comp.				T
Strength	6 AA	6 MxS		4 MES	4 MxS	4 MEM	4 MxS	6 MEM	10 Maint.: MEM, MES, MxS			4 Compens.
Energy systems	O_2 cap.	O_2 cap., O_2 P		O_2 P, lactic cap., alactic P, O_2 cap.	O_2 P, lactic P, lactic cap., alactic P, O_2 cap.			O_2 P, lactic cap., alactic P, lactic P, O_2 cap.				

Figure 6.36 Periodization model for rowing.

The suggested order of energy systems training also implies the priority of training for each training phase.

Key: AA = anatomical adaptation, cap. = capacity, comp. = competitive, compens. = compensation, maint. = maintenance, MEM = muscular endurance medium, MES = muscular endurance short, MxS = maximum strength, O_2 = aerobic, P = power, prep. = preparation, T = transition

RUGBY

Rugby is a game of high energy, power, and intricate skills performed in rhythm. For a sample periodization model for an amateur rugby team, see figure 6.37. For a sample model for a professional rugby team, see figure 6.38.

- Dominant energy systems: anaerobic alactic, lactic, aerobic
- Ergogenesis: 10% alactic, 30% lactic, 60% aerobic
- Main energy substrates: creatine phosphate, glycogen
- Limiting factors: power, power endurance, acceleration power
- Training objectives: power, maximum strength

Periodization	Sept.	Oct.	Nov.	Dec.	Jan.	Feb.	Mar.	Apr.	May	June	July	Aug.
	Prep.						Comp.				T	
Strength	4 AA	12 MxS			8 Conv. to P		16 Maint.: P, MxS				8 Compens.	
Energy systems	O_2 cap., O_2 P	O_2 P, alactic P, lactic P short, O_2 compens.			Alactic P, lactic P short, O_2 P, O_2 compens.						O_2 cap.	

Figure 6.37 Periodization model for an amateur rugby team.

O_2 training refers mostly to performing specific tactical drills of longer duration (three to five minutes nonstop). The suggested order of energy systems training also implies the priority of training for each training phase.

Key: AA = anatomical adaptation, cap. = capacity, comp. = competitive, compens. = compensation, conv. = conversion, maint. = maintenance, MxS = maximum strength, O_2 = aerobic, P = power, prep. = preparation, T = transition

Periodization	July	Aug.	Sept.	Oct.	Nov.	Dec.	Jan.	Feb.	Mar.	Apr.	May	June
	Prep.			Comp.							T	
Strength	3 AA	9 MxS		4 Conv. to P	26 Maint.: P, MxS						6 Compens.	
Energy systems	O_2 cap., O_2 P	O_2 P, alactic P, lactic P short, O_2 compens.		Alactic P, lactic P short, O_2 P, O_2 compens.							O_2 cap.	

Figure 6.38 Periodization model for a professional rugby team.

Key: AA = anatomical adaptation, cap. = capacity, comp. = competitive, compens. = compensation, conv. = conversion, maint. = maintenance, MxS = maximum strength, O_2 = aerobic, P = power, prep. = preparation, T = transition

SKIING: ALPINE

Alpine skiers must be able to react quickly to the course flags. Over the long preparation phase, maximum strength development alternates with power development. For a sample periodization model, see figure 6.39.

- Dominant energy systems: anaerobic lactic, anaerobic alactic
- Ergogenesis: 10% alactic, 40% lactic, 50% aerobic
- Main energy substrates: creatine phosphate, glycogen
- Limiting factors: reactive power, power endurance
- Training objectives: maximum strength, power endurance, muscle endurance short

Periodization	May	June	July	Aug.	Sept.	Oct.	Nov.	Dec.	Jan.	Feb.	Mar.	Apr.
	Prep.						Comp.					T
Strength	4 AA	4 MxS	4 PE	4 MxS	4 PE	4 MxS	6 Conv. to MES	14 Maint.: MES, MxS, PE				4 Compens.
Energy systems	O$_2$ cap.	O$_2$ P, lactic cap.	Lactic P, lactic cap., O$_2$ P									Alternative activities

Figure 6.39 Periodization model for alpine skiing.

The aerobic training (O$_2$) can be the cumulative effect of longer-duration specific drills.

Key: AA = anatomical adaptation, cap. = capacity, comp. = competitive, compens. = compensation, conv. = conversion, maint. = maintenance, MxS = maximum strength, O$_2$ = aerobic, P = power, prep. = preparation, T = transition

SKIING: CROSS-COUNTRY AND BIATHLON

Cross-country races require strong aerobic endurance. Maximum strength is converted to muscular endurance toward the end of the preparation phase so that the skier is primed to withstand the demands of a long race. For a sample periodization model, see figure 6.40.

- Dominant energy system: aerobic
- Ergogenesis: 5% lactic, 95% aerobic
- Main energy substrates: glycogen, free fatty acid
- Limiting factor: muscular endurance long
- Training objectives: muscular endurance long, power endurance, maximum strength

Periodization	May	June	July	Aug.	Sept.	Oct.	Nov.	Dec.	Jan.	Feb.	Mar.	Apr.
	Prep.								Comp.			T
Strength	4 AA	8 MxS		6 MEL	3 MxS	11 Conv. to MEL			12 Maint.: MEL			4 Compens.
Energy systems	O_2 cap.	O_2 cap., O_2 P	O_2 cap., O_2 P, lactic cap.									O_2 cap.

Figure 6.40 Periodization model for cross-country and biathlon skiing.

The suggested order of energy systems training also implies the priority of training for each training phase.

Key: AA = anatomical adaptation, cap. = capacity, comp. = competitive, compens. = compensation, conv. = conversion, maint. = maintenance, MEL = muscular endurance long, MxS = maximum strength, O_2 = aerobic, P = power, prep. = preparation, T = transition

SOCCER

The most popular sport in the world is a game of great technical and physical demands, in which the result is determined by power, speed, agility, and specific endurance. The accompanying figures provide sample periodization models for an amateur American soccer team (figure 6.41), a professional American soccer team (figure 6.42), a European season for an amateur soccer team (figure 6.43), a European season for a professional soccer team (figure 6.44), and a European season for a goalkeeper (figure 6.45).

- Dominant energy systems: aerobic, anaerobic lactic, anaerobic alactic
- Ergogenesis: alactic 2%, lactic 23%, aerobic 75%
- Main energy substrates: creatine phosphate, glycogen
- Limiting factors: power, starting power, power endurance short, acceleration power, deceleration power, reactive power
- Training objectives: power, maximum strength

Periodization	Oct.	Nov.	Dec.	Jan.	Feb.	Mar.	Apr.	May	June	July	Aug.	Sept.
	Prep.						Comp.				T	
Strength	4 AA	8 MxS		4 P, MxS	2 T	6 Conv. to P	16 Maint.: P, MxS				8 Compens.	
Energy systems	O_2 cap., O_2 P	O_2 P, alactic P		O_2 P, alactic P, lactic P short	O_2 P	Alactic P, lactic P short, O_2 P					Compens.	

Figure 6.41 Periodization model for an amateur American soccer team.

The energy systems can be trained via tempo training, interval training, or repetition training, as well as by means of specific drills and short-sided matches. The suggested order of energy systems training also implies the priority of training for each training phase.

Key: AA = anatomical adaptation, cap. = capacity, comp. = competitive, compens. = compensation, conv. = conversion, maint. = maintenance, MxS = maximum strength, O_2 = aerobic, P = power, prep. = preparation, T = transition

Periodization	Aug.	Sept.	Oct.	Nov.	Dec.	Jan.	Feb.	Mar.	Apr.	May	June	July
	Prep.		Comp. I			T	Comp. II					T
Strength	2 AA	6 MxS, P	12 Maint.: P, MxS			2 T	20 Maint.: P, MxS					6 Compens.
Energy systems	O_2 cap., O_2 P	O_2 P, alactic P, lactic P short, O_2 compens.	Alactic P, lactic P short, O_2 P, O_2 compens.			O_2 P	Alactic P, lactic P short, O_2 P, O_2 compens.					O_2 cap.

Figure 6.42 Periodization model for a professional American soccer team.

Key: AA = anatomical adaptation, cap. = capacity, comp. = competitive, compens. = compensation, maint. = maintenance, MxS = maximum strength, O_2 = aerobic, P = power, prep. = preparation, T = transition

Periodization	Aug.		Sept.		Oct.	Nov.	Dec.		Jan.	Feb.	Mar.	Apr.	May	June	July
	Prep. I		Comp. I				T	Prep. II	Comp. II					T	
Strength	2 AA	4 MxS, P	13 Maint.: P, MxS,				1 Cess.	3 MxS, P	19 Maint.: P, MxS					10 Compens.	
Energy systems	O_2 cap., O_2 P	O_2 P, alactic P, lactic P short, O_2 compens.	Alactic P, lactic P short, O_2 P, O_2 compens.				Cess.	Alactic P, lactic P short, O_2 P, O_2 compens.						Games, O_2 cap.	

Figure 6.43 Periodization model for an amateur soccer team (European season).

Key: AA = anatomical adaptation, cap. = capacity, cess. = cessation, comp. = competitive, compens. = compensation, maint. = maintenance, MxS = maximum strength, O_2 = aerobic, P = power, prep. = preparation, T = transition

Periodization	July	Aug.	Sept.	Oct.	Nov.	Dec.		Jan.	Feb.	Mar.	Apr.	May	June
	Prep. I		Comp. I				T	Prep. II	Comp. II				T
Strength	2 AA	6 MxS, P	15 Maint.: P, MxS				1 Cess.	3 MxS, P	19 Maint.: P, MxS				6 Com-pens.
Energy systems	O_2 cap., O_2 P	O_2 P, alactic P, lactic P short, O_2 com-pens.	Alactic P, lactic P short, O_2 P, O_2 compens.				Cess.	Alactic P, lactic P short, O_2 P, O_2 compens.					O_2 cap.

Figure 6.44 Periodization model for a professional soccer team (European season).

Key: AA = anatomical adaptation, cap. = capacity, cess. = cessation, comp. = competitive, compens. = compensation, maint. = maintenance, MxS = maximum strength, O_2 = aerobic, P = power, prep. = preparation, T = transition

Periodization	July	Aug.	Sept.	Oct.	Nov.		Dec.	Jan.	Feb.	Mar.	Apr.	May	June
	Prep. I		Comp. I			T	Prep. II	Comp. II				T	
Strength	2 AA	6 MxS, P	15 Maint.: P, MxS			1 Cess.	3 MxS, P	19 Maint.: P, MxS				6 Compens.	
Energy systems	Alactic P, O_2 compens.					Cess.	Alactic P, O_2 compens.					Games, O_2 cap.	

Figure 6.45 Periodization model for a soccer goalkeeper (European season).

Key: AA = anatomical adaptation, cap. = capacity, cess. = cessation, comp. = competitive, compens. = compensation, maint. = maintenance, MxS = maximum strength, O_2 = aerobic, P = power, prep. = preparation, T = transition

SPRINTING

A sprinter requires frequent strides that are long and powerful. His or her velocity correlates directly with the amount of force applied during the very short ground contact of each step (200 milliseconds out of the blocks and 80 milliseconds at maximum velocity). For the 60-meter event, endurance is not as important as acceleration because the sprinter needs to move as fast as possible over a short distance. For the 100-meter and 200-meter events, however, speed endurance (lactic power) is fundamental; in fact, it makes the difference between elite and sub-elite sprinters. A sample periodization model for sprinters is presented in figure 6.46.

- Dominant energy system: 60-meter—anaerobic alactic; 100-meter and 200-meter—anaerobic lactic
- Ergogenesis: 60-meter—80% alactic, 20% lactic; 100-meter—53% alactic, 44% lactic, 3% aerobic; 200-meter—26% alactic, 45% lactic, 29% aerobic
- Main energy substrate(s): 60-meter—creatine phosphate; 100-meter and 200-meter—creatine phosphate and glycogen
- Limiting factors: 60-meter—acceleration power; 100-meter and 200-meter—power endurance; all—starting power, reactive power
- Training objectives: 60-meter—power; 100-meter and 200-meter—power endurance; all—maximum strength

Periodization	Oct.	Nov.	Dec.	Jan.	Feb.	Mar.	Apr.	May	June	July		Aug.	Sept.
	Prep. I			Comp. I		T	Prep. II			Comp. II	T	Prep. III	Comp. III	T
Strength	3 AA	9 MxS		4 Conv. to P	4 Maint.: P and MxS	1 A A	6 MxS	5 Conv. to PE		6 Maint.: PE and MxS	1 AA	3 MxS, PE	4 Maint.: PE and MxS	4 Compens.
Energy systems	O_2 P	Lactic cap., alactic P, and O_2 P		Alactic and lactic P		Alactic P and lactic cap.	Alactic and lactic P			Alactic P and lactic cap.	Alactic and lactic P			Games play

Figure 6.46 Periodization model for sprinters.

Aerobic (O_2) training for a sprinter represents the cumulative effect of tempo training (repetitions of 600-meter, 400-meter, and 200-meter).

Key: AA = anatomical adaptation, cap. = capacity, comp. = competitive, compens. = compensation, conv. = conversion, maint. = maintenance, MxS = maximum strength, O_2 = aerobic, P = power, PE = power endurance, prep. = preparation, T = transition

SWIMMING: LONG DISTANCE

Long-distance swimmers must train for muscular endurance. A long race taxes the aerobic energy system, and proper muscular endurance training gives the swimmer an endurance edge. For a sample periodization model, see figure 6.47. The model assumes two competitive phases—one beginning in January and the other beginning in late spring.

- Dominant energy system: aerobic
- Ergogenesis: 10% lactic, 90% aerobic
- Main energy substrates: glycogen, free fatty acid
- Limiting factor: muscular endurance long
- Training objectives: muscular endurance medium, muscular endurance long

Periodization	Sept.	Oct.	Nov.	Dec.	Jan.	Feb.	Mar.	Apr.	May	June	July	Aug.
	Prep. I				Comp. I		T	Prep. II		Comp. II		T
Strength	4 AA	4 MxS	4 MEM	4 MxS	4 Conv. to MEL	4 Maint.: MEL, MxS	1 AA	4 MxS	4 Conv. to MEL	8 Maint.: MEL, MxS		4 Compens.
Energy systems	O$_2$ cap.	O$_2$ cap., O$_2$ P	O$_2$ P, O$_2$ cap.	O$_2$ P, lactic cap., O$_2$ cap.			O$_2$ cap., O$_2$ P	O$_2$ P, O$_2$ cap.	O$_2$ P, lactic cap., O$_2$ cap.			O$_2$ compens.

Figure 6.47 Periodization model for a national-class long-distance swimmer.

Key: AA = anatomical adaptation, cap. = capacity, comp. = competitive, compens. = compensation, conv. = conversion, maint. = maintenance, MEL = muscular endurance long, MEM = muscular endurance medium, MxS = maximum strength, O$_2$ = aerobic, P = power, prep. = preparation, T = transition

SWIMMING: SHORT DISTANCE BY A MASTER ATHLETE

The dominant training factor for a master athlete is power. Developing both power and maximum strength requires a long preparation phase. For a sample periodization model for a master swimmer, see figure 6.48. The model assumes only one competitive phase—from May through late August.

- Dominant energy systems: anaerobic lactic, anaerobic alactic, aerobic
- Ergogenesis: 50-meter—18% alactic, 45% lactic, 37% aerobic; 100-meter—15% alactic, 25% lactic, 60% aerobic
- Main energy substrates: creatine phosphate, glycogen
- Limiting factors: 50-meter—power endurance; 100-meter—muscular endurance short; all —power
- Training objectives: 50-meter—power endurance; 100-meter—muscular endurance short; all—maximum strength

Periodization	Oct.	Nov.	Dec.		Jan.	Feb.	Mar.	Apr.	May	June	July	Aug.	Sept.
	Prep.								Comp.			Transition	
Strength	8 AA		3 MxS	3 P	3 MxS	3 P	3 MxS	5 Conv. to PE	12 Maint.: PE, MxS			8 Compens.	
Energy systems	O_2 cap., O_2 P		O_2 P, O_2 cap.		Lactic cap., O_2 P	Lactic P, O_2 P, lactic cap., alactic P			Lactic P, alactic P, O_2 P			O_2 cap.	

Figure 6.48 Periodization model for a master athlete (short-distance) swimmer.

Key: AA = anatomical adaptation, cap. = capacity, comp. = competitive, compens. = compensation, conv. = conversion, maint. = maintenance, MxS = maximum strength, O_2 = aerobic, P = power, PE = power endurance, prep. = preparation

SWIMMING: SPRINT

Sprint swimmers use mainly the lactic acid system. They must generate quick, powerful strokes to move efficiently through the water for an extended time. For a sample periodization model, see figure 6.49, which presents a bi-cycle for a nationally ranked sprinter.

- Dominant energy systems: anaerobic lactic, aerobic, anaerobic alactic
- Ergogenesis: 50-meter—20% alactic, 50% lactic, 30% aerobic; 100-meter—19% alactic, 26% lactic, 55% aerobic
- Main energy substrates: creatine phosphate, glycogen
- Limiting factors: 50-meter—power endurance; 100-meter—muscular endurance short; all—power
- Training objectives: 50-meter—power endurance; 100-meter—muscular endurance short; all—maximum strength

Periodization	Sept.	Oct.	Nov.	Dec.	Jan.	Feb.	Mar.		Apr.	May	June	July	Aug.
	Prep. I				Comp. I	T	Prep. II			Comp. II			T
Strength	4 AA	8 MxS		4 Conv. to specific str.	8 Maint.: specific str., MxS	2 AA	6 MxS			4 Conv. to specific str.	7 Maint.: specific str., MxS		5 Compens.
Energy systems	O_2 cap.	Lactic cap., O_2 P	Lactic P, O_2 P, lactic cap., alactic P	Lactic P, alactic P, O_2 compens.		O_2 P, lactic cap.	Lactic P, O_2 P, lactic cap., alactic P		Lactic P, alactic P, O_2 compens.				O_2 cap.

Figure 6.49 Periodization model for a national-class sprinter in swimming (bi-cycle).

The suggested order of energy systems training also represents the priority of training for each phase.

Key: AA = anatomical adaptation, cap. = capacity, comp. = competitive, compens. = compensation, conv. = conversion, maint. = maintenance, MxS = maximum strength, O_2 = aerobic, P = power, prep. = preparation, specific str. = specific strength, T = transition

THROWING EVENTS:
SHOT PUT, DISCUS, HAMMER, AND JAVELIN

Training for throwing events in track and field requires great power (based on improvement of maximum strength) and hypertrophy (especially for shot put and to some degree for discus). Specifically, a high level of muscular strength is required in the legs, torso, and arms for generating acceleration through the range of motion and maximum throwing power. A sample periodization model for throwing events is presented in figure 6.50.

- Dominant energy system: anaerobic alactic
- Ergogenesis: 95% alactic, 5% lactic
- Main energy substrate: creatine phosphate
- Limiting factor: throwing power
- Training objectives: maximum strength, power

Periodization	Oct.	Nov.	Dec.	Jan.	Feb.	Mar.	Apr.		May	June	July	Aug.	Sept.
	Prep. I			Comp. I			T	Prep. II		Comp. II			T
Strength	3 AA	3 Hyp.	6 MxS, hyp.	4 Conv. to P	8 Maint.: MxS, hyp., P		1 A A	3 Hyp.	4 MxS, hyp.	2 Conv. to P	10 Maint.: MxS, P		3 Compens.
Energy systems	Lactic and alactic cap.		Alactic P and cap.				Alactic P	Alactic P and cap.					Games play

Figure 6.50 Periodization model for throwing events.

Hypertrophy training follows AA and must be maintained during the maximum strength macrocycles but at a ratio of one hypertrophy set for every three maximum strength sets (the back-off set method can be used in this case).

Key: AA = anatomical adaptation, cap. = capacity, comp. = competitive, compens. = compensation, conv. = conversion, hyp. = hypertrophy, maint. = maintenance, MxS = maximum strength, P = power, prep. = preparation, T = transition

TRIATHLON

Triathlon, which requires proficiency in three athletic skills, presents a great challenge to both physical and psychological endurance. Paramount to success in triathlon is the body's efficiency in using the main fuel-producing source: free fatty acid. For a sample periodization model, see figure 6.51.

- Dominant energy system: aerobic
- Ergogenesis: 5% lactic, 95% aerobic
- Main energy substrates: glycogen, free fatty acid
- Limiting factor: muscular endurance long
- Training objectives: muscular endurance long, maximum strength

Periodization	Oct.	Nov.	Dec.	Jan.	Feb.	Mar.	Apr.	May	June	July	Aug.	Sept.
	Prep.						Comp.					T
Strength	4 AA	8 MxS		12 Conv. to MEL			20 Maint.: MEL, MxS					4 Compens.
Energy systems	O_2 cap.	O_2 cap., O_2 P		O_2 P, O_2 cap., lactic cap.								O_2 cap.

Figure 6.51 Periodization model for triathlon.

The suggested order of energy systems training also implies training priorities for each training phase.

Key: AA = anatomical adaptation, cap. = capacity, comp. = competitive, compens. = compensation, conv. = conversion, maint. = maintenance, MEL = muscular endurance long, MxS = maximum strength, O_2 = aerobic, prep. = preparation, T = transition

VOLLEYBALL

A volleyball player must react quickly and explosively off the ground in order to spike, block, or dive. Maximum strength and power are required for carrying a player through the long competitive phase with stable performance and confidence. For a sample periodization model for American college volleyball, see figure 6.52. For a sample model for a European season, see figure 6.53.

- Dominant energy systems: anaerobic alactic, anaerobic lactic
- Ergogenesis: 70% alactic, 20% lactic, 10% aerobic
- Main energy substrates: creatine phosphate, glycogen
- Limiting factors: reactive power, takeoff power, power
- Training objectives: power, maximum strength

Periodization	June	July	Aug.	Sept.	Oct.	Nov.	Dec.	Jan.	Feb.	Mar.	Apr.	May
	Prep.					Comp.					T	
Strength	4 AA	6 MxS	4 P	3 MxS	3 P	20 Maint.: MxS, P					8 Compens.	
Energy systems	O_2 P, alactic P, lactic P short	Alactic P, lactic P short									Alternative activities (e.g., beach volleyball)	

Figure 6.52 Periodization model for college volleyball (American season).

The suggested order of energy systems training also implies training priorities for each training phase.

Key: AA = anatomical adaptation, comp. = competitive, compens. = compensation, maint. = maintenance, MxS = maximum strength, O_2 = aerobic, P = power, prep. = preparation, T = transition

Periodization	Aug.	Sept.	Oct.	Nov.	Dec.	Jan.	Feb.	Mar.	Apr.	May	June	July
	Prep.			Comp.		T	Comp			T		
Strength	2 AA	4 MxS	4 Conv. to P	8 Maint.: MxS, P		2 AA	18 Maint.: MxS, P			10 Compens.		
Energy systems	O_2 P, alactic P, lactic P short	Alactic P, lactic P short								Alternative activities (e.g., beach volleyball)		

Figure 6.53 Periodization model for volleyball (European season).

The suggested order of energy systems training also implies training priorities for each training phase.

Key: AA = anatomical adaptation, comp. = competitive, compens. = compensation, conv. = conversion, maint. = maintenance, MxS = maximum strength, O_2 = aerobic, P = power, prep. = preparation, T = transition

WATER POLO

Water polo requires high energy expenditure, using the aerobic system, interspersed with fast acceleration and powerful shooting actions. Passing and shooting precision are essential skills to learn during the many hours of training. For a sample periodization model, see figure 6.54.

- Dominant energy systems: anaerobic lactic, aerobic
- Ergogenesis: 10% alactic, 30% lactic, 60% aerobic
- Main energy substrate: glycogen
- Limiting factors: muscular endurance medium, power endurance, acceleration power, shooting power
- Training objectives: muscular endurance medium, power endurance, maximum strength

Periodization	Aug.	Sept.	Oct.	Nov.	Dec.	Jan.	Feb.	Mar.	Apr.	May	June	July
	Prep.							Comp.			T	
Strength	4 AA	8 MxS		6 PE	4 MxS	6 Conv. to MEM		12 Maint.: MEM, MxS, PE			8 Compens.	
Energy systems	O_2 cap., O_2 P	O_2 P, lactic cap., alactic P, O_2 cap.			O_2 P, lactic P, alactic P, O_2 cap.		O_2 P, lactic cap., alactic P				O_2 cap.	

Figure 6.54 Periodization model for a national league water polo team.

Aerobic training implies also using tactical drills of longer duration (two to four minutes).

Key: AA = anatomical adaptation, cap. = capacity, comp. = competitive, compens. = compensation, conv. = conversion, maint. = maintenance, MEM = muscular endurance medium, MxS = maximum strength, O_2 = aerobic, P = power, PE = power endurance, prep. = preparation, T = transition

WRESTLING

A wrestler's success is determined by technique and tactical skills as well as by power, power endurance, and flexibility. For a sample periodization model, see figure 6.55.

- Dominant energy systems: anaerobic alactic, anaerobic lactic, aerobic
- Ergogenesis: 30% alactic, 30% lactic, 40% aerobic
- Main energy substrates: creatine phosphate, glycogen
- Limiting factors: power, power endurance, flexibility
- Training objectives: power, power endurance, maximum strength, muscular endurance short

Periodization	1	2	3	4	5	6	7	8	9	10	11	12
	Prep. I			Comp. I		T	Prep. II		Comp. II		T	
Strength	4 AA	8 MxS, P, PE		8 Maint.: P, PE, MxS		2 Compens.	4 AA	6 MxS, P, MES	10 Maint.: P, MES, MxS		6 Compens.	
Energy systems	O_2 cap.	O_2 P, lactic cap., alactic P		O_2 P, alactic P, lactic P		O_2 cap.	O_2 cap.	O_2 P, lactic cap., alactic P	O_2 P, alactic P, lactic P		O_2 compens.	

Figure 6.55 Periodization model for wrestling.

This is a bi-cycle geared to national championships and an international competition. Aerobic training can be achieved via sport-specific drills of longer duration (two to three minutes). The suggested order of energy systems training also implies training priorities for each training phase.

Key: AA = anatomical adaptation, cap. = capacity, comp. = competitive, compens. = compensation, maint. = maintenance, MES = muscular endurance short, MxS = maximum strength, O_2 = aerobic, P = power, PE = power endurance, prep. = preparation, T = transition

Periodization of Loading Pattern per Training Phase

Loading patterns in training are not standard or rigid. Just as they vary according to the sport or level of performance, they also change according to the type of strength sought in a given training phase. To make this concept easier to understand and implement, figures 6.56 through 6.62 show how it is applied in several sports. The examples illustrate the dynamics of loading pattern per training phase for a monocycle in amateur baseball, softball, or cricket (figure 6.56), for college basketball (figure 6.57), for American college football linemen (figure 6.58), for an endurance-dominant sport such as canoeing (figure 6.59), and for bi-cycles for sprinting in track and field (figure 6.60), and sprint and long-distance swimming (figures 6.61 and 6.62).

The charts indicate (from top to bottom) the number of weeks planned for a particular training phase, the type of training sought in that phase, and the loading pattern (high, medium, or low). Even if your chosen sport is not addressed in the examples, you will be able to apply the concept to your own case once you understand it. In addition, the examples are so varied that they are applicable through association.

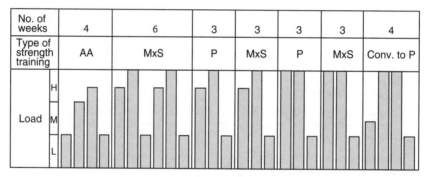

Figure 6.56 Variations of loading pattern for strength training phases for an amateur baseball, softball, or cricket team. To maximize the level of power development, the last three macrocycles involve two adjacent high loads followed by regeneration cycles (low loads).

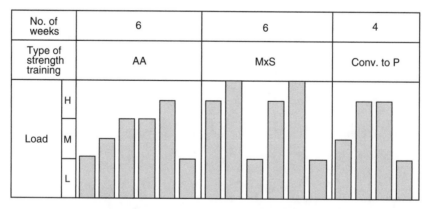

Figure 6.57 Suggested loading pattern for a college basketball team in which the preparation phase must be performed from early July through late October.

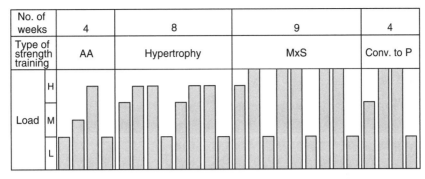

Figure 6.58 Variations of loading pattern for periodization of strength in American college football linemen. A similar approach can be used with throwers in track and field and for the heavyweight category in wrestling.

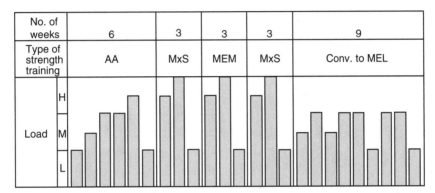

Figure 6.59 Variations of loading pattern for marathon canoeing, in which muscular endurance long is the dominant ability. A similar approach can be used for cycling, Nordic skiing, triathlon, and rowing.

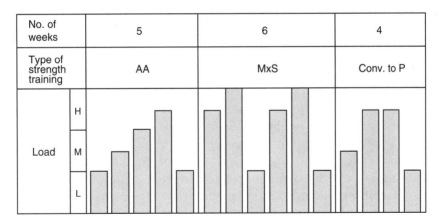

Figure 6.60 Variations of loading pattern for the first part of a bi-cycle annual plan for sprinting in track and field.

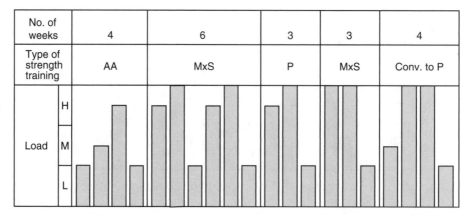

Figure 6.61 Variations of loading pattern for a sprinter in swimming (first part of a bi-cycle annual plan). Training demand for the last two phases is high since the load is high for two adjacent weeks.

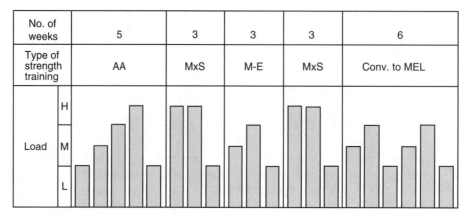

Figure 6.62 Variations of loading pattern for a long-distance swimming event. The load for maximum strength should not exceed 80% of 1RM. Similarly, the load for muscular endurance is low (30%-40%), but the number of repetitions is very high.

Periodization Effects on the Force-Time Curve

In chapter 2, we analyzed the force–time curve and pointed out the various components of strength it depicts. We also showed how different loads affect the neuromuscular system's adaptations and explained how an athlete needs to train the nervous system to display the highest amount of force in the shortest amount of time. Because of the influence of bodybuilding, strength training programs often include a high number of reps (12-15) performed to exhaustion. Such programs mainly develop muscle size, not quickness of contraction. As illustrated in figure 6.63, the application of force in sports is performed very quickly—specifically, in a period lasting from a bit less than 100 milliseconds to 200 milliseconds. The only type of strength that stimulates the highest development of such quick application of force is a sequential application of maximum strength training and power training (Bompa 1993; Verkhoshansky 1997).

The opposite is true if training employs a variant of bodybuilding work. In that case, the repetitions per set are higher than for maximum strength and power training, so the force application takes longer (more than 250 milliseconds). Therefore, it is not specific to the needs of most sports. Because the application of force in sports is usually very fast, the main purpose of strength training for sports is to shift the force–time curve to the left—or as close as possible to the typical sport-specific time of force application (less than 200 milliseconds)—through the use of maximum strength and power training applied sequentially. See figure 6.64.

This shift toward the sport-specific time of application of force is not achieved quickly. Indeed, the whole point of periodization of strength is to use phase-specific strength training to shift the force–time curve to the left—that is, to decrease execution time—before the start of a major competition. This is when athletes need the quick application of strength and when they benefit from gains in power.

As explained earlier, each training phase of the periodization of strength focuses on certain objectives. By plotting the force–time curve for each training phase, both coaches and athletes can see from another angle how the curve is influenced by training. Figure

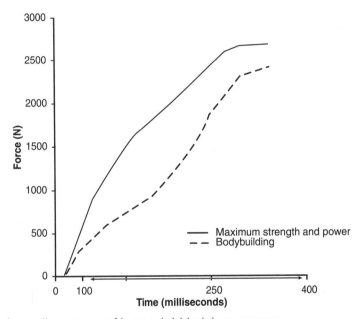

Figure 6.63 The force–time curve of two weight training programs.

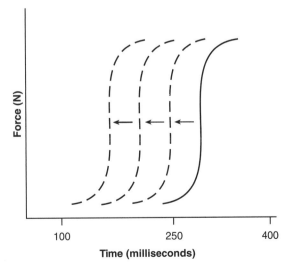

Figure 6.64 The purpose of strength training is to shift the force–time curve to the left, to the quickest contraction time.

6.65 shows the periodization of strength when a hypertrophy phase is included. Certainly, only athletes in some sports use this model, whereas those in many other sports exclude hypertrophy from the annual plan.

As figure 6.65 shows, the type of program performed during the anatomical adaptation phase has little effect on the force–time curve. At most, it may shift it slightly to the right (i.e., increase execution time). Typical hypertrophy training methods make the curve shift to the right because each set is performed to exhaustion, and thus the power output per rep gets lower and lower. Therefore, the resulting gains in muscle size do not translate into gains in the fast application of strength.

The use of heavy loads in the maximum strength phase might or might not increase explosiveness, depending on the ratio between general and specific work, as well as the total volume of maximum strength training. If the maximum strength phase falls in the general preparation phase and a high volume of strength training is programmed to give priority to the increment of this biomotor ability, the force–time curve might shift to the right. On the other hand, if the maximum strength phase falls in the specific preparation, where many high-velocity specific training means are used, then a lower volume of maximum strength training is granted and the force–time curve shifts to the left.

During the conversion of maximum strength to power phase, there is certainly a shifting of the curve to the left, as desired. As this type of strength training is continued during the maintenance phase, the curve should remain to the left.

A high level of power, or explosiveness, cannot be expected before the start of the competitive phase. Power is maximized only as a result of implementing the conversion phase; therefore, a high level of power should not be expected during the hypertrophy phase or even during the maximum strength phase. However, gains in maximum strength are vital if increments in power are expected from year to year because power is a function of maximum strength. Periodization of strength, then, offers the best road to success for both muscular endurance and power development.

Preparatory				Competitive
AA	Hypertrophy	MxS	Conv. to P	Maintenance
100 250 400	100 250 400	100 250 400	100 250	100 250
Remains unchanged	Shifts to the right	Shifts to the left or right	Shifts to the left	Remains shifted to the left

Figure 6.65 Influence of the specifics of training for each phase on the force–time curve.

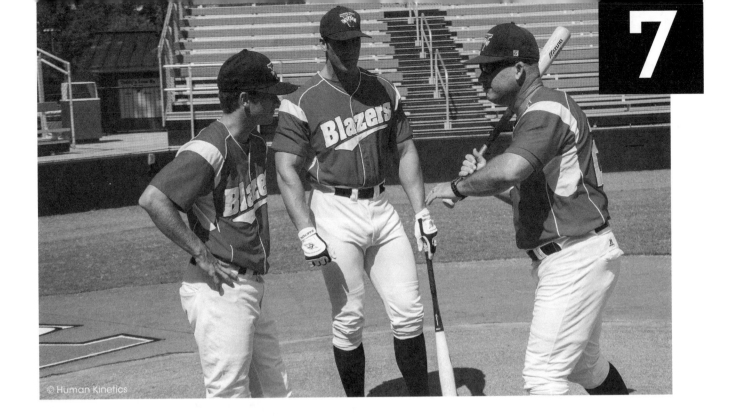
© Human Kinetics

Long-Term Planning for Team Sports

The interest to observe how young athletes are trained is an old-time concern. It has become a real hobby to observe and write about the type of training young athletes are exposed to in some clubs. If the specific needs of children are seen as superficial and disorganized, their rate of growth and development tends to be overlooked when a training program is designed for them. Long-term planning is recognized as necessary, but rarely is anything done about it.

There is also a clear discrepancy between the information available in the scientific literature and the actual training in some clubs for young athletes. Quite often, coaches still design their training programs based on what they remember doing during their own late teens. Innovations are rare, almost nonexistent. It is quite disturbing to note that in some cases training programs for children seem to imitate what professional players do. In the following few pages, we will try to offer an outline regarding a long-term training progression for children involved in team sports.

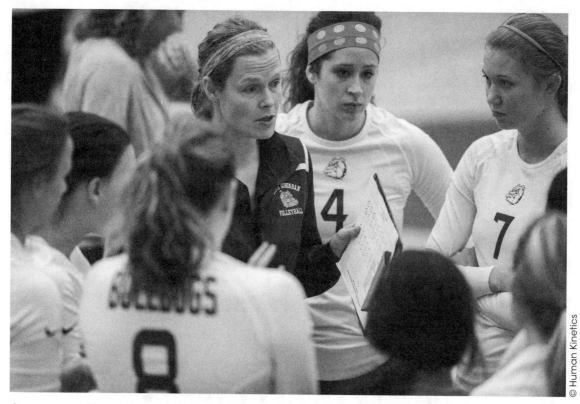

Coaches working with age-group athletes need to have an in-depth knowledge of the athletes' development stage and training requirements.

Figure 7.1 illustrates a long-term training plan for young team sport players. We have chosen to address only team sports because most of the errors are observed in some of these sports. Individual sports have a slightly better progression than team sports for junior athletes.

Often the training for juniors follows, almost literally, what top professional players do, with children under 12 (U12) participating like professional players in basketball, volleyball, and ice hockey tournaments. Sometimes these psychologically and physiologically undeveloped children even play two or three games a day during weekend tournaments. The organizers of such tournaments make good money without even knowing (or caring) that they are exposing these young players to the physical stress of many games, to emotional and psychological stress, and possibly even to mental and psychological harassment. This is why the progression proposed by figures 7.1 and 7.2 should be considered by everyone involved in children's training.

The concept promoted in figure 7.1 relies on two basic phases:

1. Make a child a player.

2. Make a player an athlete.

During the first phase—making the child a player—the scope of training involves initiating the child into the technical fundamentals of the game. Use lighter balls, lower baskets and nets, and a smaller field so that children can feel comfortable playing and learning fundamental skills. All children should learn simple technical elements. Remember that teaching always requires a great deal of tolerance and patience. These are the years when children learn the fundamental skills of the sport, and they are bound to make many mistakes. The better they acquire the fundamental elements of the main skills, the more easily they will eventually reach the stage of technical finesse and perfection.

Age	Scope of training
U12	• Technical initiation, fun via varied plays and games, occasional games from outside of the selected sport • Simple tactics • Games for weekend fun • No stressful tournaments
U15	• Make a child a player. • Stress the technical fundamentals of the game: ball control, dribbling, passing, and shooting. • Make the athlete very comfortable, especially toward the end of this phase, with the key technical skills in both offense and defense. • Teach all the essential elements of the tactics of the game in both offense and defense. • Teach the fundamentals of physical training: overall flexibility, anatomical adaptation (AA) using light implements, and exercises with own body weight. • Foster progressive adaptation and strengthening of ligaments and tendons with lighter implements and low loads on training machines.
U17	• Transition from player to top athlete. • Perfect all the fundamental skills of the game. • Improve precision passing and shooting. • Improve all the intricate elements of the tactics of the game (offense and defense). • Build the foundation of physical training (e.g., AA with different training equipment and loads). • Prepare the athletes for the next training stage, in which heavier loads are used. • Strengthen ligaments and tendons, mostly of the legs (ankle and knees).
U19	• Perfect all technical/tactical skills of the game under fatigued conditions. • Improve all physical abilities required by the game. • Improve power/agility/maximum speed. • Increase all elements of athleticism related to the chosen sport (e.g., quickness, power, and resistance).
U21	• Make a player an athlete. • Stress the finesse/perfection of all technical skills of the game under the fatigue/exhausting conditions. • Improve maximum strength (MxS). • Maximize power, speed, agility, and specific endurance. • Perfect athleticism: the ability dominant in the chosen sport. • Understand that when a team sport is played by top athletes, the game will look different.

Figure 7.1 A proposed long-term progression of training for team sport athletes.

Key: U = under

During the second phase—making a player an athlete—your players aim to reach technical and tactical perfection. You should devote time to helping your players to become top athletes and to reach the highest level of athleticism: fast, powerful, resistant, and able to effectively tolerate fatigue without it affecting their technical and tactical efficiency. Emphasize precision of passing and shooting under game conditions, fatigue, and exhaustion.

When the game is played by athletes, it will look different. If you do not use a well-organized progression, such as suggested by figure 7.1, your training will be nothing but a disorganized, confusing guessing game.

Training phases	Technical initiation		Make a child a player		Transition: from a child player to an athlete player				Make a player an athlete		
Ability/age	6-8	9-10	11-12	13-14	15	16	17	18	19-20	21-23	>24
Flexibility	In	→	De	→	Mx	→	→	→	P	→	→
Strength: • AA <50%			In	→	→	→	→				
• OBW			In	→	→	→	→				
AA 50-60					In	De	→	→	→	→	→
MxS: • 60%-70%						In	→	De	→		
• 80%-90%								In	De	Mx	P
Power: • MB <3 kg			In	De	→	→	→	Mx	→	P	→
• MB >3 kg						In	→	De	Mx	→	P
• Plyometrics				In	→	→	De	→	Mx	P	→
• Power-endurance								In	De	Mx	P
Agility: • Phosphagen			In	→	→	→	De	→	Mx	P	→
• Glycolytic					In	→	De	→	Mx	P	→
• Oxidative							In	De	Mx	P	→
Speed: • Phosphagen			In	→	→	De	Mx	→	→	P	→
• Glycolytic					In	→	De	→	Mx	P	→
• Oxidative							In	→	De	→	→
Endurance • Short: 1-2 min					In	→	De	→	Mx	P	→
• Medium: 3-5 min						In	De	→	Mx	P	→

Figure 7.2 A long-term training program for all the abilities necessary to transform a child into a top-class player.

Key: AA = anatomical adaptation, In = initiation; De = development; MB = medicine ball, Mx = maximization; p = perfection; → = Repeat the type of training suggested in the previous box; OBW= own-body-weight exercises; % = percentage of 1RM, which represents 100% of an athlete's maximum capacity at that stage; < = below the suggested load or weight; > = above the suggested load or weight

Figure 7.2 illustrates a progression of the methodology of developing all the physical attributes and abilities that are essential to making a player a top athlete. These are the years when a high level of athleticism has to be accomplished. Use specific training sessions to try to improve speed, strength, power, and agility.

We use the following terms for the different stages of athletes' development.

- Initiation (In): progressively expose children to stressless training, such as overall flexibility, light loads of AA, and other types of strength-related implements (medicine balls, dumbbells, etc.).

- Development (De): require a higher level of development of physical abilities in the chosen game.

- Maximization (Mx): reach high levels of physical development of a specific ability.

- Perfection (P): reach the highest level of physical refinement and potential appropriate to the needs of the athlete and the game.

In applying our specific suggestions regarding age and type of training, please be advised to use them just as guidelines. Use your common sense, professionalism, and knowledge regarding your athletes' capacity to adapt our suggestions. In this way, you will be able to avoid anatomical stress and prevent injuries.

The top of figure 7.2 illustrates the main training phases of a long-term training program and the corresponding age from age 6 to over 24. Next, we discuss the development of each motor ability in more detail.

Flexibility Training

You can start simple, overall flexibility exercises from an early age since at this stage all the joints of the body are relatively loose and mobile. Overall flexibility refers mostly to the main joints of the body used in sports: ankles, knees, hips, and shoulders. Keep in mind that at this age the muscles are not strong yet, and, therefore it is easy to stretch them. For athletes in team sports, it is essential to develop ankle flexibility, since many moves of the body are initiated from the ankle and up. A rigid ankle will be an impediment to many athletic actions. During flexibility training, your attitude should be relaxed, without pushing or creating a stressful environment. Be gentle, relaxed, and cheery. Kids will enjoy such an environment. So will you. Flexibility training is a relatively easy, simple training method. Do not complicate it. Instead, learn specific exercises for the principal joints and repeat them at the end of most warm-up sessions.

Strength Training

Any strength training program has to observe essential elements of training as prerequisites for an injury-free athlete: a long-term progression and adaptation and a good lifting technique as well as an adequate selection of exercises. We suggest considering the following regarding the number of exercises for different age groups.

- U15 players: a greater number of exercises (12-15) for every part of the body to build the foundation of strength training
- U17 players: a medium number of exercises (8-12) addressed to the main muscle groups of the body with an emphasis on the core area of the body and legs
- U19 and above: a lower number of exercises (6-8) but a higher number of sets and total repetitions, focusing mostly on the prime movers of the selected sport

Anatomical Adaptations

- For U12 players, you can initiate simple strength training via games using light medicine balls. During games and relays the children can carry, roll, and throw medicine balls (overhead, side, between the legs, backward). In addition, you can use dumbbells of a very low weight (5-10 lb [2-5 kg]), and easy-to-perform, simple own-body-weight (OBW) exercises: pull-ups, push-ups, abdominal exercises, and low back and leg exercises, such as straddling in different directions, and so on.
- For U15, simple implements and strength training machines can also be used but without exposing children to challenging loads and a stressful number of repetitions

and sets. During this age, anatomical adaptation (AA) training can be introduced, where the scope of training should be adaptation of muscles, ligaments, and tendons to lower loads strength training. Injury prevention should be an important goal of strength training. To achieve this, you need to use low loads exercises such as the following:

- Ankle plantar flexion and dorsiflexion
- Knee flexions and extensions (half squats, leg curls)
- Abdominal (core) exercises
- Trunk extensions and rotations for the lumbar muscles
- Trunk rotations, side bends, and trunk extensions for the intervertebral muscles
- Side, over-the-shoulder, adduction, and abduction lifts for the shoulders
- Arm flexions and extensions

• From U17 on, the AA training can become slightly more demanding by using loads of 50% to 60% of 1RM. Once again, the scope of training should be to build a solid foundation of strength training by using the methodology specific to adaptation and injury prevention (see chapter 8). This training objective can be achieved via a stressless training environment; therefore, the number of repetitions and sets should not be close to maximum. Why? A maximum number of repetitions exposes the young athletes to anatomical stress, meaning it challenges the muscles, ligaments, and tendons beyond the needs of stressless adaptation training.

Maximum attention should be constantly paid to the technique used in the exercises for strength training. The technique of lifting or using strength training machines is essential in order to avoid injuries.

Maximum Strength (MxS)

Based on the AA strength training that has been used from U15, from U17 years on you can introduce elements of MxS with lower loads: 50% to 60%. Once again, be sure to observe a careful progression. Your motto should be *Do not push!* Also, do not follow other coaches' rigid methodology of training. Make sure to allow a longer rest interval between sets than suggested by most programs on the Internet or in some strength training books. Remember, you are still working with young athletes. Unfortunately, much of the information available online and in some training books is still influenced by the motto of the 1960s to 1980s: *No pain, no gain!* This might be valid for experienced athletes, but it is far too unrealistic and dangerous for young athletes of U15-U17. Pay maximum attention to the core area of the body, such as the abdomen and the lumbar and intervertebral muscles. The time you spend at this age on core muscles will be advantageous to your athletes as they mature. Equally important, you should eliminate a stressful environment. Do not overlook a good and methodical *progression*. After the age of U17, you can progressively initiate MxS loads of 70%, while from U19 you can carefully introduce heavier loads (80%) but with a low number of repetitions and sets and longer rest intervals. Always remember that high performance is achieved at the age of maturation, which in many sports can be over the age of 23 or 24. Maximum strength is a stressful type of training, taxing the nervous system, where maximum concentration is a necessity. Muscles, ligaments, and tendons are under constant anatomical stress during MxS. It is your obligation to apply a well-planned training program with good progression and an appropriate rest interval.

Power Training

Strength training planned from childhood to the mid-teens represents the foundation on which you can build power, or the ability to apply force quickly against a given resistance in order to move faster, or to throw an implement a longer distance. If the objective of MxS is to recruit the highest possible number of fast-twitch muscle fibers, the objective of power training is to increase the discharge rate of those same muscle fibers. In this way, you have applied an important physiological law: One cannot be fast and powerful unless one first trains MxS. You can introduce simple, stressless power training from U12 on. Light medicine balls, light implements, and simple plyometrics can be applied in training sessions intended for the development of power. During relays, so popular in physical education classes, children can carry, roll, throw, or hold a ball while performing simple repetitive jumps.

Later on, from the age of U15 on, you can use heavier medicine balls, especially balls with a handle. At about the same age you can expose children to simple plyometrics, such as jumping on a box, jumping down from the same box, and immediately making a short jump forward, sideways, or backward. Your progression, imagination, and inventiveness will be important assets in both plyometrics and agility training.

Difficult types of plyometrics (reactive jumps, drop jumps from 27 to 40 inches [70-100 cm]) can be introduced from the late teens on (U21), with reactive jumps being used also from the same age on but with heights of 15 to 20 inches (40-50 cm). By now, young athletes already have five or six years' background in strength training and are ready for difficult MxS and power training. Power endurance (PE), or the capacity to repeat several powerful and quick actions, can be introduced in your training from U17 on. In combat, racket, and team sports the ability to perform a quick and powerful action repetitively is an important asset and has to be introduced after a good background of strength and power training. For maximum athletic adaptation you can use the concept of energy systems training to organize your PE training, such as these:

- Phosphagen system: sets of 5 to 10 seconds of nonstop repetitions, with a rest interval of 1 to 2 minutes
- Glycolytic system: sets of 30 to 90 seconds nonstop, with a rest interval of 2 to 3 minutes. To best facilitate the adaptations for PE, the rest interval can be progressively reduced to 45 to 90 seconds.

Agility Training

An athlete's ability to change direction rapidly and to move swiftly from one position to another position has a determinant role in their success. Once again, for maximum physiological and position-specific benefits, the duration and intensity of an agility course has to be organized according to the concept of energy systems.

- Phosphagen system (ATP-PC): repetitions of 5 to 10 seconds with a rest interval of 1 to 2 minutes
- Glycolytic system: repetitions of 30 to 120 seconds with a rest interval of 2 minutes or longer
- Oxidative (aerobic) system: repetitions of 2 to 3 minutes with a rest interval of 1 to 2 minutes

Unfortunately, most coaches select agility courses without observing the preceding suggestions. Some just perform certain agility courses mechanically, in disregard of the needs of the sport, of the position played by the athlete, and of the practical application of the three energy systems. If you want to organize an effective sport- or position-specific training, you should design your agility training based on the specifics of the energy system.

Speed Training

Short-distance speed training can be initiated by the U12 level. Most children enjoy doing short repetitions with high velocity (taxing the phosphagen energy system), provided you respect the following principles:

- Do not push children for sprints longer than 5 to 8 seconds.
- Since high velocity sprints are very taxing, allow longer rest intervals for full recovery (2 to 3 minutes).
- Stress the form rather than the child's speed. At this age, form is more important than maximum velocity, simply because it will teach children from an early age to use an efficient running technique.
- Do not expect children to be very fast at this age. Speed will increase only after they use a good technique and have increased strength (from U15 on).
- Children enjoy competitions, so you can use relays, assuming you respect the following duration and rest interval suggestions because speed training has to be organized corresponding to the energy system they will use during training:
  - Phosphagen system (ATP-CP): repetitions of 5 to 8 seconds, stressing good form, with a rest interval of 2 to 3 minutes
  - Glycolytic system: repetitions of 15 to 45 seconds, with a rest interval of 3 to 4 minutes

Endurance Training

Endurance training for team sports is often misunderstood. Some coaches still use jogging as a form of endurance training. To best adapt specific endurance for team sports, you can use specific, technical, and tactical drills of 1 to 5 minutes. Players will prefer this type of training over jogging, which they might find boring. Please consider the following options.

- Create tactical drills for each group of players under both defense and offense conditions (as called for by the specifics of the game).
- Create tactical drills for specific durations, from faster (counterattack) speed and shorter duration (1 to 2 minutes).
- Create tactical drills of longer duration (3 to 5 minutes) with specific tactical goals.
- Set the tempo of running according to the interval of specific drills
- Determine the duration of a drill: faster velocity for shorter drills and medium velocity for longer drills.
- Use your imagination and creativity to mimic specific game conditions, keeping physiological guidelines in mind.
- Use jogging mostly during the warm-up and during the preparatory phase itself but only three to four times during the league season. By being selective, you can increase training efficiency and lower the athlete's overall fatigue.

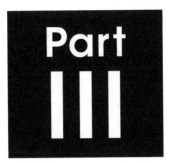

Part III

Periodization of Strength

*You will never produce a top athlete
without the determinant contribution
of strength training.*

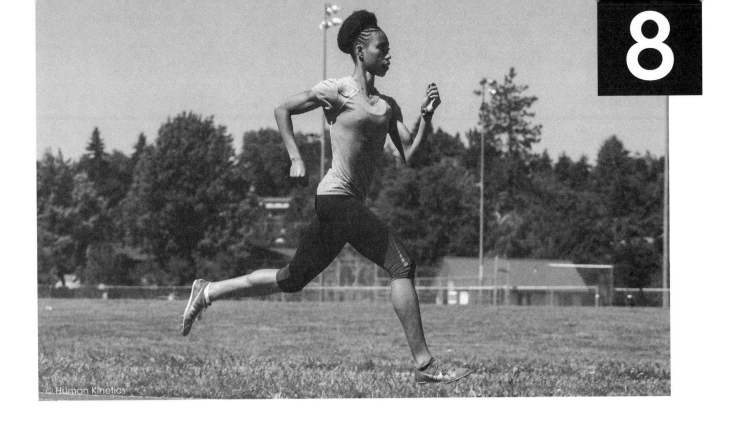
© Human Kinetics

Anatomical Adaptation

Have you ever watched how homes are built? From the foundation up to the roof? Do you know that the solidity of the foundation dictates how many floors you can build? We can use this as an analogy for the methodology of producing top athletes: to start with a strong foundation, the anatomical adaptation (AA), and progressively reach the highest level of strength, power, agility, maximum speed, and sport-specific endurance. The AA is essential to building a strong base of progressive adaptation and, as a result, to ensure an injury-free athlete.

The selected rules for the AA phase are as follows.

- Always start slowly, especially during the first two weeks, and increase the load progressively from low to medium.
- Do not push, especially with young athletes who have not yet been involved in strength training. Remember the Roman adage: *festina lente* (hurry up . . . slowly).
- Allow time for a good anatomical adaptation of muscles, ligaments, and tendons.
- Develop an overall and specific flexibility, particularly for the ankles and the hips.

Injuries and Their Causes

Traditionally, sporting activities are an important means for socializing but also for improving health and well-being. Many millions of people are active, especially children. The sports industry has earned $17 billion in the United States alone (*The Atlantic*, November 6, 2018). Although youth participation in sports is very high (30 million in the United States), the rate of attrition is also very high: 70% (*Washington Post*, January 1, 2016). Reasons for drop-out include that it is not fun anymore, that there is too much emphasis on winning, and that there is physical discomfort, including many injuries. Most injuries occur in American football, bicycling, basketball, baseball and softball, soccer, trampoline, and the like.

Sports injuries among youth have reached 3.5 million. Of these, 775,000 age 14 and younger were treated in hospitals (Stanford Children's Health 2019). Treatment in hospitals has increased by 78% per year among youth 7 to 17 (National Children's Hospitals 2016). In 2017, the National Collegiate Athletic Association (NCAA) reported 45,000 injuries. The NCAA has also reported that 65.6% of these injuries occurred in the lower limbs: ankle sprains, anterior cruciate ligament (ACL) tears, meniscus injuries, and hamstring strains. In Spain, the same injuries have reached 81% (García-Fernández et al. 2017). A study of 10 years of high school soccer injuries concluded that sports professionals show the need for injury prevention programs (*British Journal of Sports Medicine*, March 2017).

In Italy, there are more injuries per hour of practice in soccer than in rugby, a more physical game than soccer. Why is that? Could it be that rugby players have better strength training and, as a result, are more able to prevent injuries than soccer players? Is soccer such a dangerous sport? Or might it be that ignorance in training is higher in some sports?

> The new gimmicks used in soccer should also raise the question of inappropriate physical training (strength and flexibility training). Similarly, the increase of overuse injuries has drastically increased in the past few years.

How is it possible to have so many injuries in sports, mostly in team and racket sports? In the case of soccer, other team sports, and contact sports, most injuries have common causes, including the following.

- There are far too many games. Professional players (soccer, basketball, American football) are very highly paid. Team owners translate this to mean, "I pay you, but you have to produce for me by playing as often as possible." In Europe, soccer players have games year-round. Many professional players rarely have a vacation longer than two weeks. They are under constant stress, especially anatomical and mechanical stress on specific parts of the body, particularly the ankles and knees.

- Professionalism among some strength and conditioning (S&C) instructors is lower than ever. There are S&C coaches who have a limited education and a poor understanding of sports science and methodology, and consider themselves certified after attending a one-week summer course. To be truly competent and professional, a full, science-based S&C education is needed.

- Strength training is rarely used as a tool for injury prevention, especially for the foot and for the ankle and knee joints.

- Not surprisingly, most injuries are recorded in August and January, prior to and at the beginning of the new league games: 37.6% from running or sprinting; 16.6% from overuse (Prof. Jan Ekstrand, MD, UEFA Medical Committee).

- Do S&C coaches know that sprinting must be preceded by good strength training? High velocity in sprinting is possible only if you can apply increased force against the ground.

- Three times as many injuries occur during games. (See the following section on injury prevention.)

- Commercialism, with many gadgets and gimmicks invading the market, seems to have made good physical training a part of the past.

- Most injuries do not occur at the muscle level but rather at the level of the ligaments and tendons, the connective tissues. And yet, instructors rarely address the need to prevent injuries via strengthening the ligaments and tendons.

- The ankles are the most neglected joints. This is why so much discomfort and so many injuries are recorded in racket and team sports. To prevent injury, the ankle joint formed by the foot bones (the tarsals and the metatarsals) and ligaments has to be strengthened by using flexion-extension and side-to-side movements, and rotations against resistance.

- Since ligaments and tendons are not properly trained, they are not able to withstand the high mechanical stress specific to most athletic movements.

- Preparatory strength training, particularly the AA phase, is too superficial.

- Flexibility training is often inadequate in many athletes.

Injury Prevention

In strength training programs for youth, and even for some professional sports, injury prevention is often overlooked. More specifically, programs frequently omit the training of ligaments and tendons because the AA training is simply inappropriate or nonexistent. That is why injury prevention has to be a major concern for all athletes, and of significant interest to coaches, athletes, and club owners. In the latter case, club owners lose some of their investment because injured players cannot play.

For maximum athletic benefit, injury prevention should consider the following two fundamental training rules.

1. *Flexibility training.* Maximum angle or degrees of flexibility required during the contest or game has to be the minimum angle or degrees trained during workouts. In other words, flexibility should be worked at the highest acute angles possible during each training session, mostly at the end of warm-up and at the end of training. If this is done, the incidence of injuries will decrease drastically.

2. *Strength training.* Maximum force applied against resistance, ground or water, during competitions and games has to be the minimum load used during training the MxS phase. Once again, we emphasize that the force (load) used during high-velocity running during the game, say 685 N (70 kg [154 lb]) during the push-off phase, has to be a minimum load used during strength training. This is a very safe and effective method of preventing injuries. The loads in strength training are usually quite low, however, so do not increase the force application against the ground during the push-off phase. If you want your athletes to run faster and to change direction

quickly, then improve the force of their prime movers (the push-off, the propulsion phase of the running step).

Ligaments and Tendons

The mechanical work done by muscles, the force of contraction, depends on the actions of actin-myosin coupling, but also on the capacity of the ligaments and tendons to withstand stress. When a muscle contracts to perform work, the force of the muscles is transmitted to the bone via a tendon and, as a result, the limb moves to perform a sporting skill. Therefore, if a tendon is a transmitter of force, the ligaments keep together the anatomical integrity of a joint. The stronger the ligaments, the more stable the joints. The more stable the joints, the easier it is to prevent injuries.

Well-trained, strong tendons can withstand great mechanical stress. If the strength capability of tendons and ligaments is inappropriate, they may become a limiting factor for performance, a weak link in a stronger chain. As a result, every time these connective tissues are exposed to high mechanical strain, they may produce anatomical discomfort or even injury.

Coaches should remember that unlike muscle tissue adaptation, which takes a shorter time, connective tissue (ligaments and tendons) adaptation often takes several weeks (McDonagh and Davies 1984; Enoka 2015). This time requirement justifies why we suggest a longer AA for most athletes, especially for the younger ones. The AA training must focus not only on strengthening the muscles but also on fortifying the connective tissues.

Figure 8.1 illustrates the location of the gastrocnemius muscle on the calf and the place where the Achilles tendon is inserted on the heel, or calcaneus bone. In the coaches' strategy to prevent injuries to this big and strong tendon, they also have to be aware of the equally important anatomical element, the size of the area of the insertion of the Achilles tendon on the bone. Strong tendons always have a larger area where the tendon is attached to the bone, in this case, 65 mm^2 or more (Enoka 2015). For well-trained sprinters, this area is much larger. The larger the size of the Achilles tendon and the larger the attachment area to the bone, the better insurance against injuries.

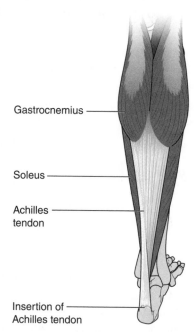

Gastrocnemius

Soleus

Achilles tendon

Insertion of Achilles tendon

Figure 8.1 An illustration of the calf where the gastrocnemius, soleus, and insertion of the Achilles tendon on the calcaneus bone (the heel) are shown (based on information from Neto et al. 2004; Enoka 2015).

The gastrocnemius is the strongest skeletal muscle of the human body, the powerhouse of speed and agility. Other features of the gastrocnemius are the following.

- It has, by far, the highest number of muscle cells, meaning that for any forward push-off actions, it can recruit the highest number of muscle cells of all the skeletal muscles of the human body. Therefore, it can generate the highest force of all muscles. Keep in mind that increased force = high velocity.

- It has the highest number of end plates (~2,000) that innervate muscle cells. The higher the number of innervated (stimulated) muscles, the higher the force and velocity capabilities of an athlete.

- The Achilles tendon can transmit the highest maximal force, 4900 N/510 kg, from the gastrocnemius to the foot (Enoka 2015). When the foot can apply higher force against the ground, the athlete can reach higher velocity and changes of direction.

- For all sports performed on the ground—track, team sports, the martial arts, and so on—the gastrocnemius is the most potent muscle. Strengthening this muscle via AA and MxS should be a major goal of training to enable athletes to be fast and quick in changing directions and performing agile motions.

The Importance of Range of Motion

Another essential element in your strategies to prevent injuries is the range of motion (ROM) of the major joints of the body. Although a good overall flexibility is important, you should emphasize sport-specific ROM, and particularly for team sports, at the ankles, the knees, and the hips. Effective flexibility training, with acute angles between two segments, will always result in stretching the muscles and the ligaments and tendons alike. Any flexibility training should start with a good warm-up and a slow and progressive decrease of the angle between two segments.

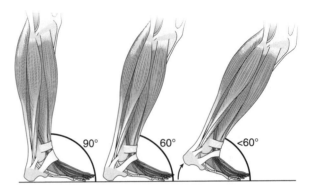

Figure 8.2 The degrees of ankle flexion in three different positions: standing = 90 degrees; maximum dorsiflexion without lifting the heel = 60 degrees. When flexion is intended at a more acute angle (beyond 60 degrees), inadequate flexibility makes the athlete lift the heel and lose 30% of the applied maximum force (Bompa 2006).

Figure 8.2 illustrates the degrees of ankle flexibility in different body positions. In the first case, the left part of the figure, standing position, the angle between the foot and the calf, is 90 degrees. As the athlete inclines forward to start running, the mean maximum degrees of flexion without lifting the heel is 60 degrees. As the runner inclines forward toward maximum flexion, for lack of better flexibility than 60 degrees the runner is forced to lift the heel. When this happens, the force of the gastrocnemius muscle decreases by 30% (Bompa 2006).

Most flexibility training programs grossly neglect ankle flexibility, even though the ankle is an extremely important joint in any type of running, particularly in sprinting, and in jumping. You should test your athletes' dorsiflexion (bringing the toes toward the calf) frequently, using a goniometer.

Muscles that limit ROM, or span between two joints, such as the gastrocnemius, the rectus femoris (quadriceps), the long head of the biceps femoris (hamstrings), the triceps, and the pectoralis, seem to be more prone to injuries. Pay maximum attention during eccentric actions with heavy loads because these moves can result in injuries.

Why is it important to assess maximum dorsiflexion? Because maximum push-off, the propulsion phase of the running step, is reached at degrees of higher flexion than 60 degrees. The more acute angle an athlete can reach without lifting the heel off the ground, the higher the force exerted by the gastrocnemius muscle. To increase your athlete's propulsion force, improve his or her ankle dorsiflexion.

Figure 8.3 shows the mean of dorsiflexion flexibility between the calf and the foot (60 degrees). It also implies that the scope of training is to improve ankle flexibility; to progressively reach a more acute angle between the two parts of the leg in order to be able to apply a higher propulsion force: 27.5 to 39 newtons; mean 33.3 newtons (2.8-4.1 kg; mean 3.4 kg).

This finding demonstrates that there is a direct relationship between the ankle's dorsiflexion and the propulsion force of the gastrocnemius and soleus. A coach who wishes to improve propulsion force must also improve the degree of dorsiflexion. Therefore, coaches should develop not only overall flexibility, but in the case of team sports and sprinting, for the maximization of the propulsion of force of the gastrocnemius and soleus muscles, a prime concern should be to develop ankle dorsiflexion flexibility.

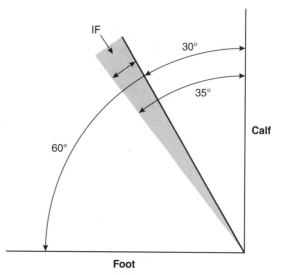

Figure 8.3 The relationship between the ankle's flexibility and propulsion force. For every degree of dorsiflexion, propulsion force increases by 2.8 to 4.1 kilograms (Bompa 2006). (IF = improved flexibility).

Strength Training During the Anatomical Adaptation Phase

All athletes involved in competitive sports follow a yearly program intended to enable peak performance in major competition. Peak performance requires athletes to build a proper physiological foundation, and one key factor in doing so is strength training, an essential element in a coach's quest to produce good athletes.

General athletic training must be planned and periodized in a way that ensures performance improvement from phase to phase and enables peak performance during the competitive season. The same is true of strength training. Like general athletic ability and skill, strength can be refined through various methods and phases of training to create the desired final product: sport-specific strength.

Strength training should be performed throughout the annual plan, following the concept of periodization of strength, and based on the physiological needs and specifics of each sport. Athletes can transform strength into a sport-specific quality by applying periodization of strength and by using training methods specific to the needs of each strength training phase. Thus, an athlete's training methods must change as the training phase changes.

This chapter and the next four discuss all available training methods as they relate to the periodization of strength. Each training phase is treated separately in order to show which method best suits a particular phase and the needs of the athlete. The discussions also address positive and negative aspects of most methods and how to apply them, as well as training programs using particular methods.

Circuit Training and the Anatomical Adaptation Phase

During the early stages of strength training, especially with entry-level athletes, almost any strength training method or program results in strength development to some degree. As the athlete develops a strength foundation, however, the coach should create a specific, periodized strength training program to maximize the athlete's natural abilities. Coaches must bear in mind the fact that each athlete has a unique rate of adaptation to a given method—and therefore a different rate of improvement.

Strength training is a long-term proposition. Athletes reach their highest performance level not after four to six weeks of a strength training program but rather during the competitive phase, which comes months after the anatomical adaptation (AA) phase. The goal of the AA phase is to progressively adapt the muscles, and especially their attachments to bone (tendons), so that they can cope more easily with the heavier loads used in the ensuing training phases. As a result, the overall training load must be increased without causing the athlete to experience much discomfort.

The simplest method to consider for AA is circuit training, mainly because it provides an organized structure and alternates muscle groups. Circuit training can be used not only to develop the foundation of strength for future training phases but also to develop nonspecific cardiorespiratory endurance by combining strength and endurance training.

Some authors suggest that combining aerobic endurance with strength training during the same phase may seriously compromise the development of maximum strength and power. They claim that strength training is incompatible with long-distance aerobic training because fast-twitch muscle fibers may adapt to behave like slow-twitch muscle

During the AA phase, you have to select exercises that involve most muscle groups of the body, emphasizing, at the same time, the prime movers. Maximum attention should refer to:

- *Core muscles, the back and the abdominals.* Remember that the trunk is a transmitter of force from the legs to the arms and from the arms to the legs. This is why it has to be strong, to represent a support for most exercises and actions performed during contests. Concentrate on the intervertebral muscles (trunk extensions, rotations), lumbar (trunk extensions), abdominals (flexions, rotations).
- *Legs (ankles, hips, and knees).* Concentrate on *toe raises, hip thrusts, hip flexion, knee flexion, and knee extension.* Focus also on the foot side motions on the sagittal plane, such as eversion (lifting the inner side up) and inversion (lifting the outer side up). The strengthening of the foot using the above motions against resistance represents an injury-prevention of the foot for most sports, particularly racket and team sports.
- *Arms and shoulders.* Focus on flexions and extensions, pull and push, adductions, abductions, and so forth. Use own body weight, light to medium loads, medicine ball, simple apparatus, training machines.

fibers. These studies scientifically validate the theory that adaptation in speed and power sports is negatively affected by combining an aerobic activity with maximum strength or hypertrophy training on the same day. Short-term adaptation suffers.

However, athletes in sports for which both strength and aerobic endurance are equally important (e.g., soccer, rowing, kayaking, canoeing, and cross-country skiing) have no choice but to train both during the preparatory phase. In addition, the argument against such combined training is based mostly on research that was conducted for just a few weeks, whereas training is a long-term endeavor. Has the full adaptation to such training actually occurred? Indeed, some research suggests the opposite—that a certain compatibility exists between strength and endurance training performed at the same time. As shown by the following examples, the type of endurance training suggested in this text for the AA phase differs considerably from long- and slow-duration activities.

Circuit training was first proposed by Morgan and Adamson (1959) of Leeds University as a method for rehabilitating World War II veterans and developing general fitness. Their initial circuit training routine consisted of several stations arranged in a circle (hence the term *circuit training*) so as to work muscle groups alternately from station to station. As circuit training grew in popularity, other authors began to modify it.

A wide variety of approaches can be used in a circuit training routine, such as body weight, medicine balls, light implements, dumbbells, barbells, and strength training

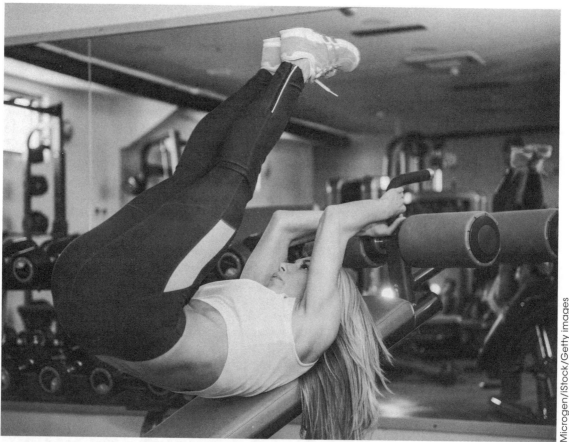

Microgen/iStock/Getty images

Body-weight exercises can strengthen the torso muscles during the anatomical adaptation phase.

machines. A circuit may be short (6-9 exercises), medium (10-12 exercises), or long (13-15 exercises) and may be repeated a certain number of times, depending on the number of exercises involved; the more exercises, the fewer circuit repetitions. The number of circuits should be no more than two for a long circuit and no more than four for a short circuit. The number of reps per station should start higher (say, at 20) and decrease over time (say, down to 8-10). For advanced athletes, with a periodized strength training experience of at least three years, fewer reps (5 or 6) can be used for the fundamental exercises starting with a high number of repetitions in reserve that is decreased over time.

In determining the number of reps per station, the number of circuit repetitions, and the load, the coach must consider the athlete's work tolerance and fitness level. Total workload during the AA phase should not be so high as to cause the athlete pain or great discomfort. Athletes themselves should help determine the amount of work to perform.

Circuit training is a useful, though not magical, method for developing the foundation of strength during the AA phase. Other training methods (e.g., jump sets) can be equally beneficial if they alternate the muscle groups.

As the following examples show, the training methodology used for the AA phase must be adapted to the physiological profile of the sport (e.g., speed or power versus endurance) and the needs of the athlete. The methodology must also develop most of the muscles used in the chosen sport. More specifically, in line with the overall purpose of the preparatory phase—and particularly the goal of anatomical adaptation—exercises should be selected to develop the core area of the body as well as the prime movers.

The alternation of muscle groups in circuit training facilitates recovery. The rest interval can be 30 to 90 seconds between stations and one to three minutes between circuits. Circuit training also enables a wide variety of routines to be created because most gyms contain many apparatuses, workstations, and strength training machines. This variety constantly challenges an athlete's skills while also keeping him or her interested.

Program Design for the Circuit Training Method

Circuit training may be used from the first few weeks of the AA phase. The coach should select the workstations according to the equipment available. Athletes should follow a certain progression, depending on their classification and training background. Younger athletes with little or no strength training background should start with exercises using their own body weight or lower loads (e.g., medicine balls, small dumbbells, empty barbells). Over time, they can progress the load using heavier medicine balls, loaded barbells, and strength machines. Again, exercise during this phase must be selected to involve most muscle groups, irrespective of the needs of the specific sport; in other words, the coach should implement a multilateral approach. However, the prime movers should also be targeted. After all, they are the engines for effective performance of sport-specific skills.

The three circuits presented in figure 8.4 do not come close to exhausting the available possibilities in a gym, but they are typical for entry-level or junior athletes. Young athletes who are new to circuit training may want to split circuits into two phases. As adaptation occurs, an athlete can begin progressively adding exercises from phase 2 to the end of phase 1 until he or she can perform all of the exercises nonstop. Start with two groups of four, as presented in circuit B; as the athlete adapts to the program, bring the fifth exercise into phase 1, and so on. This approach keeps the athlete motivated to reach the goal and keeps the body open to new challenges and levels of adaptation.

Circuit A: body weight	1. Squat to parallel 2. Push-up 3. Bent-knee sit-up 4. Quad hip extension 5. Back extension 6. Toe raise 7. Plank

Circuit B: body weight (combination of two minicircuits)	Phase 1
	  1. Squat to parallel
	  2. Push-up (wide stance)
	  3. Bent-knee sit-up
	  4. Quad hip extension
	Phase 2
	  1. Push-up (narrow stance)
	  2. Back extension
	  3. Toe raise
	  4. Front plank

Circuit C: dumbbells and medicine ball	1. Squat to parallel 2. Floor press 3. Quad hip extension 4. Bent-over row 5. Toe raise 6. Military press 7. Upright row 8. Medicine ball forward throw 9. Jump squat 10. Medicine ball overhead throw 11. Bent-knee sit-up 12. Plank

Figure 8.4 Sample circuit training programs.

Note: The suggested exercises in this chapter may be changed to conform to the needs of the athlete and the specifics of the selected sport (prime movers).

Entry-level athletes should individualize the load for the prescribed number of reps by working up to the point of feeling either slight discomfort or actual discomfort. For *slight discomfort*, read uneasiness. *Discomfort*, on the other hand, refers to the threshold at which the athlete is maintaining good technique but must stop the exercise due to pain.

Table 8.1 shows how to plan a circuit training program, including duration, frequency of training sessions per week, and other parameters for both novice and experienced athletes. As you can see, training parameters for experienced athletes are quite different from those for novices. For example, it makes good sense for novice athletes to use a longer AA phase because they need more time for the adaptation itself and for creating a good base for the future. On the other hand, extending this phase much longer than four weeks does not produce visible gains for experienced athletes.

Similar differences apply to the number of stations per circuit. Because novice athletes must address as many muscle groups as realistically possible, they use more stations, and their circuits are longer. Advanced athletes, however, can reduce the number of stations to focus on exercises for the prime movers, on compensation, and on core exercises, which results in shorter circuits that are repeated more times.

Both load and the total physical demand per circuit must be increased progressively and individually. The example shown in figure 8.5 illustrates that both the load and the pattern of increase differ between novice and experienced athletes. Of course, as the number of repetitions goes down, the load goes up, and the load changes from cycle to

Table 8.1 Training Parameters for Circuit Training

Training parameter	Novice athlete	Experienced athlete
Duration of anatomical adaptation	6-9 (multiples of 3, to facilitate step loading) weeks	2-4 weeks
Load (if applicable)	20 reps down to 8 throughout the entire phase	12-15 reps down to 8 throughout the entire phase
Number of stations per circuit	9-12	6-8
Number of circuits per session	2 or 3	3 or 4
Total time of circuit training session	35-60 minutes	40-60 minutes
Rest interval between exercises	30-90 seconds	30-120 seconds
Rest interval between circuits	2-3 minutes	1-2 minutes
Frequency per week	2 or 3	3 or 4

Novice athlete (performing sets to *slight discomfort*)	20 reps, 2 circuits	15 reps, 3 circuits	12 reps, 2 circuits	12 reps, 3 circuits	10 reps, 3 circuits	8 reps, 2 circuits
Experienced athlete (performing sets to *discomfort*)	15 reps, 2 circuits	12 reps, 3 circuits	10 reps, 2 circuit	12 reps, 3 circuits	10 reps, 3 circuits	8 reps, 2 circuits
Microcycle	1	2	3	4	5	6

Figure 8.5 Suggested pattern for load increments during circuit training for novice and experienced athletes.

cycle. For exercises performed against resistance, lower loads are used for entry-level athletes, and slightly heavier loads (and lower reps per set) are used for advanced athletes.

Standard Training Program During the Anatomical Adaptation Phase

Circuit training is not the only possible way to organize strength training during the AA phase. A standard, horizontal execution strength training program can be used as well. In a horizontal approach, all the planned warm-ups and work sets of an exercise are performed before switching to the next one in the program. As long as the methodological characteristics of the AA phase are respected (such as starting with a high number of exercises, short rest intervals, and a higher number of reps per set, and progressing to a lower number of reps and higher loads over the course of the phase), the horizontal approach is just as valid as circuit training and is actually more indicated for intermediate and advanced athletes.

The following list shows how to plan a standard training program during the AA phase, including duration, frequency of training sessions per week, and other parameters that are valid for intermediate and advanced athletes.

Training Parameters for Standard Training

Duration (of anatomical adaptation): 2 to 4 weeks

Load: 12 to 20 reps down to 6 to 8 throughout the entire phase

Number of exercises: 6 to 8

Number of sets: 2 to 4

Total time of training session: 40 to 60 minutes

Rest interval between exercises: 30 to 120 seconds

Frequency per week: 3 or 4

Figures 8.6 through 8.10 illustrate standard and circuit training in various sports for four and seven weeks of anatomical adaptation training. A seven-week cycle gives the athlete time to build a stronger base and offers the physiological benefits of longer and better adaptation. These programs should be adapted to each athlete's classification and abilities.

Toward the end of the AA phase, the load reached allows athletes to make an immediate transition to the maximum strength phase, as shown in figure 8.6. This approach can be used for all athletes except those requiring increased muscle mass, such as throwers and American football linemen. For these athletes, a hypertrophy phase must be planned between the AA phase and the MxS phase. Figure 8.7 illustrates a four-week AA program appropriate for athletes with a very short preparatory phase, especially those in racket and combat sports that require three or four major peaks per year. Because this AA phase is so short, the load in training is increased very quickly to ready the athlete for the maximum strength phase. Detraining poses less of a concern in these sports because their transition phase is much shorter than those of most other sports. Figure 8.8 illustrates standard

Exercise	WEEK						
	1	2	3	4	5	6	7
1. Leg press	2 × 15	3 × 12	3 × 10	2 × 10	3 × 8	3 × 6	2 × 6
2. Chest press	2 × 15	3 × 12	3 × 10	2 × 10	3 × 8	3 × 6	2 × 6
3. Dumbbell stiff-leg deadlift	2 × 15	3 × 12	3 × 10	2 × 10	3 × 8	3 × 6	2 × 6
4. Military press	2 × 15	3 × 12	3 × 10	2 × 10	3 × 8	3 × 6	2 × 6
5. Leg curl	2 × 12	3 × 10	3 × 8	2 × 8	3 × 8	3 × 6	2 × 5
6. Upright row	2 × 15	3 × 12	3 × 10	2 × 10	3 × 8	3 × 6	2 × 6
7. Toe raise	2 × 15	3 × 12	3 × 10	2 × 10	3 × 8	3 × 6	2 × 6
8. Bent-knee sit-up	2 × 12	3 × 12	3 × 15	2 × 15	3 × 18	3 × 20	2 × 20
LOADING PATTERN							
	Low	Medium	High		Low	Medium	High / Low

Figure 8.6 Example of a standard strength training program for the anatomical adaptation phase.

Exercise	WEEK 1	WEEK 2	WEEK 3	WEEK 4	Rest interval
1. Rope skipping	3 min	2 × 3 min	4 × 2 min	2 × 2 min	30 sec
2. Half squat	2 × 10	3 × 8	3 × 6	2 × 5	2 min
3. Bench press	2 × 10	3 × 8	3 × 6	2 × 5	2 min
4. Back hyperextension	2 × 15	3 × 12	3 × 10	2 × 8	2 min
5. Front lat pull-down	2 × 10	3 × 8	3 × 6	2 × 5	2 min
6. Toe raise	2 × 15	3 × 12	3 × 10	2 × 8	1 min
7. Ab crunch	2 × 15	3 × 20	3 × 30	2 × 30	1 min
8. Trunk side bend (each side)	2 × 10	3 × 8	3 × 6	2 × 5	1 min
9. Medicine ball chest throw (4 kg)	2 × 8	3 × 8	3 × 10	2 × 8	1 min
10. Low-impact plyometrics	2 × 10	3 × 10	3 × 12	2 × 12	1 min

LOADING PATTERN

Low — Medium — High — Low

Figure 8.7 Sample suggested circuit training for sports with a short preparatory phase.

Rope skipping aids in cardiorespiratory training.

Exercise	WEEK 1	WEEK 2	WEEK 3	WEEK 4	WEEK 5	WEEK 6	WEEK 7	Rest interval
1. Cardio	10 min	10 min	2 × 5 min	2 × 5 min	3 × 3 min	4 × 2 min	2 × 2 min	1 min
2. Half squat	2 × 15	3 × 12	3 × 10	2 × 10	3 × 8	3 × 6	2 × 6	2 min
3. Dumbbell press	2 × 15	3 × 12	3 × 10	2 × 10	3 × 8	3 × 6	2 × 6	1 min
4. Leg curl	2 × 12	3 × 12	3 × 10	2 × 10	3 × 8	3 × 6	2 × 5	2 min
5. Dumbbell row	2 × 15	3 × 15	3 × 12	2 × 12	3 × 10	3 × 8	2 × 8	1 min
6. Toe raise	2 × 15	3 × 15	3 × 12	2 × 12	3 × 10	3 × 8	2 × 8	1 min
7. Ab crunch	2 × 20	3 × 20	3 × 25	2 × 20	3 × 25	3 × 30	2 × 25	1 min
8. Medicine ball backward throw (4 kg)	2 × 6	3 × 8	3 × 10	2 × 8	3 × 10	3 × 10	2 × 8	2 min
9. Low-impact plyometrics	2 × 8	3 × 10	3 × 12	2 × 10	3 × 12	3 × 12	2 × 10	1 min
10. Power ball side throw (10 kg)	2 × 6	3 × 8	3 × 10	2 × 8	3 × 10	3 × 10	2 × 8	1 min
11. Cardio	5 min	7 min	7 min	2 × 5 min	3 × 3 min	3 × 3 min	2 × 2 min	1 min

LOADING PATTERN

Low — Medium — High — Low — Medium — High — Low

Figure 8.8 Sample suggested circuit training program for team sports in which cardiorespiratory endurance is an important component.

The cardio component in this example could include any of various options (e.g., running, using a stair-stepper, riding a bicycle ergometer).

strength training for team sports with a high-endurance component; cardio repetitions are placed both at the beginning and at the end of the strength workout. Figure 8.9 illustrates a circuit training program with a higher number of unilateral lower-body exercises for athletes in team sports such as soccer, basketball, rugby, lacrosse, water polo, and hockey. Figure 8.10 illustrates standard training for baseball, softball, and racket sports. To enable maximum adaptation in these sports, certain specific exercises are introduced early on in the AA phase for trunk and hip rotation—specifically, abdominal rainbows, incline trunk rotations, and power ball side throws.

Exercise	REPS					
	Week 1	Week 2	Week 3	Week 4	Week 5	Week 6
1. Leg press	20	15	12	10	8	6
2. Supine dumbbell press	20	15	12	10	8	6
3. One-leg hip bridge	20	15	12	10	8	6
4. Dumbbell row	20	15	12	10	8	6
5. Deadlift	20	15	12	10	8	6
6. Seated dumbbell press	20	15	12	10	8	6
7. Standing calf raise	20	15	12	10	8	6
8. Dumbell upright row	20	15	12	10	8	6
9. Bent-knee sit-up	20	15	12	10	8	6
10. Front plank	45 sec	60 sec	75 sec	75 sec	90 sec	60 sec with weight
No. of circuits	2	3	2	2	3	2
Rest interval between exercises	1 min					
Rest interval between circuits	2 min		1 min	2 min		1 min
Workout duration (approximate)	50 min	65 min	40 min	35 min	50 min	30 min
	LOADING PATTERN					

Loading pattern: Medium, High, Low, Medium, High, Low

Figure 8.9 Sample suggested circuit training program for team sports (using unilateral exercises and dumbbells).

Exercise	WEEK							Rest interval
	1	**2**	**3**	**4**	**5**	**6**	**7**	
1. Side or diagonal lunge (each side)	2 × 15	3 × 12	3 × 10	2 × 10	3 × 8	3 × 6	2 × 6	2 min
2. Cable crossover	2 × 15	3 × 12	3 × 10	2 × 10	3 × 8	3 × 6	2 × 6	1-2 min
3. Back extension	2 × 15	3 × 15	3 × 12	2 × 12	3 × 10	3 × 8	2 × 8	1-2 min
4. Front lat pull-down	2 × 15	3 × 12	3 × 10	2 × 10	3 × 8	3 × 6	2 × 6	2 min
5. Dumbbell external rotator	2 × 15	3 × 15	3 × 12	2 × 12	3 × 10	3 × 8	2 × 8	1 min
6. Toe raise	2 × 15	3 × 15	3 × 12	2 × 12	3 × 10	3 × 8	2 × 8	1-2 min
7. Bent-knee sit-up	2 × 20	3 × 20	3 × 25	2 × 20	3 × 25	3 × 30	2 × 25	2 min
8. Ab rainbow (each side)	2 × 20	3 × 20	3 × 25	2 × 20	3 × 25	3 × 30	2 × 25	1-2 min
9. Power ball side throw (10 kg)	2 × 6	3 × 8	3 × 10	2 × 8	3 × 10	3 × 10	2 × 8	1-2 min
10. Low-impact plyometrics	2 × 8	3 × 10	3 × 12	2 × 10	3 × 12	3 × 12	2 × 10	2-3 min

LOADING PATTERN

		High			High	
	Medium			Medium		
Low			Low			Low

Figure 8.10 Sample suggested circuit training program for baseball, softball, and racket sports.

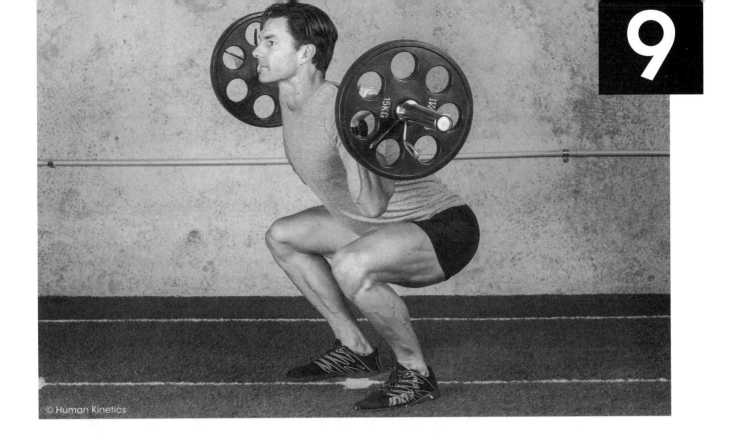

9

© Human Kinetics

Hypertrophy Training

Many people think that the larger a person is, the stronger that person is. This is not always the case. For example, a weightlifter may be capable of lifting heavier loads than a larger, bulkier bodybuilder can lift. That is why athletes should seek an increase of lean body mass that is functional for their sport, because some hypertrophy (increase in muscle size), especially of the fast-twitch muscle fibers, contributes to an increase in force expression.

As the preceding distinctions imply, bodybuilding hypertrophy and sport-specific hypertrophy differ in important ways. In bodybuilding hypertrophy, the bodybuilder generally uses loads of 60% to 80% of 1RM for sets of 8 to 15 reps taken to failure. Some bodybuilders, however, attribute their success to using fewer reps and high training loads taken beyond failure with forced and negative reps, while others believe in performing high reps (usually up to 20). Given that all these types of bodybuilders are massively built and share similar records and number of wins, we may infer that in professional bodybuilding, it is not only training that makes a difference.

In any case, athletes and coaches of other sports must keep in mind that the purpose of bodybuilding is not optimal performance but optimal symmetry and maximal muscle mass. Aesthetic symmetry, however, is irrelevant to many sports in which function is the main priority. And although bodybuilders do increase muscle mass, the functionality of that mass is questionable, whereas functionality—that is, improved performance—is the goal of training in other sports.

Sport-Specific Hypertrophy

Hypertrophy training is intended for athletes whose sport performance will be helped by an increase in muscle size. To name a few, such athletes include football linemen, shot-putters, discus throwers, and heavy weight categories in contact sports (for a detailed periodization-of-strength model for your sport, refer to chapter 6). For most other sports, a hypertrophy phase is not necessary, as the fast-twitch muscle fibers of the prime movers will eventually hypertrophy (hypertrophy of myosin filaments) as a result of maximum strength training. This will also allow a better strength-to-body-weight ratio (relative strength) than a general hypertrophy program.

For athletes, hypertrophy should be achieved by applying a sport-specific training methodology. In other words, whereas bodybuilding focuses on enlarging overall musculature, hypertrophy training for sports focuses mainly on increasing the size of the specific prime movers without neglecting the neural component of force expression.

This kind of hypertrophy—sport-specific hypertrophy—is achieved by other than bodybuilding methods. Specifically, training for sport-specific hypertrophy requires heavy loads and a high number of sets to increase the density (thickness) of, and amount of protein in, the prime movers. Hypertrophy training for sports is long lasting because the increase in muscle size is based on the increase in strength.

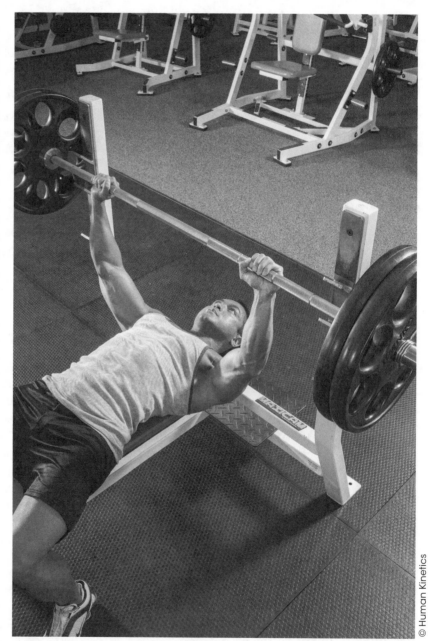

© Human Kinetics

Athletes increase muscle mass using sport-specific training methodology, not bodybuilding.

Athletes and coaches should be cautious when incorporating hypertrophy methods into a training program. Specifically, they must take into consideration the athlete's physical maturity and the timing in relation to the yearly training program. During the early preparatory season, hypertrophy methods work very well to help stimulate the highest increase in lean muscle mass. The majority of the program should consist of multijoint exercises, such as squats, leg presses, bench presses, back rows, chin-ups, dips, and core exercises, to stimulate muscle growth and strengthen the prime movers integrated in a complex kinetic chain, as happens in sporting activities. Isolation exercises should be kept to a minimum.

The hypertrophy phase can last six to eight or nine weeks, depending on the type of macrocycles used (how many 2+1 and 3+1 have been planned) and microcycles, depending on the needs of the athlete and the sport or event. Again, hypertrophy training methods should be used early in the preparatory phase. The total length of the preparatory phase is also important because the longer it is, the more time the athlete has to work on hypertrophy as well as on maximum strength.

The end of the hypertrophy phase does not mean that an athlete who needs to build muscle mass must stop this training. As illustrated in the example for a lineman in figure 9.1, hypertrophy training, if needed, can be maintained and even further developed during the maximum strength phase. Depending on the needs of the athlete, the ratio of MxS training and hypertrophy training can be three to one, two to one, or even one to one. During the maintenance phase, however, only certain athletes—such as shot-putters and linemen in American football—should continue hypertrophy training, and then only during the first half. As the most important competitions approach, power and maximum strength training should prevail.

Preparatory				Competitive
3 AA	6 Hyp.: 3 or 4 sessions	6 MxS: 2 or 3 sessions Hyp.: 1 or 2 sessions	5 Conv. to P: 2 sessions MxS: 1 session Hyp.: 1 session	Maint.: P, MxS, hyp.

Figure 9.1 Suggested proportions of hypertrophy, maximum strength, and power training for American football linemen.

Key: AA = anatomical adaptation, conv. = conversion, hyp. = hypertrophy, maint. = maintenance, MxS = maximum strength, P = power

Program Design for Sport-Specific Hypertrophy Training

Once the anatomical adaptation (AA) phase has readied and strengthened the connective tissue (tendons and ligaments), hypertrophy training can begin with a test for 1RM. In that case, the 1RM test must be performed at the end of the last microcycle (unloading) of the AA phase. Athletes then start with a 60% load, or one that allows them to perform 12 reps. The load is then increased in each microcycle until it reaches a level at which the athlete can perform only 6 reps. For training parameters of the hypertrophy phase, see table 9.1.

To achieve maximum training benefits, the athlete must reach the highest number of reps possible in each set. This means reaching a degree of exhaustion that prevents him

Table 9.1   Training Parameters for the Hypertrophy Phase

Duration of hypertrophy phase	6-8 weeks
Load	60%-80% of 1RM
Number of exercises	6-9
Number of reps per set	12 down to 6
Number of sets per session	Split* or full-body; up to 8 sets for prime movers
Rest interval	2-5 minutes
Speed of execution	Slow eccentric (3-5 seconds), possible pause between eccentric and concentric (1-5 seconds), fast concentric (1 second or less—explosive)
Frequency per week	2-4 times

*Exercises for the lower body are trained on separate days from the exercises for the upper body. A usual split routine for sports during the hypertrophy phase is as follows: Monday, lower body; Tuesday, upper body; Wednesday, rest; Thursday, lower body; Friday, upper body; Saturday and Sunday, rest.

or her from doing another rep even when applying maximum contraction. Without performing each set to exhaustion, the athlete does not achieve the expected level of muscle hypertrophy because the first reps do not produce enough stimulus to maximize muscle mass. The key element in hypertrophy training is not just exhaustion per set but the cumulative effect of exhaustion in the total number of sets. This cumulative exhaustion stimulates the chemical reactions and protein metabolism necessary for optimal muscle hypertrophy. Because sets are taken to failure during the hypertrophy phase, you may decide not to test the 1RM, and just increase the load week by week by doing 12RM on the first week of loading, 10RM on the second, unloading, and continuing the progression in the ensuing macrocycle (e.g., 8RM, 6RM, unload).

Hypertrophy exercises should generally be performed at low to moderate speed of execution in order to maximize the muscles' time under tension (increased time under tension is favorable for enlarging muscle size). However, athletes in speed- and power-dominant sports are strongly advised against slow concentric speed of execution, especially if the hypertrophy phase is longer than six weeks. The primary reason for this advice is that the neuromuscular system adapts to slow execution and therefore does not stimulate the immediate recruitment of fast-twitch muscle fibers that is crucial for speed- and power-dominant sports.

As compared with bodybuilding, hypertrophy training for sports involves fewer exercises in order to focus mainly on the prime movers rather than on all muscle groups. The benefit of this approach is that more sets are performed per exercise (3 to 6, or even as many as 8), thus stimulating better muscle hypertrophy for the prime movers.

Depending on the microcycle, the rest interval between sets can vary from two to five minutes. The closer the athlete gets to switching to a maximum strength phase of training, the longer the rest interval must be between sets. For instance, in a six- to nine-week hypertrophy phase of training, the first three weeks can be used to stimulate maximum hypertrophy gains by using short rest periods (60-90 seconds between sets) thus increasing the volume possible for the duration of the session, and the last three or four weeks can use longer rest periods.

VARIATIONS OF HYPERTROPHY TRAINING METHODS

The main factors responsible for hypertrophy are not fully understood, but researchers increasingly believe that increased muscle size is stimulated mainly by the mechanical stress to the muscle fibers (Owino et al. 2001; Goldspink 2005; Ahtiainen et al. 2001; Liu et al. 2008; Hameed et al. 2008; Roschel et al. 2011; Goldspink 2012; Schoenfeld 2012), mainly determined by the load used, the total time under tension, especially of the eccentric phase, and the total volume in terms of reps; the metabolic stress (Sjøgaard 1985; Febbraio and Pedersen 2005; Hornberger et al. 2006), mainly determined by the set duration that should be preferable in the anaerobic lactic energy system domain (30-60 seconds), and, again, the total volume in terms of reps. Because taking a set to concentric failure represents the main element of success in achieving muscle hypertrophy, several variations of the original bodybuilding method have been developed. Most of them pursue the same objective: When exhaustion is reached, a few more reps must be performed through hard work. The expected result is greater muscle growth, or increased hypertrophy. Of all the variations (there are more than 20), the following are most representative.

- *Split routine.* Athletes perform two or three exercises per muscle group. Because they address every muscle of the body, they may be in the gymnasium for almost two hours to finish the entire program. Even if athletes have the energy to do this, the physiological response to such endurance does not favor the maximization of hypertrophy. The solution is to divide the total volume of work into parts and address one part of the body on each day—hence the term *split routine.* This approach means that even if an athlete trains four times per week, any given muscle group is worked only twice per week.
- *Forced repetitions.* As an athlete performs a set to concentric failure, a partner assists by providing sufficient support to enable one or two more reps.
- *Rest-pause.* An athlete reaches concentric failure in a set, then rests only 10 to 20 seconds before starting again until concentric failure is reached (usually after one to three reps). This approach increases the set's duration and the hypertrophic stimulus.
- *Drop sets.* An athlete reaches concentric failure in a set, then quickly lowers the load by 5% to 10% (depending on how many more reps the trainer expects the athlete to perform, or whether an additional drop set is programmed), starts again, and continues until concentric failure. This technique also increases the set's duration and the hypertrophic stimulus.

The initial load in the rest-pause and drop-set approaches can be higher than in the usual bodybuilding programs because the set's duration is increased via micropauses (in rest-pause) or small deloading (in drop sets). This characteristic makes these two techniques particularly useful for hypertrophy training because it increases the fast-twitch muscle fibers' time under tension during a set. Bodybuilding books and magazines often refer to many other methods, some of which are said to work miracles. Coaches and athletes should take care to recognize the fine line that separates fact from fantasy.

At the end of a training session, an athlete should stretch the muscles that have been worked. Because of the many contractions, the muscles shorten. This results in reduced muscle range of motion and decreased quickness of contraction, which in turn affects joint positioning and overall body posture, as well as neurally facilitating the agonist and neurally inhibiting the antagonist, reducing, over time, the overall performance ability of the affected muscles. In addition, a shortened muscle has a slower rate of regeneration because only the normal anatomical length facilitates active biochemical exchanges. These exchanges provide nutrients to the muscles and remove metabolic wastes, facilitating better recovery between sets and after training sessions.

Figure 9.2 shows a sample eight-week program developed for a heavyweight wrestler. The program suggested in each box is repeated three times per week. Figure 9.3 shows a sample six-week program for a female college volleyball player who has a relatively large disproportion between height and weight. Figure 9.4 shows a sample six-week program for a power and speed athlete who wants to gain muscle mass. The first seven exercises for the lower body are performed on days 1 and 4, and the next seven exercises for the upper body are performed on days 2 and 5. Figure 9.5 shows a sample hypertrophy program designed in jump-set format to save time. Figure 9.6 shows a sample split routine (upper and lower body) where bodybuilding intensification methods are employed to further elicit hypertrophy. When such methods are employed, a lower number of sets per

Exercise	WEEK								Rest interval
	1	2	3	4	5	6	7	8	
Deadlift	2×12	3×12	3×10	2×10	3×8	3×6	3×5	2×5	2 min (weeks 1-4) 3 min (weeks 5-8)
Bench press	2×12	3×12	3×10	2×10	3×8	3×6	3×5	2×5	2 min (weeks 1-4) 3 min (weeks 5-8)
Squat	2×12	3×12	3×10	2×10	3×8	3×6	3×5	2×5	2 min (weeks 1-4) 3 min (weeks 5-8)
Pulley row	2×12	3×12	3×10	2×10	3×8	3×6	3×5	2×5	2 min (weeks 1-4) 3 min (weeks 5-8)
Hip thrust	2×12	3×12	3×10	2×10	3×8	3×6	3×5	2×5	1 min (weeks 1-4) 2 min (weeks 5-8)
Floor press	2×12	3×12	3×10	2×10	3×8	3×6	3×5	2×5	1 min (weeks 1-4) 2 min (weeks 5-8)
Good morning	2×12	3×12	3×10	2×10	3×8	3×6	3×5	2×5	1 min (weeks 1-4) 2 min (weeks 5-8)
Farmer's walk (weight on one side; time in sec)	30+30 × 2 sets	40+40 × 2 sets	50+50 × 2 sets	30+30 × 2 sets	40+40 × 2 sets	50+50 × 2 sets	60+60 × 2 sets	40+40 × 2 sets	1 min
LOADING PATTERN									
			High				High		
		Medium				Medium			
	Low			Low	Low			Low	

Figure 9.2 Sample training program for a heavyweight wrestler in the hypertrophy phase.

session must be planned because they heavily tax both the muscles and the CNS. In the following figures, you find the repetitions decreasing from week to week. Each decrease of repetitions corresponds to an increase of load so that each set is taken to failure. Because of the residual fatigue, the load might be adjusted downward in the second and third set to fulfill the required number of reps per set.

Bodybuilding workouts, even those using the split routine, are very exhausting; often, in fact, 120 to 180 reps are performed in a single training session. Such high muscle loading requires a long recovery. Because of the type of work specific to bodybuilding, the ATP-CP and glycogen stores are greatly taxed after a demanding training session. Although ATP-CP is restored very quickly, liver glycogen (if tapped) requires 40 to 48 hours to replenish. Thus, heavy workouts to complete exhaustion should not be performed more than two times per microcycle for the same muscle groups.

Some may argue that athletes who use the split routine train a given group of muscles on every second day, thus leaving 48 hours between the two training sessions, which is sufficient for the restoration of energy fuels. However, though this may be true for local muscle stores, it ignores the fact that when muscle glycogen is exhausted, the body starts tapping the glycogen stores in the liver. If the liver source is tapped every day, 24 hours may be insufficient to restore glycogen. This deficit may result in the *functional*

Exercise	WEEK						Rest interval
	1	2	3	4	5	6	
Half squat	2×12	3×12	3×10	2×10	3×8	3×6	1 min (weeks 1-4) 2 min (weeks 5-8)
Incline dumbbell press	2×12	3×12	3×10	2×10	3×8	3×6	1 min (weeks 1-4) 2 min (weeks 5-8)
Dumbbell walking lunge	2×20	2×15	2×12	1×12	3×10	3×8	1 min (weeks 1-4) 2 min (weeks 5-8)
Mid-pronated lat pull-down	2×12	3×12	3×10	2×10	3×8	3×6	1 min (weeks 1-4) 2 min (weeks 5-8)
Back hyperextension	2×12	2×12	2×10	1×10	2×8	2×6	1 min (weeks 1-4) 2 min (weeks 5-8)
Dumbbell shoulder press	2×12	3×12	3×10	2×10	3×8	3×6	1 min.
Standing calf raise	2×12	2×12	3×10	2×10	2×8	2×6	1 min.
Dumbbell triceps extension	2×12	2×12	2×10	1×10	2×8	2×6	1 min.
Dumbbell external rotator	2×12	2×12	2×10	1×10	2×8	2×6	1 min.
Weighted crunch	2×12	2×12	2×10	1×10	2×8	2×8	1 min.
LOADING PATTERN							
			High			High	
		Medium			Medium		
	Low			Low			

Figure 9.3 Sample training program for a female college volleyball player in the hypertrophy phase.

Exercise	Week 1 Days 1 and 4	Week 2 Days 1 and 4	Week 3 Days 1 and 4	Week 4 Days 1 and 4	Week 5 Days 1 and 4	Week 6 Days 1 and 4	Rest interval
Squat (day 1) or deadlift (day 4)	2×8	3×8	3×6	2×6	3×5	4×5	2 min (weeks 1-4) 3 min (weeks 5-8)
Hip thrust	2×12	3×12	3×10	2×10	3×8	3×6	1 min (weeks 1-4) 2 min (weeks 5-8)
Back hyperextension	2×12	3×12	3×10	2×10	3×8	3×6	1 min (weeks 1-4) 2 min (weeks 5-8)
Leg curl	2×8	3×8	3×6	2×6	3×5	4×5	1 min (weeks 1-4) 2 min (weeks 5-8)
Standing calf raise	2×12	3×12	3×10	2×10	3×8	3×6	1 min.
Weighted crunch	2×12	3×12	3×12	2×10	3×8	3×6	1 min.
Exercise	**Week 1** Days 2 and 5	**Week 2** Days 2 and 5	**Week 3** Days 2 and 5	**Week 4** Days 2 and 5	**Week 5** Days 2 and 5	**Week 6** Days 2 and 5	**Rest interval**
Bench press	2×12	3×12	3×10	2×10	3×8	3×6	2 min (weeks 1-4) 3 min (weeks 5-8)
Mid-pronated lat pull-down	2×12	3×12	3×10	2×10	3×8	3×6	2 min (weeks 1-4) 3 min (weeks 5-8)
Military press	2×12	3×12	3×10	2×10	3×8	3×6	1 min (weeks 1-4) 2 min (weeks 5-8)
Dumbbell curl	2×8	3×8	3×6	2×6	3×5	4×5	1 min.
French press	2×12	3×12	3×10	2×10	3×8	3×6	1 min.
Land mine (reps, left and right)	12+12	14+14	16+16	14+14	16+16	18+18	1 min.
Farmer's walk (time in seconds, left and right)	30+30	40+40	50+50	40+40	50+50	60+60	1 min.

LOADING PATTERN

		High			High
	Medium			Medium	
Low			Low		

Figure 9.4 Sample training program for an ice hockey player in the hypertrophy phase.

Sequence*	Exercise	Rest interval	Week 1	Week 2	Week 3	Week 4	Week 5	Week 6
A1	Squat	2 min.	3×12	4×10	2×10	3×8	4×6	2×6
A2	Hip thrust	2 min.	3×12	4×10	2×10	3×8	4×6	2×6
B1	Bench press	2 min.	3×12	4×10	2×10	3×8	4×6	2×6
B2	Barbell row	2 min.	3×12	4×10	2×10	3×8	4×6	2×6
C1	Semi-stiff-leg deadlift	1 min.	2×12	2×10	1×10	2×8	2×6	1×6
C2	Standing calf raise	1 min.	2×12	2×10	1×10	2×8	2×6	1×6
D1	Narrow dip	1 min.	2×12	2×10	1×10	2×8	2×6	1×6
D2	Dumbbell curl	1 min.	2×12	2×10	1×10	2×8	2×6	1×6
E	Weighted crunch	1 min.	2×12	2×10	1×10	2×8	2×6	1×6
			LOADING PATTERN					
				High			High	
			Medium			Medium		
					Low			Low

Figure 9.5 Sample loading pattern for a six-week training program for a heavyweight wrestler in the hypertrophy phase.

Note: All sets are taken to failure, so the weight might be adjusted downward in the second set in order to fulfill the required number of reps per set.

*Jump-set format: Do one set of exercise A1, take rest interval, do one set of exercise A2, take rest interval, and repeat the sequence. Then pass to the next pair (B1 and B2) and continue until finished.

overreaching phenomenon (localized neuromuscular fatigue that prevents the normal force expression of the muscle group). Moreover, many of the routines and methods used by bodybuilders, such as four- or five-day split routines or two workouts per day, do not allow for nervous system recovery or the recruitment of the fast-twitch muscle fibers that are integral to sport performance.

In addition to exhausting energy stores, constant intense training puts wear and tear on the contractile proteins, exceeding their *anabolism* (the myosin's protein-building rate). Such overloading can cause the muscles involved to no longer increase in size; in other words, there may be no gains in hypertrophy.

When this happens, coaches should reassess the application of the overloading principle and start using the step-type method, as suggested by the principle of progressive increase of load in training. They should also consider inserting an unloading microcycle more frequently in order to facilitate regeneration, which is just as important as training. A workout is only as good as the athlete's ability to recover from it. Athletes can perform lower-volume split sessions—working two or three muscle groups for a total of 12 to 18 sets, tapping less into the liver's glycogen, and generating less muscle breakdown (*catabolism*)—up to four times per week, with at least 72 hours of recovery between trainings of the same muscle group. For example, an athlete could devote Monday and Thursday to the lower body and Tuesday and Friday to the upper body.

Exercise	Week 1 Days 1 and 4	Week 2 Days 1 and 4	Week 3 Days 1 and 4	Week 4 Days 1 and 4	Week 5 Days 1 and 4	Week 6 Days 1 and 4	Rest interval
Leg press	2×8	2×8+ds	2×6+ds	2×8	3×5	4×5	2 min (weeks 1-4) 3 min (weeks 5-8)
Dumbbell walking lunge	2×10	2×12+rp	2×14+rp	2×10	3×8	3×6	2 min.
Semi-stiff-leg deadlift	2×12	3×10	3×8	2×10	3×8	3×6	1 min (weeks 1-4) 2 min (weeks 5-8)
Leg curl	2×8	2×8+rp	2×6+rp	2×6	3×5	4×5	2 min.
Standing calf raise	2×8	2×+ds	2×6+ds	2×10	3×8	3×6	2 min.
Weighted crunch	2×12	3×12	3×10	2×10	3×8	3×6	1 min.
Exercise	**Week 1** Days 2 and 5	**Week 2** Days 2 and 5	**Week 3** Days 2 and 5	**Week 4** Days 2 and 5	**Week 5** Days 2 and 5	**Week 6** Days 2 and 5	**Rest interval**
Bench press	2×8	2×+ds	2×6+ds	2×6	3×5	4×5	2 min (weeks 1-4) 3 min (weeks 5-8)
Pulley row	2×8	2×8+ds	2×+ds	2×6	3×5	4×5	2 min (weeks 1-4) 3 min (weeks 5-8)
Dumbbell shoulder press	2×12	3×10+ds	3×8+ds	2×10	3×8	3×6	1 min (weeks 1-4) 2 min (weeks 5-8)
Dumbbell curl	2×8	2×8+rp	2×6+rp	2×6	3×5	4×5	1 min.
Cable push-down	2×12	3×10+ds	3×8+ds	2×10	3×8	3×6	1 min.
Plank (sec.)	40	50	60	40	60	70	—

LOADING PATTERN						
		High			High	
	Medium			Medium		
Low			Low			

Figure 9.6 Sample split routine using bodybuilding intensification methods to elicit hypertrophy.
Key: ds = drop sets; rp = rest pause

Because improperly used bodybuilding techniques can handicap most athletes, they are used sparingly in sport training. Even so, bodybuilding methods may benefit some athletes in a certain phase of strength development. For instance, because bodybuilding is relatively safe and employs moderately heavy loads, some novice athletes can use its methods, provided that they do work just short of exhaustion in each set. The techniques may also benefit athletes who want to move up a weight class in sports such as boxing, wrestling, and the martial arts.

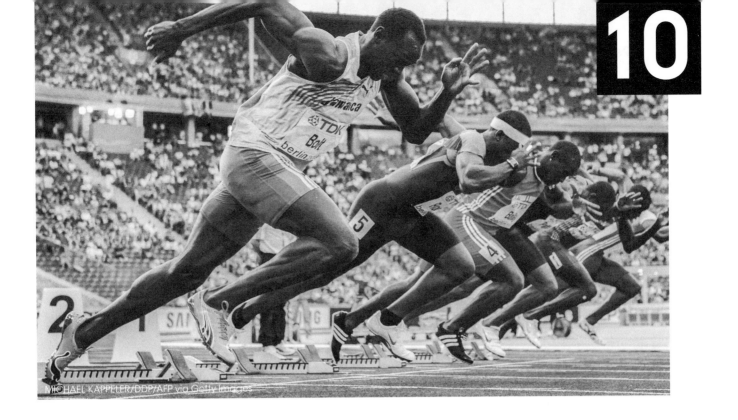

MICHAEL KAPPELER/DDP/AFP via Getty Images

10

Maximum Strength

Please imagine two cars side by side. One is an ordinary car; the other, a sports car. Do you know which is faster? You certainly do. However, do you know why? The engine! The stronger the engine, the fastest the car. In the same way, maximum strength is the engine of an athlete. The stronger the athlete's engine, the better they will perform.

Nearly every sport requires strength, but what each sport really calls for is sport-specific strength. In creating sport-specific strength, an important role (if not the determinant one) is played by maximum strength. The specific role played by maximum strength varies between sports and determines the length of the MxS training phase for a given sport. The more important the role—for example, it is quite important for throwers in track and field and for American football linemen—the longer the maximum strength phase. Similarly, the phase is shorter for sports in which maximum strength contributes less to final performance (e.g., golf, table tennis). Do not be surprised to see table tennis included. What is significant is not the light weight of the ball or what happens above the table but rather what happens below table level: the stronger and more powerful the legs, the faster and more reactive the player. That is why the coach must know the physiology behind the increase of maximum strength as well as the methods to apply during each training phase to maximize the final outcome: the highest possible level of specific strength.

Physiology of Strength Training

Until a few years ago, we believed that strength was determined mainly by the muscles' cross-sectional area (CSA). For this reason, weight training was used to increase "engine size"—in other words, to produce muscular hypertrophy. Now, we see it differently. CSA remains the single best predicting factor of an individual's strength, but the main factors responsible for strength increase (especially in advanced athletes) are in fact the neural adaptations to strength training, such as improvements in inter- and intramuscular coordination and the disinhibition of inhibitory mechanisms (refer back to chapter 2 for further explanation on the neural adaptations to strength training).

> Of all types of strength training, maximum strength makes the highest contribution to high performance.

Briefly, an athlete's ability to generate high forces depends to a great extent on the following factors.

- Intermuscular coordination: the ability to synchronize all muscles of a kinetic chain involved in an action
- Intramuscular coordination: the capacity to voluntarily recruit as many motor units as possible and send nerve impulses at high frequencies
- Hypertrophy: the diameter or cross-sectional area of the muscle involved

Improving intermuscular coordination—coordination between muscle groups—depends strictly on learning (technique), which requires many reps of the same exercise using a moderate load (40%-80% percent of 1RM) and performed dynamically with perfect technique (MxS-I). Intramuscular coordination—the capacity to recruit fast-twitch muscle fibers—depends on training content, in which high loads (80%-90% of 1RM) are moved explosively (MxS-II). Both types of strength training, MxS-I and MxS-II, activate the powerful fast-twitch motor units.

Overall muscle mass depends on the duration of the hypertrophy phase, but an athlete does not necessarily have to develop large muscles and high body weight to become significantly stronger. Throughout maximum strength and power training, athletes learn to better coordinate the relevant muscle groups and use loads that result in higher recruitment of fast-twitch muscle fiber (loads greater than 80% of 1RM). By using the methods outlined in this chapter for the maximum strength phase, athletes can improve their maximum strength with some gains in functional muscle mass.

Of the three types of muscle contraction, eccentric contractions create the highest tension (up to 140% of concentric 1RM strength). The second-highest tension is created by isometric contractions (up to 120% of concentric 1RM strength). Still, concentric strength must be developed at the highest levels because most sport actions are concentric. Indeed, the direct application of other forms of contraction—isometric and especially eccentric—directly benefits athletic performance by supporting further improvements in concentric force.

Exercises used to develop maximum strength should never be performed under conditions of exhaustion, as they are in bodybuilding, except when the goal is to achieve absolute strength gains (strength plus hypertrophy). Because MxS training engages maximum activation of the central nervous system—including factors such as concentration and moti-

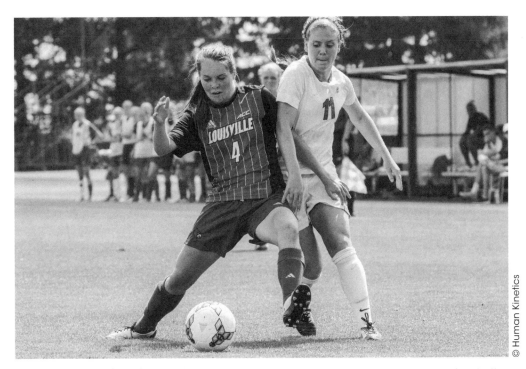

Maximum strength, increased via intramuscular coordination methods, transfers to the athlete's specific skills.

vation—it improves intermuscular and intramuscular coordination. High CNS adaptation (e.g., improvement of neuromuscular coordination) also results in adequate inhibition of the antagonist muscles. This means that when maximum force is applied, these muscles are coordinated in such a way that the antagonists do not contract to oppose the movement.

The CNS normally prevents the activation of all the motor units available for contraction. Eliminating this inhibition is one of the main objectives of MxS-II training—that is, intramuscular coordination training with loads above 80% of 1RM. This reduction in CNS inhibition is accompanied by an increase in strength that results in the greatest improvement in specific performance potential.

Training Methods for the Maximum Strength Phase

Throughout the MxS phase a number of training methods can be used. The most commonly employed methods entail the use of moderately heavy loads during MxS-I and heavy loads during MxS-II, applied in this sequence. In certain circumstances, the eccentric method, the isometric method, or the maxex method can supplement the former, basic methods. In the following sections, you will find out what these methods are and how to implement them within a periodized training plan.

Please note that all of these methods are percentage-based, meaning that the load indicated is a percentage of the 1RM. For this reason, before the beginning of the MxS phase (be it at the end of the AA phase or the hypertrophy phase when present) and at the end of each macrocycle that constitutes it, the 1RM for the main exercises must be tested. The 1RM test serves the double purpose of assessing the maximum strength improvement of the athlete and acting as a base for the calculation of the training loads for the macrocycle to follow.

Submaximum (MxS-I) and Maximum (MxS-II) Loads Methods

In periodization of strength for sports, the submaximum and maximum load methods are probably the most effective ways to develop maximum strength. In the case of MxS-I, it should be seen as a transition from the AA phase to MxS-II, where heavy loads are utilized. Improving maximum strength is paramount for most sports for the following reasons.

- The increase in voluntary motor unit activation results in high recruitment of fast-twitch muscle fibers that transfers to any sport activity.

- Maximum strength is the determinant factor in increasing power. It enables the athlete to reach a high neural output for sports in which speed and power are dominant.

- Maximum strength is also a critical element in improving muscular endurance, especially of short and medium duration.

- Maximum strength is important for sports in which relative strength is crucial, such as the martial arts, boxing, wrestling, sprinting, jump events in track and field, and most team sports. Relative strength is the proportion between maximum strength and body weight, meaning that the higher the relative strength, the better the performance.

Submaximum and maximum load methods positively influence athletes in speed- and power-dominant sports by increasing the muscle size and recruitment of more fast-twitch fibers. Large increases in muscle size are possible for athletes who are just starting to use these methods, but they are less likely in athletes with longer training backgrounds. The latter, too, will steadily put on small amounts of functional muscle mass as their training loads increase over time. The greatest gains in maximum strength, however, result from better muscle group coordination and increased recruitment of fast-twitch motor units.

The loads used for maximum strength development—70% to 95% of 1RM for only one to five reps—result in sets of short duration and, combined with complete rest intervals, allow complete restoration of ATP. As a result, the ATP deficiency and the depletion of structural protein are too low to strongly activate the protein metabolism that stimulates hypertrophy. Consequently, when used with sufficient rest intervals, such loads result in an increase in maximum strength but not so much in hypertrophy unless total volume (i.e., high total time under tension) is high enough.

The MxS-I and MxS-II load methods also increase testosterone level, which further explains improved maximum strength. The level of testosterone in the blood appears to depend on the frequency (per day and per week) of sessions using the maximum load method. Testosterone increases when the number of these sessions per week is low and decreases when maximum load training is performed twice a day. A correct training frequency with maximum loads can lead to higher testosterone levels, while a too-high frequency may lead to depressed levels of testosterone. Such findings substantiate and further justify the suggestions made earlier regarding the frequency of high-intensity training sessions per microcycle as well as the reduced duration of high-intensity macrocycles.

The maximum load method can be used only after a minimum of one year (two years for junior athletes) of general strength training (using AA and the MxS-I load method). Strength gains can be expected even during long-term use of the MxS-I method, mainly because of the motor learning that occurs as athletes learn to better use and coordinate the muscles involved in training.

However, highly trained athletes with four to five years of MxS training are so well adapted to such training that further increases in maximum strength may be difficult to achieve. Therefore, if further maximum strength development is necessary, alternate methods enable continued improvement. Options include the following.

- If an athlete has used periodization of training for three to four years and cannot see a further positive transfer of strength to his or her specific performance, he or she can alternate various stimulations of the neuromuscular system. Following anatomical adaptation and the first phase of MxS training, the athlete should alternate three weeks of MxS training with three weeks of power training. Power training, with its explosiveness and fast application of force, stimulates the CNS.

- For power sports, mostly for throwing events in track and field, another option can be used for stimulation: alternating three weeks of hypertrophy training with three weeks of MxS training. The additional hypertrophy phases result in slight enlargement in muscle size or an increase in lean muscle mass. This additional gain in hypertrophy provides a new biological base for further improvement of maximum strength.

- Increase the ratio between eccentric and concentric types of contraction, as explained later in this chapter. The additional eccentric training produces higher stimulation for MxS improvement because eccentric contraction creates higher tension in the muscle.

Important elements of success for training with the maximum load method include load, rest interval, exercise order, the speed performing the contraction, and the loading pattern. These factors are discussed in the following sections.

> Maximum strength is important not only to overcome resistance (water, force of gravity) but equally important for absorbing the shock of landing and to successfully manage a strong contact with opponents, such as in contact sports.

Load

Maximum strength is developed only by creating the highest possible tension in the muscle. Although lower loads engage slow-twitch muscle fibers, loads of greater than 70% of 1RM, moved explosively, are necessary if most muscle fibers, especially fast-twitch fibers, are to be recruited in contraction. In fact, in terms of recruitment, loads of 80% or higher are even better. Using high loads with few reps results in significant CNS adaptation: better coordination of the muscles involved in a kinetic chain and an increased capacity to recruit fast-twitch fibers.

These changes are the reasons that maximum strength and explosive power training are also called nervous system training (Schmidtbleicher 1984; Enoka 2015). In addition, as Goldberg and colleagues (1975) and Hessel et al. (2017) suggested, the stimulus for protein synthesis is the tension developed in the myofilaments, and in the giant titin protein filament, that is further proof that MxS training should be carried out mainly with high loads (80% to 95%).

To produce the most MxS improvement that transfers to the sport-specific activity, the prime movers must do the greatest amount of work. Coaches should plan training sessions with the highest number of sets per prime mover that the athlete can tolerate (3 to 8). Because this approach is possible only with a low number of prime mover exercises (no more than 5), coaches should resist the temptation to use higher numbers of exercises.

Exercises can be classified as either prime mover or accessory. Prime mover exercises lie at the core of the strength program, and their loading parameters are those of the MxS phase. Accessory exercises are isolation exercises aimed at addressing individual weaknesses or supporting the strength increase in a prime mover exercise—for example, using an adductor machine for an athlete deficient in adductor strength or the French press to increase an athlete's bench-press strength. Given the nature of accessory exercises, their loads are lower, and their rep counts higher, than those of the prime mover exercises.

Table 10.1 provides the training parameters for the submaximum load method (MxS-I) and table 10.2 provides the training parameters for the maximum load method (MxS-II). Note: Training the accessory muscles is suggested mostly for medium-level athletes, such as U19 and U21. For high class/international level athletes, accessory exercises have very limited benefits since many accessory muscles are activated during training for prime movers via a physiological principle of irradiation (Enoka 2015). When prime movers are stimulated and do contract, the activation of these muscles spreads to the entire area of a joint, innervating the accessory muscles as well.

When using a high load, the number of reps per set is kept low (1 to 5), and the suggested total number of reps per exercise for a training session is between 6 and 25. The number

Table 10.1   Training Parameters for the Submaximum Load Method (MxS-I), Suggested Mostly for U19 and U21

Load	70%-80% (up to 100% for 1RM testing every 3 or 4 weeks)
Number of exercises	2-5 prime mover 2 or 3 accessory
Number of reps per set	3-6 prime mover 8-12 accessory
Number of sets per exercise	3-8 prime mover 1-3 accessory
Rest interval	2-3 minutes prime mover 1-2 minutes accessory
Total sets per session	16-24
Frequency per week	2-4 (usually 3)

Table 10.2   Training Parameters for the Maximum Load Method (MxS-II), Suggested for National- and International-Level Athletes

Load	80% to 95% of 1RM (up to 100% for 1RM testing every 3 or 4 weeks)
Number of exercises	2-5 prime mover
Number of reps per set	1-3 prime mover
Number of sets per exercise	3-8 prime mover
Rest interval	3-5 minutes prime mover
Total sets per session	16-24
Frequency per week	2-4 (usually 3)

of reps per exercise varies depending on the athlete's classification, training background, and training phase. To stimulate the necessary physiological and morphological CNS changes, a higher number of sets should always take precedence over a higher number of reps. See table 10.3 for the number of reps per exercise proposed per training session.

The number of prime mover exercises dictates whether to use the lower or higher number of total reps (see table 10.3). Athletes performing five fundamental exercises should use the lower number, whereas those performing two fundamental exercises should use the higher number. If the number of total reps is much lower than recommended, maximum strength benefits decline seriously. These suggestions should reinforce the wisdom of selecting a low number of exercises—the fewer the exercises, the more sets and reps the athlete can perform, and the greater the maximum strength improvement will be for the prime movers.

Figure 10.1 shows a sample nine-week progression, passing from the submaximum load method to the maximum load method. The notation of load, number of reps, and number of sets is expressed as follows: For example, under week 1 in figure 10.1, the numerator (e.g., 72.5) refers to the load as a percentage of 1RM, the denominator (e.g., 5) represents the number of reps, and the multiplier (e.g., 4) indicates the number of sets.

During each of the low steps, a 1RM testing session is planned for the latter part of the week, when the athlete has better recovered from the strain of the preceding high step. For the low step, the load is always decreased (by 5%-10%), and the number of total reps per exercise is reduced (50%).

Table 10.3 Proposed Number of Reps per Exercise per Training Session in the Maximum Strength Phase (MxS)

Percent of 1RM	Reps per set	Suggested range of reps and sets per session	Range of total reps per session
70-75	5-8	4×3 to 5×5	12-25
75-80	3-5	4×2 to 5×4	8-20
80-85	2-3	4×2 to 5×3	8-15
85-90	1 or 2	6×1 to 5×2	6-10
90-95	1	3×1 to 6×1	3-6

MXS-I (SUBMAXIMUM LOAD METHOD)						MXS-II (MAXIMUM LOAD METHOD)		
Week 1	Week 2	Week 3	Week 4	Week 5	Week 6	Week 7	Week 8	Week 9
$\frac{72.5}{5}$ 4	$\frac{75}{5}$ 4	$\frac{70}{5}$ 2	$\frac{77.5}{4}$ 3	$\frac{80}{3}$ 4	$\frac{75}{4}$ 2	$\frac{85}{3}$ 3	$\frac{90}{2}$ 4	$\frac{80}{2}$ 2
LOADING PATTERN								

	High				High		High	
Medium				Medium		Medium		
		Low				Low		Low

Figure 10.1 Sample nine-week progression passing from the submaximum load method to the maximum load method.

Rest Interval

The rest interval between sets is based on the athlete's fitness level and should be calculated to ensure adequate recovery of the neuromuscular system. For the submaximum load method, a rest of two to three minutes between sets is sufficient for both CNS and ATP-CP recovery. For the maximum load method, a three- to five-minute rest interval is necessary because maximum loads heavily tax the CNS, which therefore takes longer to recover. If the rest interval is much shorter, CNS participation could plummet in terms of maximum concentration, motivation, and the power of nerve impulses sent to the contracting muscles (Robinson et al. 1995; Pincivero, Lephart, and Karunakara 1997; Pincivero and Campy 2004; de Salles et al. 2010). Insufficient rest may also jeopardize complete restoration of the required fuel for contraction (ATP-CP).

Exercise Order

Ordering exercises to ensure better alternation of muscle groups facilitates local muscle recovery between sets. Four approaches have been developed for sequencing exercises in order to maximize muscle group involvement

- *Vertical sequence.* Our suggestion is to perform one set of each exercise from the top to the bottom of the exercise list and then repeat until all the prescribed sets are performed (vertical sequence).

- *Horizontal sequence.* Others, particularly bodybuilders, choose to perform all sets for the first exercise before moving on to the next exercise (horizontal sequence). For best hypertrophy gains, you may use the horizontal sequence

- *Jump set.* Also a preference of some bodybuilders, it is combination of the vertical and horizontal approaches. In this sequence, the athlete alternates one set each of a pair of antagonist muscle exercises until the planned number of sets per exercise has been reached, then proceeds to another pair of antagonist muscles. For example:
  - *A1*: Squat
  - *A2*: Leg curl
  - *B1*: Bench press
  - *B2*: Arm pull-down

- *Mini circuit.* This approach is mostly suitable for team sports because of the high number of athletes training simultaneously and the needs of effectively organizing training time. In this approach, the exercises are divided into groups—such as upper body, lower body, core, and plyometrics—and performed in a circuit by rotating groups of athletes, who pass from one set of stations to the next.

Compared to all the other methods, the vertical approach provides the best recovery between sets, lower local and central fatigue, and decreased hypertrophic response. The vertical approach is particularly suited for macrocycles using the maximum load method.

When an athlete performs an exercise for a given joint, say squats or leg press, targeting mainly the quadriceps (knee extensors), the bioelectrical muscle activation is sent across to the hip extensors, too, such as the semimembranosus, the semitendinosus, and the long head of the biceps femoris. The prime mover for this exercise is the quadriceps. The training effect is not beneficial just to the quadriceps, however; thanks to synergy, it also improves the strength of the hip extensors as well as the stabilizers and accessory muscles (such as the erector spinae in the case of the squat). *Synergy* is an essential concept (Enoka 2015) that instructors should consider when selecting exercises for MxS.

When planning an MxS session, try to be as selective as possible with regard to exercises, choosing a lower number of exercises that effectively target the prime movers. The lower the number of exercises, the higher the number of sets and, as a result, the higher the physiological adaptation and training benefit.

It justifies why coaches can select a lower number of exercises, to primarily target the prime movers, but also why less emphasis should be given to accessory muscle. This essential physiological concept allows athletes to be more time- and energy-efficient, to concentrate mostly on prime movers. Top athletes are already greatly taxed and in need of more time for recovery-regeneration-compensation activities.

In our era of extreme commercialism, the abundance of exercises selected for a training session seems to be more important than the quality and efficiency of the training. Once again, soccer seems to be the sport in which the main concern of instructors is how many exercises they plan for training and not necessarily how beneficial these exercises are to the needs of the athlete. Many exercises are variations of agility types of exercises. Strength training, the prerequisite for developing power, maximum speed, and agility, has an incredibly low significance. Yet, some instructors seem to miss an essential law of training: the higher the number of exercises, the lower the benefits for individual muscles, particularly the prime movers.

Speed of Contraction

Speed of contraction plays an important role in submaximum and maximum load training. Athletic movements are often performed fast and explosively, and for this reason athletes should perform explosive concentric actions almost all year long during strength training (the AA phase could be an exception). To maximize speed, the entire neuromuscular system must adapt to quickly recruiting fast-twitch muscle fibers—a key factor in all sports dominated by speed and power. Therefore, even with the maximum loads typical of the maximum load method, the athlete's force application against resistance must be exerted as quickly as possible, even explosively. The will to apply as much force as possible in the shortest amount of time, or to accelerate the bar or training machine as much as possible, is fundamental for the transfer of the neuromuscular adaptations to strength training to the specific sport activity. That is why maximum strength and power training require a high level of motivation in each repetition.

To achieve dynamic or explosive force, the athlete must maximize concentration and motivation before each set, concentrating on contracting or activating the muscles quickly. Only a high speed of contraction performed against a submaximum or maximum load will quickly recruit fast-twitch fibers, resulting in the highest increase in maximum strength and power (González-Badillo et al. 2014). For maximum training benefits, athletes must mobilize all strength potentials in the shortest time possible from the early part of the lift.

In the case of maximum loads, such as 90% 1RM, the speed of contraction looks slow but the application of concentric force against resistance has to be maximal in order to recruit the highest number of fast-twitch muscle fibers necessary to overcome the load.

Loading Pattern

Considering the high demand placed on the neuromuscular system, most athletes should perform submaximum and maximum load training no more than two to three times a week. Only elite athletes, particularly shot-putters and American football linemen, should do this training four times a week. During the competitive phase, this can be reduced to one to two maximum load sessions per week, often performed in combination with other strength components, such as power.

Figure 10.2 shows the MxS phase of a strength training program for Olympic-class sprinters. To better exemplify the step method for load increment, the step loading pattern is illustrated graphically at the bottom of the chart. This nine-week program is repeated twice a year because sprinters usually follow a bi-cycle annual plan. A testing session is planned in each of the low steps and is performed in the latter part of the week, when the athlete has better recovered from the strain of a high step. For the low step, the load is always decreased (by 10%-20%), and the number of sets is reduced (by 30%-50%). The goal of the test, of course, is to determine the new 100% (1RM) so that it can be used to calculate the load for the following three-week cycle. The discrepancy in the number of sets results from the fact that prime movers are given high priority, whereas accessory exercises are of relatively low concern. In this way, most of the athlete's energy and concentration is focused on the high-priority exercises.

Figure 10.3 shows a sample six-week maximum strength program for a college-level women's volleyball team. In the program, force was applied aggressively without jerking or snapping. During the rest interval, the limbs used were shaken to relax the muscles. Dumbbells were used for deadlifts. The program was repeated three times a week.

Figure 10.4 illustrates a flat loading pattern used for a world heavyweight boxing champion. The training strategy was designed to address the fact that the boxer was not very fast in initiating attacks against his opponents, nor did he throw enough punches to overcome his rivals. Therefore, a strategy to correct his shortcomings was designed: (1) to stimulate his aggressiveness and initiate constant charges during the match, and (2) to increase his ability to throw more punches to dominate his opponents.

Because in boxing, tactical charges against the opponents are initiated by the ankles (gastrocnemius and soleus) and the knees (quadriceps), an MxS program was designed to improve the force of these muscles (see figure 10.4).

Exercise	Rest interval (min.)	WEEK								
		1	2	3	4	5	6	7	8	9
1. Half squat	3	$\frac{75}{3}$ 4	$\frac{80}{3}$ 3	$\frac{75}{2}$ 3	$\frac{85}{3}$ 3	$\frac{90}{3}$ 4	$\frac{70}{1}$ 4	$\frac{85}{2}$ 3	$\frac{90}{2}$ 4	$\frac{70}{1}$ 4
2. Bench press	3	$\frac{75}{3}$ 4	$\frac{80}{3}$ 3	$\frac{70}{1}$ 4	$\frac{80}{3}$ 3	$\frac{85}{3}$ 3	$\frac{70}{1}$ 4	$\frac{85}{2}$ 3	$\frac{90}{2}$ 3	$\frac{70}{1}$ 4
3. Lat pull-down	2	$\frac{75}{3}$ 3	$\frac{80}{4}$ 3	$\frac{80}{3}$ 3	$\frac{85}{3}$ 3	$\frac{85}{4}$ 4	$\frac{80}{3}$ 3	$\frac{85}{3\text{-}4}$ 3	$\frac{90}{4}$ 2-3	$\frac{75}{3}$ 3
4. Leg curl	2	3 × 10	3 × 10	1 × 10	3 × 8	3 × 8	1 × 8	3 × 6	3 × 6	1 × 6
5. Standing calf raise	2	$\frac{80}{5}$ 3	$\frac{85}{4}$ 4	$\frac{80}{3}$ 3	$\frac{85}{4}$ 4	$\frac{90}{4}$ 4	$\frac{80}{3}$ 3	$\frac{90}{4}$ 2-3	$\frac{95}{2}$ 4	1 × $\frac{80}{3}$ 3

LOADING PATTERN

				High			High	
	Medium		Medium			Medium		
Low		Low			Low			Low

Figure 10.2 Sample maximum strength phase of an Olympic-class sprinter.

Exercise	WEEK					
	1	2	3	4	5	6
1. Half squat	$\frac{70}{5}$ 3	$\frac{75}{4}$ 3	$\frac{80}{3}$ 3	$\frac{75}{2}$ 2	$\frac{85}{3}$ 3	$\frac{90}{2}$ 3
2. Lat pull-down	$\frac{70}{5}$ 3	$\frac{75}{4}$ 3	$\frac{80}{3}$ 3	$\frac{75}{2}$ 2	$\frac{85}{3}$ 3	$\frac{90}{2}$ 3
3. Romanian deadlift	$\frac{70}{5}$ 3	$\frac{75}{4}$ 3	$\frac{80}{3}$ 3	$\frac{75}{2}$ 2	$\frac{85}{3}$ 3	$\frac{90}{2}$ 3
4. Incline dumbbell press	$\frac{70}{5}$ 3	$\frac{75}{4}$ 3	$\frac{80}{3}$ 3	$\frac{75}{2}$ 2	$\frac{85}{3}$ 3	$\frac{90}{2}$ 3
5. Calf raise	2 × 12	2 × 10	1 × 10	2 × 8	2 × 6	1 × 6
6. External rotator (sagittal)	2 × 15	2 × 12	1 × 12	2 × 10	2 × 8	1 × 8
7. Weighted crunch	2 × 12	2 × 10	1 × 10	2 × 8	2 × 6	1 × 6

LOADING PATTERN

		High			High
	Medium			Medium	
Low			Low		

When selecting the Romanian deadlift exercise, please make sure the athletes have a decent background, particularly for the intervertebral or extensor muscles of the back

Figure 10.3 Sample six-week maximum strength phase for a college-level women's volleyball team.

Number	Exercises	Week 1	Week 2	Weeks 3-6	Rest interval
1	Half squat or chinbone squat	$\frac{75}{8}$ 3	$\frac{80}{6}$ 4	$\frac{85}{4}$ 4	4
2	Bench press	$\frac{70}{8}$ 3	$\frac{80}{6}$ 4	$\frac{85}{4}$ 4	4
3	Calf raise/calf press	$\frac{80}{7}$ 4	$\frac{85}{8}$ 4	$\frac{85}{4}$ 4	3

Figure 10.4 An example of a six-week MxS using the flat loading pattern.

Isometric Method

The isometric training method was known and used for some time before Hettinger and Müller (1953) and again Hettinger (1966) scientifically justified the merits of static contractions in the development of maximum strength. This method's popularity peaked in the 1960s, then faded. Although static contraction has little functional effect overall, it is still useful for the development of maximum strength and can be used in strength training by fighters in grappling, Brazilian jujitsu, mixed martial arts, sailboat racing, windsurfing, or any other sport where the activity requires repeated or prolonged isometric contractions. Static conditions can be realized through two techniques: (1) attempting to lift a weight heavier than one's potential and (2) applying force (by pushing or pulling) against an immobile object.

An isometric contraction produces high tension in the muscle, which makes this method most useful during the MxS phase, although it can be used for specific muscular endurance, too, if required. Even if, as some enthusiasts claim, isometric training can increase maximum strength by 10 to 15% more than other methods, however, it has clear limitations in the development of power. In fact, maximum strength gains obtained through the isometric method cannot be applied readily to dynamic contractions because they do not shift the force–time curve to the left, a disadvantage that must not be ignored.

As isometric force is applied against a given resistance, the tension in the muscle builds progressively, reaching maximum in about two or three seconds and, toward the end, decreasing in a much shorter time (one or two seconds). Because training benefits are angle specific, each invovled muscle group must be trained at sport-specific angles. For instance, if the range of motion of a joint is 180 degrees, and the isometric actions usually encountered during the sport-specific activity are at 180 and 45 degrees, then those are the angles at which the isometric contractions must be performed in training, either in isolation or interspersed in the eccentric–concentric motion of an exercise (this approach is referred to as *functional isometrics*).

The isometric method can also be used to rehabilitate injured muscles. Because no joint motion occurs, "the athlete may continue training even with a joint or bone injury" (Hartmann and Tünnemann 1988). This approach can certainly reduce the risk of muscular atrophy.

As stated previously, strength development is angle specific. In fact, to be more precise, strength increases in a range of 15 degrees—7.5 above and below the angle at which the isometric contraction is performed. Athletes with heart, blood pressure, or circulation problems are strongly discouraged from engaging in isometric training because blood flow is temporarily stopped in the isometrically contracted muscle, which increases blood pressure and might have severe consequences for people with such health conditions.

Achieving maximum transferable gains with isometric training requires the athlete to perform exercises that are as similar as possible to the sport-specific angle of force application. The isometric method should be used primarily by advanced athletes in combination with other maximum strength methods. See table 10.4 for training parameters.

Isometric contraction can be performed with all the limbs using angles ranging from completely open to fully bent. The following issues should be considered.

- Isometric training is most effective when contraction is near maximum (80%-100%).

- For maximum strength at sport-specific angles, a single contraction can range from 6 to 8 seconds, for a total of 30 to 50 seconds per muscle per training session.

- The training load is intensified by increasing either the load or the number of sets—not the duration of contraction.

Table 10.4 Training Parameters for the Isometric Method

Load	80%-100% of 1RM
Number of exercises	2-4
Number of sets per session	6-8
Duration of contraction per set	6-8 seconds for maximum strength; longer for specific muscle endurance
Total duration of isometric contractions per session	30-50 seconds for maximum strength; longer for specific muscle endurance
Rest interval	60-90 seconds
Frequency per week	2 or 3

- During the 60- to 90-second rest interval, relaxation and breathing exercises are recommended. Performance of breathing exercises is a compensatory necessity because static contraction is performed in a state of apnea (holding the breath). In addition, this training increases intrathoracic pressure, which restricts circulation and thus oxygen supply.

- For a more effective program, static contractions should be alternated with isotonic contractions, especially in sports that require speed and power.

- A more effective variant of the isometric method is the functional isometric contraction, which involves free weights. This variant combines isometric with isotonic exercises. The athlete executes the lift to a certain angle, then holds it for 3 to 6 seconds. While working through the entire range of motion, the athlete may stop two to four times at sport-specific angles and for sport-specific durations, thus combining the isotonic and isometric methods. This variant provides better physiological benefit (hence the term *functional*), especially for sports that have repeated isometric actions.

Eccentric Method

Any strength exercise performed with free weights, or with most isokinetic equipment, employs both concentric and eccentric actions. During the concentric phase, force is produced while the muscle shortens; during the eccentric phase, force is produced as the muscle lengthens.

Both practice and scientific research on the physiology of eccentric training have demonstrated that the eccentric phase always seems to be easier than the concentric phase. For example, when performing a bench press, the return of the barbell to the chest (the eccentric part of the lift) always seems easier than the lift itself. One could logically conclude that because an athlete can work with heavier loads during the eccentric action, strength is improved to higher levels by using the eccentric method alone. Researchers have indeed concluded that eccentric training creates higher tension in the muscles than isometric or isotonic contractions do. In turn, because higher muscle tension normally means higher strength development (Goldberg et al. 1975), eccentric training is considered a superior training method than concentric and isometric (Roig et al. 2009; Hassel et al. 2017; Franchi et al. 2017).

Other researchers have found that gains in maximum strength appear to result mostly from changes in neural activation rather than from hypertrophic response (Dudley and Fleck 1987; Mallinson et al. 2020).

This finding means that MxS improvements do not result mainly from gains in muscle mass but rather from specific neural adaptations, such as an increase in fast-twitch muscle fiber recruitment (intramuscular coordination), increased strength with little or no hypertrophy, and modifications in the neural commands used to control movement (intermuscular coordination), resulting in increased strength with little or no hypertrophy.

The CNS commands the eccentric contraction differently from the concentric one. This process occurs mostly as grading, or ranking, the amount of muscle activation necessary to complete a task (Enoka 1996 and 2015). Specifically, the amount of muscle activation and the number of fibers involved are proportional to the training load. The neural command for eccentric contraction is unique in that it decides (1) which motor units should be activated, (2) how much they need to be activated, (3) when they should be activated, and (4) how the activity should be distributed within a group of muscles (Abbruzzese et al. 1994).

Because muscles resist fatigue and prevent muscle soreness during eccentric action, such activity can be maintained longer than concentric (Tesch et al. 1978; Hody et al. 2019), possibly because of the altered recruitment order of motor units. In addition, the load in eccentric training can be much higher than the load in the maximum concentric contraction (up to 140% of the concentric 1RM).

When using supermaximum loads (for very advanced athletes, and only for one or two exercises, for a limited amount of time), one or two spotters (depending on the exercise and the athlete's strength level) are needed to help the athlete lift the barbell for the concentric phase because the load for eccentric training is higher than 1RM. The spotters should also ensure that as the bar is lowered, the athlete does not let it drop, which can cause injury. The need for careful assistance as the bar is slowly lowered makes it impossible to perform the exercise quickly.

During the first few days of eccentric training, athletes may experience muscle soreness. This is to be expected because higher tension provokes more muscle damage. As athletes adapt, the muscle soreness disappears (in 5-7 days). Short-term discomfort can be avoided by increasing the load in steps.

As expected, the eccentric method shifts the force–time curve to the left. Heavy loads that generate high tension in the muscles improve strength because they result in high recruitment of the powerful fast-twitch motor units. The eccentric method is particularly useful for strengthening muscle groups whose peak of activation is encountered during an eccentric phase, such as the biceps femoris in the sprinting cycle.

The supramaximum eccentric training method should be used only by athletes with at least five years of strength training because it employs the heaviest loads (110%-140% of 1RM). The eccentric method should always be limited to one or two muscle groups and should be combined with other methods, especially the maximum load method. Eccentric contractions should not be used excessively. Every time an athlete uses maximum or supramaximum loads, maximal mental concentration is required, which can be psychologically wearing. Therefore, athletes should use the eccentric method carefully—no more than twice a week—in combination with MxS training. In addition, the use of active recovery techniques eliminates discomfort, reduces soreness, and encourages faster regeneration.

Training parameters for the eccentric method are shown in table 10.5. The range of the load is presented as the percentage of maximum strength capacity for the concentric contraction and suggests a resistance between 110% and 140%. Athletes at all levels should be progressed from lower loads up to the highest load allowed by their capabilities.

ECCENTRIC TRAINING PROGRESSION FOR THE HAMSTRINGS

For an advanced athlete using a leg curl machine, a coach can plan the maximum strength development of the hamstrings this way:

- MxS-I (3+1) $\frac{77.5}{5}$ 3 $\frac{80}{4}$ 4 $\frac{82.5}{3}$ 4 $\frac{80}{3}$ 2 (ecc-conc)

- MxS-II (3+1) $\frac{85}{3}$ 3 $\frac{87.5}{3}$ 4 $\frac{90}{3}$ 4 $\frac{85}{3}$ 2 (ecc-conc)

- MxS-II (2+1) $\frac{100}{3}$ 3 $\frac{110}{3}$ 4 $\frac{90}{3}$ 2 (ecc only)

Because the load is supramaximum, the speed of contraction is slow. Such loads should be used only after at least four seasons of MxS training.

The rest interval is also an important element in the athlete's capacity to perform highly demanding work. If an athlete does not recover well enough between sets to complete the next set at the same level—insufficient recovery is indicated by the inability to perform the eccentric phase in the time allowed—the rest interval must be increased accordingly. Other important factors include the athlete's motivation and concentration capacity. Because eccentric actions involve such heavy loads, athletes must be highly motivated and able to concentrate in order to perform them effectively.

The eccentric method should never be performed in isolation from the other MxS methods. Even during the maximum strength phase, the eccentric method is used with the maximum load method; therefore, only one eccentric training session per muscle group is suggested per week.

Figure 10.5 shows the last three weeks of a nine-week program developed for an international-class shot-putter. A three-week conversion-to-power phase followed, then two weeks of unloading prior to an important competition.

Table 10.5 Training Parameters for the Eccentric Method

Load	110%-140% of 1RM
Number of exercises per session	1 or 2
Number of reps per set	1-5
Number of sets per exercise	2-4
Rest interval	2-8 minutes, depending on the size of the muscle group
Speed of execution	Slow (3-6 seconds, depending on the range of motion of the exercise)
Frequency per week	1 or 2

Exercise	WEEK		
	7	8	9
1. Squat (eccentric)	$\frac{110}{5}$ 3	$\frac{120}{4}$ 3	$\frac{130}{3}$ 3
2. Incline bench press (eccentric)	$\frac{110}{5}$ 3	$\frac{120}{4}$ 3	$\frac{130}{3}$ 3
3. Back hyperextension	$\frac{80}{3}$ 3	$\frac{85}{2}$ 3	$\frac{90}{1}$ 3
4. Calf raise	$\frac{80}{5}$ 3	$\frac{85}{3}$ 3	$\frac{90}{3}$ 3
5. Jump squat	$\frac{70}{5}$ 3	$\frac{70}{5}$ 3	$\frac{70}{5}$ 3

Figure 10.5 Last three weeks of a nine-week program for an international-class shot-putter.

Maxex Training

Maximum tension exercises can be combined with exercises requiring dynamic contraction, or explosiveness. This method, which combines maximum strength exercises with high loads with exercises for explosiveness, is called *maxex training*.

Motor unit force is determined by the rate at which the CNS sends firing signals, called *action potentials*, from the motor neuron to the muscle fibers. A higher rate means a greater magnitude of motor unit force. As the frequency of the action potentials increases, tetanus (a state of continuous muscle contraction) changes from an irregular force profile to a *fused tetanus*, or plateau profile (Enoka 2002, Enoka 2015). The peak force of a fused tetanus represents the maximum force that a motor unit can exert.

The goal of maximum strength exercises with very high loads performed before explosive exercises, then, is to create a period in which the motor units of the prime movers are maximally activated to produce the greatest possible force. This is really the only way to physiologically produce maximum force output. To this end, the maxex training discussed here, at its best, can be used to combine maximum force with exercises for explosiveness. More specifically, it can elicit a high level of motor unit recruitment and force production before the athlete performs a high-discharge-rate power exercise such as plyometrics. MxS methods can be combined with plyometrics for all team sports; for sprinting, jumping, and throwing events in track and field; for the martial arts, boxing, and wrestling; for alpine skiing and ski jumping; for fencing; for diving; for figure skating; and for sprint events in swimming.

The variations of training proposed here need not be performed year-round. They can be planned at the end of the preparatory phase or, in the case of a long maximum strength phase, during the last macrocycle, as well as during the maintenance phase, where the maxex method excels at maintaining the strength and power levels reached in the previous phases. A maximum strength phase is still necessary before any power/maxex training because power is a function of maximum strength. The incorporation of power training during the maximum strength phase enhances speed, agility, and explosiveness to ready the athlete for the competitive phase.

However, combining maximum strength with power must be done carefully and conservatively. Although many combinations are possible, training must be simple so that athletes can focus on the main task of the workout or training phase. The more variations coaches use, the more they may confuse their athletes and disrupt the way their athletes' bodies adapt.

The concept of maxex training relies on science—specifically, manipulating two physiological concepts to produce speed, agility, and explosiveness, and thereby improve athletic performance. The first part of the maxex routine is performed against a heavy (85%-95% of 1RM) load, which stimulates high recruitment of fast-twitch muscle fibers. The follow-up explosive or quickness movements increase the firing rate of the fast-twitch muscle fibers, preparing the athlete for the quick, explosive actions required for all speed and power sports during the competitive phase.

Maxex training is suggested for the prime movers only via multijoint exercises. Because this training method can be quite stressful mentally and physically, only athletes with a good background in strength training should use it. The duration of maxex training should be approximately two to three weeks, depending on the athlete's background. Maxex training should follow a maximum strength phase in which eccentric–concentric contraction has been used. One or two training sessions per week with at least 48 hours of rest between bouts are suggested.

Maxex training applies to the upper body as well as to the lower body. Strong arms and shoulders are essential in various sports, including basketball, baseball, ice hockey, football, lacrosse, the martial arts, boxing, wrestling, rowing, kayaking, squash, European handball, water polo, wrestling, and throwing events in track and field. Without exhausting all options, exercises that can be applied in these sports for maxex training include drop jumps, jump squats, drop push-ups, short sprints, hurdle jumps, and medicine ball throws.

During the maximum strength phase, athletes can combine maximum strength methods with some of the following variations or with plyometrics (either low or medium impact). Coaches should consider the following methods.

- *Isometric-dynamic.* This is a near-maximal or maximal isometric contraction immediately followed by a plyometric contraction for the same kinetic chain. Perform 1 or 2 sets of 3 to 4 reps of four to six seconds per isometric contraction. Each set is followed by a very short sprint or by 3 to 5 plyometric reps (reactive jumps). Take at least three minutes of rest between reps and five minutes between sets.

- *Complex drill.* For better exemplification, we use the squat exercise (for sprinters, jumpers, throwers, volleyball spikers, and the contact and martial art). The athlete performs 1 or 2 sets using a load of 80% to 85% of 1RM in the following sequence: (1) slow eccentric contraction, (2) isometric contraction for one or two seconds in the deepest part of the squat, and (3) concentric contraction with maximum acceleration. Immediately afterward, the athlete does a very short sprint or 3 to 5 plyometrics. Alternatively, the athlete uses the quarter squat for 2 sets of two dymamic reps with 150% of the full-squat 1RM, followed immediately by a very short sprint or 3 to 5 plyometrics.

Both these techniques increase speed, reactivity, explosive strength, and especially the discharge rate of fast-twitch muscle fibers.

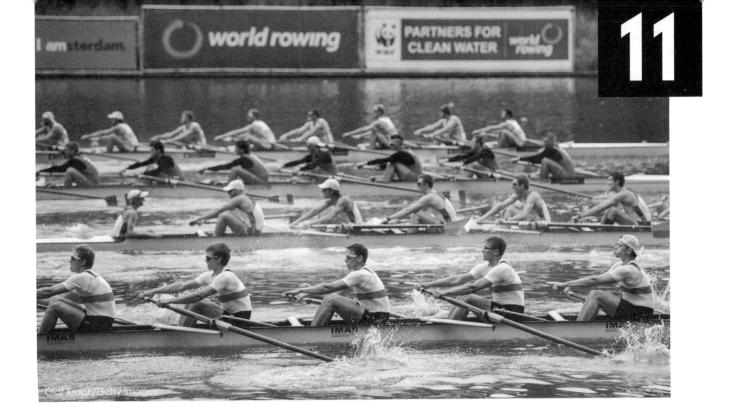
Olaf Kraak/Getty Images

Conversion to Specific Strength

Today, almost every athlete uses some sort of strength training program to improve performance. Most strength programs, however, fail to transform the strength gains made during the MxS training phase into sport- or event-specific strength, such as power or muscular endurance. This failure prevents athletes from maximizing their athletic potential in order to increase their sport performance in tasks requiring speed, agility, or prolonged effort. Periodization of strength, on the other hand, is designed precisely to produce such transformations during the conversion phase so that the athlete achieves peak performance during main competitions.

The loading parameters used in the conversion stage should reflect the characteristics of the sport, particularly the relationship between strength and the dominant energy system. Table 11.1 shows how an event's duration and intensity of effort determine the energy systems, and therefore the specific strength, that must be trained.

During the year, the goals of strength training and their consistent methods vary depending on the characteristics of the sport, the characteristics of the athlete, and the competition calendar. The ultimate goal, however, is the maximization of specific strength. In relation to this final objective of strength training periodization, we can distinguish two main types of sports:

Table 11.1 Event Duration and Specific Strength Conversion

Event duration	Event intensity	Main energy system	Specific strength
<10 seconds	Maximum	ATP-CP	Power
10-30 seconds	Maximum to very high	Anaerobic glycolysis (power)	Power endurance
30 seconds to 2 minutes	High	Anaerobic glycolysis (capacity)/ aerobic glycolysis (power)	Muscular endurance short
2-8 minutes	Moderately high	Aerobic glycolysis (power)	Muscular endurance medium
>8 minutes	Moderately high to low	Aerobic glycolysis (power to capacity)/fat oxidation (capacity)	Muscular endurance long

1. Sports that require power (a synonym for what is sometimes called "speed-strength," or starting strength and explosive strength in the force–time curve)—that is, the ability to apply force as quickly as possible, as in the jumps, throws, and sprints in athletics, most team sports, and all sports in which power strongly influences performance.

2. Sports that require muscular endurance—that is, the ability to apply less force for a longer time, as in most events in swimming, rowing, kayaking, triathlon, cross-country skiing, and middle- and long-distance running.

The human body can adapt to any environment and therefore any type of training. If an athlete is trained with bodybuilding methods, which is often the case in North America, the neuromuscular system adapts to those methods. More specifically, because bodybuilding methods focus on a slow rate of contraction, they increase muscle size (hypertrophy) but do not increase power, speed, agility, or quickness. An athlete who trains in this way should not be expected to display fast, explosive power, because his or her neuromuscular system has not been trained for it.

To develop sport-specific power, a training program must be specifically designed to achieve that objective. Such a program must be specific to the sport or event and must use exercises that simulate the physiological and biomechanical characteristics of the sport's skills as closely as possible. Because power training addresses muscles at a high degree of specificity, inter- and intramuscular coordination become more efficient and the athlete's skill performance becomes smoother, quicker, and more precise.

During the conversion phase, athletes should use more energy for technical and tactical training than they do for specific strength training. Coaches must plan training with the lowest possible number of exercises that closely relate to the skill. For maximum returns, such programs must be efficient, with two or three exercises performed dynamically over several sets. Time and energy should not be wasted on anything else.

Power Training

Power is the main ingredient for all sports that require a high rate of force, speed, and agility. Sports that are speed and power dominant include sprinting, jumping, and throwing events in track and field; team sports; racket sports; gymnastics; diving; and the martial arts. For an athlete's performance to improve, his or her level of power must improve; indeed, power is the main ingredient necessary to produce a fast, quick, and agile athlete.

People use different terms for power, including *dynamic strength* and the aberrant and confusing terms *strength-speed* (which is, in fact, power training with high loads) and *speed-strength* (which is power training with low loads). If we are committed to employing science in sport training, the correct term should be borrowed from physics and physiology, both of which use the term *power*, which is defined as

- the rate of producing force,
- the product of force and velocity ($P = F \times V$, or force times velocity),
- the amount of work done per time unit, or
- the rate at which muscles can produce work (Enoka 2002).

For athletic purposes, any increase in power must be the result of improvements in either strength, speed, or a combination of the two. An athlete can be very strong, with a large muscle mass, yet be unable to display power because of an inability to contract already strong muscles in a very short time. To overcome this deficiency, the athlete must undergo power training to improve his or her rate of force development.

The advantage of explosive, high-velocity power training is that it trains the central nervous system (CNS). Improvements in performance can be based on neural changes that help individual muscles achieve greater performance capability (Sale 1986; Roig et al. 2009). This gain is accomplished by shortening the time required for motor unit recruitment, especially of fast-twitch fibers (Häkkinen 1986; Häkkinen and Komi 1983; Ekoka 2015).

Power training exercises activate and increase the discharge rate of fast-twitch muscle fibers leading to specific CNS adaptations. Adaptation, especially in well-trained athletes, shows itself in the form of discharging a greater number of muscle fibers in a very short time. Both training practice and research have shown that such adaptations require considerable time and that they progress from year to year.

Adaptation to power training is further evidenced by better intermuscular coordination, or the ability of agonist and antagonist muscles to cooperate in order to perform a movement. This coordination is achieved through better linkage between the excitatory and inhibitory reactions of a muscle in a complex motor pattern. As a result of such adaptation, the CNS learns when and when not to send a nerve impulse that signals the muscle to contract and perform a movement. In practical terms, improved intermuscular coordination enhances the athlete's ability to contract some muscles and relax others (e.g., to relax the antagonist muscles), which improves the speed of contraction of the prime movers—the agonist muscles.

During the conversion phase—except for the conversion to muscular endurance long—exercises must be performed quickly and explosively in order to recruit the highest number of motor units at the highest rate of contraction (in other words, at an increased discharge rate). Especially for the conversion to power, the entire program should be geared to achieving only one goal: moving the force–time curve as far to the left as possible so that the neuromuscular system is trained to display force explosively. Coaches should select only those training methods that fulfill the requirements of power development—that is, methods that enhance quickness, facilitate explosive application of force, and increase the reactivity of the relevant muscles.

The methods presented in this chapter can be used separately or in combination. When they are combined, the total work per session must be distributed among them.

Physiological Strategy to Increase Power

Some sport practitioners and authors maintain the philosophy that athletes who want to increase power should do only power drills all year long, that athletes who want to be fast should do only short reps with high speed, and that athletes who want to be quick and agile should do only agility drills. This training philosophy takes to the extreme the fundamental physiological principle that a given type of work results in a specific adaptation but contradicts the methodological principle that specific adaptations are maximized on the base of general adaptations, especially for low-trainability biomotor abilities such as speed.

Athletes who maintain the same type of work for longer periods of time experience a plateau, a stagnation of improvement, or even a slight detraining, which results in performance deterioration. To prevent this outcome, and to ensure that athletes consistently improve their power in order to benefit their performance during the competitive phase, they must constantly stimulate their neuromuscular system to produce the highest voluntary recruitment of fast-twitch muscle fibers and display higher levels of muscular strength more quickly. This stimulation can be achieved by applying the training methods of the periodization of strength.

Research shows that using lighter loads exclusively produces a more modest increase in peak power than is produced by using heavier loads. In fact, the greatest increases in power are obtained not from higher-velocity training but from a combination of high force and high velocity training (Aagaard et al. 1994; Verkhoshansky 1997; Enoka 2002). Indeed, the peak power that a muscle can produce depends directly on gains in maximum strength (Fitts and Widrick 1996).

The same is true for speed. As trainers have known since the 1950s, maximum velocity does not increase unless power is increased first. These findings validate and add more substance to the theory of periodization of strength, allowing us to draw the conclusion that speed, agility, and quickness never increase unless maximum strength is trained first and then converted to power.

With these realities in mind, we propose two training phases to maximize power, speed, agility, and quickness (see figure 11.1).

During the first phase, the scope of training is to train the CNS to recruit the highest number of fast-twitch muscle fibers. This training usually occurs during the MxS phase, in which athletes use loads of more than 70% of 1RM moved explosively. These training loads result in high stimulation of the neuromuscular system, which then recruits high numbers of fast-twitch muscle fibers. To avoid detraining and a loss in strength, maximum strength training sessions should also be planned during the conversion and maintenance phases of the annual plan.

The power exerted during athletic actions depends on the number of active motor units, the number of fast-twitch fibers recruited into the action, and the rate at which those fibers are discharged, producing a high force-to-frequency ratio (Enoka 2002). The increase in the discharge rate of fast-twitch fibers is achieved by training with lighter loads, either by using less than 50%

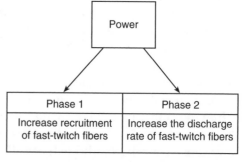

Figure 11.1 The physiological strategy used to increase power, speed, and agility.

of 1RM for novice athletes and between 50% and 60% of 1RM for advanced athletes (Moritani 1992; Van Cutsem, Duchateau, and Hainaut 1998; Enoka 2002) or by using any type of lighter implement (e.g., shots from track and field, power balls, medicine balls) or by performing plyometrics or specific drills for speed, agility, and quickness. Such exercises—performed with maximum power, speed, and quick application of force against the resistance provided by the implement, the pull of gravity, or both—facilitate activation of high-threshold motor units and high frequency of discharge. Such high-velocity exercises are necessary during the second phase when a higher discharge rate of the fast-twitch fibers is sought.

Clearly, then, the main scope of strength training for sports is to continually increase maximum strength so that 50% of 1RM is always higher. This gain, in turn, produces the maximum benefit of increasing peak performance.

Heavy Loads Versus Light Loads in Power Enhancement

Trainers and athletes often debate the rival merits of using heavy loads or light loads to improve power performance. The fact is that both play a role but at different points in training. This is the beauty of periodization: All training methods have a place in the various phases of training.

The speed at which an athlete can perform concentric (shortening) movements—such as pushing a barbell up from the chest during a bench press—depends, of course, on the load that the athlete is using. As the load is increased, the velocity of the shortening activity of the muscles decreases. However, the opposite is true for eccentric or lengthening movements. When performing an eccentric contraction, the force production is greater when the movement is performed at a high velocity. This relationship explains the positive transfer from plyometric exercises to power performance. The intrinsic elastic properties of muscles favor the absorption and reuse of stored elastic energy, which is optimized when a muscle is lengthened as quickly as possible. Therefore, to improve force expression of the full spectrum of velocity and increase the rate of force development, both heavy loads and light loads are necessary in training.

Moderate-velocity strength training (characteristic of the MxS phase) enhances intramuscular coordination because of both motor unit recruitment and the firing rate of motor units. In essence, moderate-velocity training using high resistance leads primarily to improvement in muscular strength. In contrast, high-velocity training (characteristic of power training) involves training with lighter resistances at higher velocities. This type of training increases the rate of force development, which obviously includes a speed component. The exact nature of that component may be a question in itself. One study, for instance, concluded that the *intent* to produce ballistic contractions—not the speed of movement per se—was responsible for a high-velocity training effect (Behm and Sale 1993).

However, because heavy loads cause a very slow angular speed—much lower than the sport-specific one—the transition from MxS training to sport-specific speed is vital in sports that require explosive movement. For example, a long jumper who spends hours squatting will develop a high level of strength, but that strength will not automatically transfer into jump-specific movements that synchronize the use of all prime movers. Such a transfer can be achieved only by performing maxex training, plyometrics, and sport-specific drills.

The degree of emphasis placed on heavy loads versus light loads ultimately depends on the type of sport. The periodization of strength program is characterized by a maximum strength phase (using high loads) followed by a conversion phase (using low loads). The most effective approach is a combination of both, as presented in the periodization model. To explore this issue, one study compared the training of three groups. Group 1 performed heavy squat training, group 2 performed plyometric training with a light load, and group 3 combined squats and plyometric training. Because the largest gain in indexes of power occurred in group 3, the authors concluded that optimal training benefits are acquired by combining heavy-load training with explosive movements (Adams, Worlay, and Throgmartin 1987).

An even more intriguing study, conducted by Verkhoshansky in the 1970s, also compared three groups. Group 1 performed a macrocycle of heavy squat training followed by a macrocycle of plyometrics, group 2 performed a macrocycle of plyometrics followed by a macrocycle of heavy squat training, and group 3 combined both squats and plyometrics for the two macrocycles (that is, engaged in complex training). The third method (complex training) delivered the quickest improvement, but the first sequential method resulted in the highest improvement at the end of the two macrocycles (Verkhoshansky 1997). This is the same approach that we use in the periodization of strength.

Agility Training

Agility training is one of the most misunderstood elements of sport training. Agility refers to an athlete's ability to swiftly change direction, accelerate and decelerate, and rapidly vary movement patterns. Intrinsic elements of agility include proprioception (sensors that inform the CNS regarding the position of the body), anticipation, reactive time, reactive strength, decision making abilities, dynamic flexibility, and effective rhythm and timing of movements. Another element in the efficiency of performing agility drills is learning, where improved intermuscular coordination also has an important role in injury prevention (Wojtys et al. 2001).

Agility as an ability does not exist independently. Rather, it relies on the development of a host of other abilities, such as those just listed, in which the determinant factors are relative strength and power. Without high levels of relative strength and power, no one would ever be agile or quick. The higher an athlete's maximum strength is relative to body weight—that is, the higher his or her relative strength is—the easier it is for the athlete to decelerate and accelerate his or her own body weight. By the same token, the higher the athlete's level of power is, the more quickly he or she can do it. Agility, then, is the ability to accelerate quickly by using concentric strength; to decelerate by using eccentric strength, as in stop-and-go movements; and to change direction or perform the cuts that are so important in many sports, especially team and racket sports.

Some trainers erroneously suggest that agility evolves from speed. This is an obvious misconception because maximum speed itself depends directly on the force application on the ground. Consequently, agility does not improve as expected without consistent activation and increased recruitment of fast-twitch fibers. That calls for strength training. Athletes who repeatedly perform agility drills ultimately reach a plateau and stagnate in their performance of any skills in which agility is a determinant factor. For these reasons, the periodization of agility is based on the physiological strategy suggested earlier, in figure 11.1.

For maximum efficiency of agility training, consider the following guidelines:

- *The impulse is essential in agility training* (as discussed in Part I). The stronger the gastrocnemius, soleus, tibialis anterior, and quadriceps muscles, the shorter the impulse of the stretch–shortening cycle.

- *The higher the force applied on the ground* the higher (but in the opposite direction) the ground reaction, and the more the athlete benefits from it to move more quickly.

- *Maximize propulsion force* by increasing ankle flexibility. An acute angle generates increased force and elastic energy return from the Achilles tendon.

- *Intensity.* Except for learning new drills, most agility training is performed at high intensity, taxing the neuromuscular system, being directly dependent on the neural response and reactivity (neuromuscular training).

- *Duration.* Most agility drills are of short duration, taxing the phosphagen system (5-8 seconds). In addition, for sports where the glycolytic (lactic acid) energy system is an important supplier of energy, agility drills can be extended to 20 to 60 seconds. However, to avoid the detrimental effect of fatigue on intensity and performance, a rest interval of 1 to 2 minutes is advisable for the short drills, and up to 5 minutes for the lactic drills.

- *Placement of agility training in a training session.* Since agility training is of high intensity, it should be placed immediately after the warm-up, when the CNS is still fresh, well rested, and able to respond quickly to various stimuli.

- *Detection of fatigue.* Since fatigue affects the neural reactivity of the fast-twitch muscle fibers and the effectiveness of the myotatic stretch reflex, fatigue manifests itself in the visible deterioration of technique. Players seem to be sloppy and the foot contact on the ground is noisy and of longer duration (because the heel touches the ground). If these technical disturbances are seen, the coach should stop the drill and allow for a longer rest interval.

- *The technique of the first step.* A quick performance of the first step influences athletes' quickness. This is why athletes should concentrate on how quickly they move the opposite arm. For instance, if a player initiates a forward step or a crossover with the left leg, the quickness of that step will depend on how fast the athlete moves the right arm. In both running and agility drills, the arms and legs should move in perfect alternating synchrony and coordination. The arms-legs coupling is performed in the following sequence: (1) arm action and (2) leg reaction (it is a reaction because it reacts to the arm motion). However, the interval between the arm action and the leg reaction should be minimal—a few milliseconds.

- *Watch the foot contact.* To maximize the effect of the stretch reflex, foot contact should always occur on the ball of the foot. Elastic, springy actions and short foot contact is called light feet; in contrast, hard landing on the sole constitutes heavy feet. Any lengthening of the contact phase on the ground results in slower movements. That is why athletes must perform agility exercises quickly, emphasizing light feet, maximizing the elasticity and minimizing the duration of the contact phase.

- *Listen to the step sound;* it provides the players and coaches with important feedback regarding the quality of execution of agility drills. A noisy, clapping sound is an indication that the landing is on the sole rather than on the ball of the foot, not an evidence of quick and agile motion. The quieter the contact with the ground, the more fluid and elastic the movement is performed, resulting in an improved level of power. However, a noisy landing can also be an indication of neuromuscular fatigue.

- *Observe the height of the steps.* For agility moves, changes of direction, and acceleration, the athlete's steps should always be as low as possible so the foot can get back to the ground quickly and be ready for another push-off. To enhance quickness of motions athletes should (1) try to recover the foot with the tip below the height of the ankle (any upward motions indicate loss of quickness) and (2) try to move as quickly as possible between the two points of the agility step, the push-off and the landing phase. The dynamic element of agility and quickness is the push-off or propulsion phase. The higher the frequency of pushing against the ground, the faster and more agile an athlete is.

- *Examine body mechanics.* During agility drills, athletes should maintain a correct posture: feet shoulder width apart, feet pointing forward, and body weight distributed equally on both legs. The vertical projection of the center of gravity (CG) should fall inside of the base of support, between the feet. To make some agility drills more sport-specific, they should be performed from an unbalanced position, with the vertical projection of the CG falling outside of the base of support.

Periodization of Agility and Power Training

A periodization model for agility as shown in figure 11.2 results in the greatest improvement in agility (Bompa 2005). The top of the chart lists traditional training phases of the annual plan and specific phases of the periodization of strength, which are explained in other chapters. During the AA phase, which focuses on building a foundation of strength and general conditioning, repeating agility drills will not produce visible improvement because the neuromuscular system is not yet trained to recruit fast-twitch fibers.

During the MxS phase, however, the recruitment of fast-twitch muscle fibers becomes the scope of training, and therefore agility training can be initiated in the form of repeating known drills and learning new ones. As the neuromuscular system improves its ability to recruit more motor units, and in particular a higher number of fast-twitch fibers, especially toward the end of the maximum strength phase, the athlete improves in velocity or quickness of performing agility drills. This ability is then maximized toward

Training phase	Preparation			Competitive	Transition
Periodization of strength	Anatomical adaptation	Maximum strength	Conversion to power	Maintenance: maximum strength, power	Compensation training
Periodization of agility	No agility drills	Learning phase: repeating known agility drills, learning new ones	Increasing velocity of agility drills	Increasing velocity of agility drills	No agility drills (not in scope of training for this phase)
Benefits to agility	Low	Good to high	Maximum		Low

Figure 11.2 Periodization of agility.

the end of the conversion phase and during the competitive phase, when the discharge rate of fast-twitch fibers increases as a result of increasing the velocity of agility drills and applying force against lighter implements or against the force of gravity. From this phase of training onward, and throughout the maintenance phase, agility is maximized and contributes to improvement in the athlete's performance.

Finally, many trainers still consider agility and quickness to be separate physical qualities. This view is apparent in many seminars and books on these topics. In reality, however, when the neuromuscular system is trained according to the physiological strategy suggested in figure 11.1, the final physiological product is an increased discharge rate of the fast-twitch fibers. Because of high adaptation to the periodization of strength, athletes possess more power, run faster, and can perform any type of drill with quickness. The human body doesn't care whether we use two different terms to describe the same neuromuscular quality. No matter what we call these movements, the properly trained body is capable of performing powerful actions, moving limbs fast, and changing direction quickly.

Some agility instructors or coaches have their athletes perform similar agility drills and quickness exercises throughout the year of training—disregarding the concept of periodization—and with pretty much the same duration, intensity, and number of repetitions. In addition, some inexperienced instructors take no account of an athlete's age or training background. Thus, we should not be surprised that some athletes, especially those with a superficial training background, experience anatomical discomfort or even injury. The best way to avoid injury is to apply the concept of periodization.

During the preparatory phase of the annual plan, athletes can improve their agility and quickness by using implements or types of training that include power balls, medicine balls, and plyometric exercises. For the best training organization and periodization, plyometric exercises are organized into five categories of intensity. These intensities can also be periodized, as can the weight of power and medicine balls (see figure 11.3).

Figure 11.3 shows particular activities and intensities used in the preparatory phase. During the AA portion, which emphasizes the foundation of strength, low loads are used for the implements and low intensity (level 5) is used for plyometrics. During the maximum strength portion, the athlete uses high loads for power ball and medicine ball training in order to activate a higher number of motor units. At the same time, the intensity of plyometric exercises is increased in order to heighten the reactivity of the athlete's

Training phase	Preparatory						Competitive		
Periodization of strength	Anatomical adaptation	Maximum strength	Conversion to power, maximum strength				Maintenance: maximum strength, power		
Periodization of power ball or medicine ball (weight)*	Light		Medium to heavy		Medium	Light	Light		
Periodization of plyometrics (intensity)	5	4	4	3	2	2 or 1	2 or 1	1 and 3	3

*Power balls weigh between 2 and 35 pounds (about 1 and 16 kg). Light weight ranges from 2 to 10 pounds (about 1 to 4.5 kg); medium weight ranges from 12 to 20 pounds (about 5.5 to 9 kg), and heavy weight ranges from 22 to 35 pounds (about 9 to 16 kg). Medicine balls weigh between 2 and 20 pounds (about 1 and 9 kg). For plyometric intensity level descriptions, refer to table 11.5 later in this chapter.

Figure 11.3 Periodization of plyometrics and power and medicine balls.

neuromuscular system. Finally, during the conversion portion, the loads are decreased for power ball and medicine ball training in order to maximize the benefits of quickness of force application. The intensity of plyometrics, however, is at its highest, pushing the eccentric contractions to their maximum, which results in higher force production. Under these conditions, the discharge rate of fast-twitch muscle fibers increases to ensure that the athlete reaches peak performance at the time of a major competition.

During the competitive phase, the first period features high-intensity plyometrics and is followed by alternating microcycles in which high- and medium-intensity plyometrics are used according to the macrocycle structure and the competitive calendar. In the week preceding the major competition of the year (for individual sports), medium-intensity plyometrics are used; they are then suspended during the final, competitive microcycle.

Throughout this book, illustrations of the planning of periodization and training methods use a vertical bar to separate training phases. This approach might seem to imply that a certain type of training ends on the last day of one phase and that a completely different type begins on the first day of the next phase. In fact, the transition between phases is not quite so abrupt. There is always an overlap, a transition, and a training method to be used in a given phase is introduced progressively in the previous phases. For instance, as depicted in figure 11.3, this approach is used for power training that starts from the beginning of the annual plan and gets its moment of emphasis after the maximum strength phase. Similarly, the method used in a previous phase is usually maintained in the next phase with a progressive reduction in emphasis. Thus, each training phase focuses on a dominant method (or methods) but also involves another that is progressively introduced. This training approach allows for a more effective transition from one method to the next and finally for higher levels of adaptation by the athlete.

A transition of emphasis between two training methods or phases can take place over the span of a few microcycles. Figure 11.4 shows that as the isotonic method for power development is progressively introduced, maximum strength work is progressively reduced. This transition can be accomplished by controlling the number of training sessions dedicated to each ability. An example is provided in figure 11.5, where, in the third MxS microcycle, all three training sessions are dedicated to maximum strength. In the following microcycles, however, maximum strength is decreased, whereas power is increased. As a result, during the power macrocycle, two of the three training days are dedicated to power, and one MxS session is planned to retain gains in maximum strength.

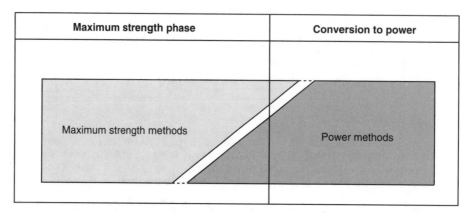

Figure 11.4 Switch of training emphasis in the preparation phase.

Macrocycle		Maximum strength		Power	
Microcycle		3	4	1	2
Training days	Maximum strength	3	2**	1***	1***
	Power	0	1	2	2

*Maximum strength is maintained via a dedicated session.

**Including one day for the 1RM test.

***Maximum strength maintenance session.

Figure 11.5 Progressive transition from a maximum strength macrocycle to a power macrocycle.

Another method of transitioning from the maximum strength phase to the conversion (power) phase is to create different combinations of sets of maximum strength and power, as illustrated in figure 11.6. This figure also depicts a different way to retain maximum strength during a power macrocycle. For easier presentation, it is assumed that each microcycle includes three strength training sessions of five sets per fundamental exercise. In this option, during the power phase, a lower number of maximum strength sets is performed in each training session in order to retain maximum strength levels.

Macrocycle		Maximum strength			Power					
		Microcycle 4			Microcycle 1			Microcycle 2		
Training day		1	2	3	1	2	3	1	2	3
Sets	Maximum strength	5	2	1RM test	3	2	1**	1**	1**	1**
	Power	0	1		2	3	4	4	4	4

*Maximum strength is maintained via maximum strength sets in each session.

**Maximum strength maintenance sets.

Figure 11.6 Progressive transition from a maximum strength macrocycle to a power macrocycle.

The transition from one type of training to another can also be planned more elaborately, as illustrated in figure 11.7. This chart shows the periodization of strength, the number of workouts per week, the duration of each phase in weeks, and the transition from one type of strength to another. In this case, the core strength for synchronized swimming—which is the strength of the hips, abdominal muscles, and low back—was emphasized or maintained throughout the annual plan. A well-organized coach also structures a plan that shows how to use a certain type of training method and for how long. In doing so, the coach plans the most appropriate methods for each training phase, showing the duration of each as well as which method is dominant.

Figure 11.8 illustrates how training methods can be planned. The example refers to hypothetical sports in which power is the dominant ability. As usual, the top of the chart shows the training phases of a monocycle, and the row below that shows the periodization of strength. The bottom part of the chart lists several methods. Three types of symbols are used, because in a given training phase one method can have a higher priority than the others. The solid line indicates the method with the highest priority, the dashed line shows the second priority, and the dotted line shows the third priority. For instance,

	Dates	Sept.	Oct.	Nov.	Dec.	Jan.	Feb.	Mar.	Apr.	May
P E R I O D I Z A T I O N	**Competition**	—			Provincial			Divisional		National
	Training phase	Preparatory			Competitive					
	Periodization of strength	AA; core strength	MxS; maint. of core strength		Conversion to P; ME; maint. of core strength				Maint.	Cessation
	Duration in weeks	4	8		4	4	4	4	4	1
	No. of workouts per week	3	3 or 4		3				2	0
	No. of workouts per type of strength	2 AA, 1 core	2 or 3 MxS, 1 core		2 ME, 1 P, 1/2 MxS, 1/2 core	2 ME, 1 P, 1/2 MxS, 1/2 core	3 ME, 1 P	2 ME, 1 P	1 ME, 1 P	

Key: AA = anatomical adaptation, maint. = maintenance, ME = muscular endurance, MxS = maximum strength, P = power

Figure 11.7 Transition to different types of strength for synchronized swimming.

during the AA phase, circuit training is the dominant training method. When the MxS phase begins, the submaximum load method prevails, and during the latter part of the maximum strength program, the maximum load method dominates.

In power training, the figure presents the ballistic method and plyometrics (explained later in this chapter). The dotted line shows that these methods are a third priority in some phases. Please bear in mind that figure 11.8 is a hypothetical example and does not show all available methods or all possibilities for using those that are presented.

	Sept.	Oct.	Nov.	Dec.	Jan.	Feb.	Mar.	Apr.
Training phase	Preparatory						Precompetitive	Competitive
Periodization of strength	Anatomical adaptation		Maximum strength (MxS)			Conversion to power (P)	Maintenance: P 70%, MxS 30%	
			MxS | P | MxS | P | MxS					
Microcycles	1 2 3 4	5 6 7 8	9 10 11 | 12 13	14 15 16 | 17 18 | 19 20 21		22 23 24 25	26 27 28 | 29 30 31	32
Circuit training	<------------------>							
MAXIMUM STRENGTH								
Submaximum load			<---------------------->				<·····························>	
Maximum load					<-->			
POWER TRAINING								
Plyometrics		<····························>	<>	<·····>	<>	<·····>	<------------------>	<·····>
Ballistic			<-->	<·->	<-->	<·->	<-->	<··············>	<--->

Figure 11.8 Hypothetical example of planning the training methods for a power-dominated sport.

DECELERATION–ACCELERATION: THE KEY TO AGILITY

To change direction quickly, the athlete must first slow down before moving quickly in another direction. In other words, the action is performed in two phases: deceleration followed by acceleration, or deceleration–acceleration. Deceleration, or slowing down almost to a stop, results from the eccentric loading (lengthening) of the knee and hip extensors (quadriceps, hamstrings, glutes) and the plantar flexors (gastrocnemii). Elastic energy stored in the muscle–tendon unit during deceleration is then used to start the acceleration.

A high level of quickness and agility can be developed by improving the strength and power of the major lower-leg muscles (particularly the gastrocnemius) and the major upper-leg muscles (the quadriceps, the semimembranosus, the semitendinosus, the long head of the biceps femoris, and the gluteals). The ability to decelerate and accelerate quickly relies heavily on the ability of these muscles to contract powerfully, both eccentrically and concentrically. In particular, deceleration (related to eccentric strength) appears to be the determinant and limiting factor for performance. Furthermore, deceleration–acceleration coupling is slow if power is not trained adequately.

An athlete should learn to perform deceleration and acceleration using a specific technique that involves not only the legs but also the arms. In the case of deceleration, the arms move in coordination with the legs but with reduced amplitude and force. In other words, the arms make a very slight action that influences deceleration. Quick deceleration, however, invariably depends on the strength of the legs. If you want to decelerate fast, improve the strength (especially the eccentric strength) of the knee and hip extensors and the plantar flexors.

Acceleration, on the other hand, is greatly influenced by arm action. In particular, for an athlete to initiate the acceleration part of a sprint, an agility movement, or one requiring quick feet, the arms must move first. If the legs are to move fast, the arms' back-and-forth drive must be very active, even powerfully performed. In addition, the stronger the push-off is against the ground (which is related to concentric strength), the more powerful the ground reaction force that works in the opposite direction. Remember Newton's third law of motion: Every action has an equal and opposite reaction. Therefore, during the propulsion phase, the athlete exerts force onto the ground and the ground simultaneously exerts a force back onto the athlete. That is why maximizing an athlete's sprinting ability requires a high level of maximum strength and the ability to display it in the shortest possible time.

Methods for Power Training

A number of training methods can be used during the power phase; normally, this phase uses a combination of the isotonic, ballistic, power-resisting, and plyometric methods. The following sections describe these methods and how to implement them in a periodized training plan.

Isotonic Method

One classic method of power training is to attempt to move a weight as rapidly and forcefully as possible through the entire range of motion. Good means for developing power include free weights and other equipment that can be moved quickly. The weight of the equipment used in the isotonic method provides the external resistance. The force necessary to defeat the inertia of a barbell, or move it, is referred to as applied force—and the more the applied force exceeds the external resistance, the faster the acceleration of the weight.

A novice athlete who applies force equal to 95% of 1RM to lift a barbell loaded with the 1RM load is incapable of generating any acceleration. However, if the same athlete works on maximum strength for one or two years, his or her strength increases so much that lifting the same weight equals only 40% to 50% of 1RM. The athlete is then capable of moving the barbell explosively and generating the acceleration that is necessary in order to increase power. This difference explains why the periodization of strength requires a maximum strength phase prior to power training. No visible increments of power are possible without clear gains in maximum strength.

A high level of maximum strength is also necessary for the early part of a lift or throw. Any barbell or implement (such as a ball) has a certain inertia, which is its mass or weight. The most difficult part of lifting a barbell or throwing an implement explosively is the early part. To overcome inertia, the athlete must build a high level of tension in the relevant muscles. Consequently, the higher an athlete's maximum strength, the easier it is to overcome inertia, and the more explosive the start of the movement can be. As an athlete continues to apply force against the barbell or implement, he or she increases its velocity. As more velocity is developed, less force is necessary to maintain it.

Increasing velocity continuously means that limb speed is also increasing. This increase is possible only if the athlete can contract the muscle quickly, which is why athletes involved in speed- and power-dominant sports need to power-train during the conversion phase. Without power training, an athlete will never be able to jump higher, run faster, throw farther, or deliver a quicker punch. In order to improve, athletes need more than just maximum strength. They must also be able to express maximum strength at a very high rate—a capacity that can be achieved only through power training methods.

During the MxS phase, the athlete gets accustomed to heavy loads. Therefore, using loads between 30% and 80% of 1RM helps the athlete develop sport-specific power and at the same time meet the challenge of creating the high acceleration needed for power performance. The load to be used to develop sport-specific power depends on the strength training experience of the athlete (beginners use lower loads), the resistance encountered in the sporting activity (linemen, for example, should use the "power high loads" method), and the type of exercise (see figures 11.9, 11.10, and 11.11).

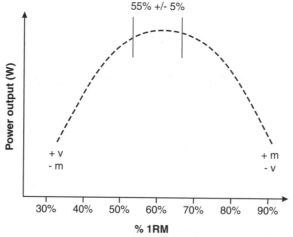

Figure 11.9 The peak mechanical power output of advanced athletes using strength exercises such as the squat, deadlift, or bench press is reached with percentages of 55%±5%.

Data from D. Santa Maria, P. Gryzbinski, and B. Hatfield, "Power as a Function of Load for a Supine Bench Press Exercise" (abstract), *NSCA Journal* 6, no. 58 (1985).

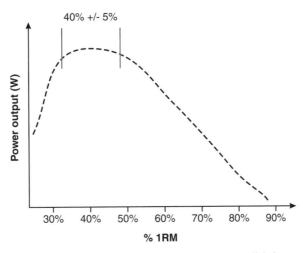

Figure 11.10 The peak mechanical power output of beginner athletes using strength exercises such as the squat, deadlift, or bench press is reached with percentages of 40%±5%.

Data from R.U. Newton, A.J. Murphy, B.J. Humphries, et al., "Influence of Load and Stretch Shortening Cycle on the Kinematics, Kinetics and Muscle Activation That Occurs During Explosive Bench Press Throws," *European Journal of Applied Physiology and Occupational Physiology* 75 (1997): 333-342.

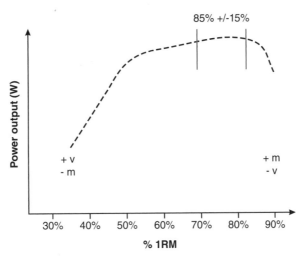

Figure 11.11 The peak mechanical power output using Olympic lifts and variants is reached with percentages of 85%±15%.

Data from R.U. Newton, A.J. Murphy, B.J. Humphries, et al., "Influence of Load and Stretch Shortening Cycle on the Kinematics, Kinetics and Muscle Activation That Occurs During Explosive Bench Press Throws," *European Journal of Applied Physiology and Occupational Physiology* 75 (1997): 333-342.

For most sports involving cyclic motions (such as sprinting, team sports, and the martial arts), the load for the isotonic method can be 30% or higher (up to 50%). For sports involving acyclic motions (such as throwing, weightlifting, and line play in American football), the load can be higher (50%-80%) because these athletes have much higher mass and maximum strength to start with and must defeat a higher external resistance. In fact, power improvements are very specific in terms of angular speed and load; as a result, the load should be chosen according to the external resistance to be defeated. See table 11.2 for a summary of training parameters.

Table 11.2 Training Parameters for the Isotonic Method

Phase duration	3-6 weeks
Load	Cyclic: 30%-50% of 1RM Acyclic: 50%-80% of 1RM
Number of exercises	3-6
Number of reps per set	Cyclic: 3-6 reps Acyclic: 3-5 reps at 50%-70%, 1-3 reps at 70%-80%
Number of sets per exercise	3-6
Rest interval	Cyclic: 2-3 min Acyclic: 3-5 min
Speed of execution	Explosive
Frequency per week	2 or 3

As a joint approaches its full extension, the nervous system would naturally activate the antagonist muscles to slow down the movement (Newton et al. 1996). At the same time, the exercise usually becomes biomechanically more advantageous as a joint "opens" (requiring less application of force). For these reasons, it is advisable to use accommodating resistance, such as bands or chains, when using lower loads (30%-50%). In fact, research has proven that accommodating resistance leads to higher increase of power when light loads are used (Rhea et al. 2009).

Please remember, however, that the use of bands in particular heavily taxes the CNS, which means that one must appropriately adjust the rest between sets and the frequency of exposure to this type of training. In addition, because the key element for power training is not how many reps are performed but the ability to activate the highest number of fast-twitch fibers, we suggest a low number of reps (1 to 8).

Athletes should also attend to safety. When a limb is extended, it should not be snapped. In other words, exercises should be performed explosively but without jerking the barbell or implement. Perfect technique is paramount.

For sport actions that require power to be performed in an explosive, acyclic manner—for example, throwing, jumping, diving, cricket actions, batting, pitching, and line play in American football—reps must be performed with some rest between them so that the athlete can concentrate maximally in order to achieve the most dynamic move. This strategy also improves fast-twitch motor unit recruitment and power output (Gorostiaga et al. 2012). The athlete can perform one rep at a time, as long as it is performed explosively in order to achieve maximum recruitment of fast-twitch muscle fibers and increased discharge rate.

When the athlete can no longer perform a repetition explosively, he or she should stop, even if the set has not been completed. Continuing the reps without explosiveness trains power endurance (discussed at the end of this chapter) rather than power. Only the combination of maximum concentration and explosive action produces the greatest fast-twitch fiber recruitment and discharge rate, and these crucial elements are attainable only when the athlete is relatively fresh.

During the rest interval, regardless of whether the athlete is working on power or on power endurance, he or she should try to relax the muscles previously involved. Relaxing during the rest interval enhances the resynthesis of ATP, thus helping resupply the working muscles with necessary fuel. This recommendation does not mean that the athlete must stretch the muscles involved, which in fact would lower the power output in the following set; therefore, stretching of agonist muscles should be avoided between sets.

Exercises for power training must be very sport specific in order to replicate the kinetic chain used in the sporting activity. From this perspective, we can see that bench presses and power cleans, despite being traditional power-training exercises, offer no built-in magic. Power cleans, which have been used to test and train the force of men since the late Bronze Age (1550-1200 BC), are useful for throwers and American football linebackers but not necessarily for, say, athletes in soccer or racket sports. These athletes can better use jumping squats and strength training machines.

Selecting the lowest number of exercises (3 to 6) allows the athlete to perform the highest number of sets realistically possible (3 to 6 per exercise for a maximum of 18 sets per session) for the most benefit to the prime movers. When deciding the number of sets and exercises, coaches should remember that power training is performed in conjunction with technical and tactical training and can therefore be given only a certain amount of energy.

A key element in developing power through the isotonic method is the speed of exertion. For maximum power improvement, exertion speed must be as high as possible. Fast application of force against an implement or weight throughout the range of motion is essential and must start from the early part of the movement. To be able to displace the barbell or other implement immediately and dynamically, the athlete must be maximally concentrated on the task.

Figure 11.12 shows a sample power training program for a college-level female basketball player with four years of strength training. Maximum mechanical power output is usually achieved at 50% of 1RM (+/-5%) in strength exercise (Baker, Nance, and Moore 2001) and around 85% for Olympic lifts (Garhammer 1989). A power loss occurs at about the sixth rep of a given set (Baker and Newton 2007).

Exercise	WEEK		
	1	2	3
1. Power clean	$\frac{80}{2}$ 4	$\frac{82.5}{2}$ 4	$\frac{85}{2}$ 4
2. Jump squat	$\frac{40}{5}$ 3	$\frac{45}{5}$ 3	$\frac{50}{5}$ 3
3. Military press	$\frac{50}{3}$ 4	$\frac{55}{3}$ 4	$\frac{60}{3}$ 4
4. Lat pull-down	$\frac{50}{3}$ 4	$\frac{55}{3}$ 4	$\frac{60}{3}$ 4
5. Weighted crunch	2 × 12	2 × 10	2 × 8

Figure 11.12 Sample power training program for a college-level female basketball player with four years of strength training.

Ballistic Method

Muscle energy can be applied in different forms and against different resistances. When the resistance is equal to the force applied by the athlete, no motion occurs; this is isometric exercise. If the resistance is less than the force applied by the athlete, the strength training equipment moves either slow or fast; this is isotonic exercise. And if the athlete's applied force clearly exceeds the external resistance (e.g., with a medicine ball), a dynamic motion occurs, in which either the athlete's body or the implement is projected; this is ballistic exercise.

For power training purposes, an athlete's muscle power can be applied forcefully against implements such as track-and-field shots, medicine balls, slam balls, or barbells. The resulting motion occurs explosively because the force of the athlete far exceeds the resistance of the implement. Employing such instruments to enhance power is therefore referred to as the ballistic method.

Some instructors and coaches believe that the use of elastic cords is beneficial for the development of power. To develop power, one has to apply force dynamically and explosively. Pulling against the cord has exactly the opposite effect. As an athlete pulls against the cord, the cord is stretched, increasing the resistance and, as a result, slowing down the dynamics of motion. This is not exactly conducive to power development.

Elastic cords have their place in the fitness industry (e.g., for developing general strength), but they are not particularly useful in sports, with the exception of endurance-dominant sports.

During a ballistic action, the athlete's energy is exerted dynamically against resistance from the beginning to the end of the motion. As a result, the implement is projected for a distance proportional to the power applied against it. Throughout the motion, the athlete must apply considerable force in order to accelerate the equipment or implement continuously, culminating in the release. To project the implement for the maximum possible distance, the athlete must achieve the highest velocity at the instant of release.

The fast ballistic application of force is possible as a result of quick recruitment of fast-twitch muscle fibers, high discharge rate, and effective intermuscular coordination of the agonist and antagonist muscles. After years of practice, an athlete can contract the agonist muscles forcefully while the antagonist muscles reach a high level of relaxation. This superior intermuscular coordination maximizes the force capabilities of the agonist muscles because the antagonist muscles exert no opposition to the agonists' quick contraction.

Depending on the training objectives, ballistic exercises can be planned to occur either after the warm-up or at the end of the training session. For example, if technical and tactical work has been planned for a given day, the development and improvement of power is a secondary goal. However, for events in which speed and power are dominant—such as sprinting, field events in track and field, and the martial arts—power work can often be planned to occur immediately after the warm-up, especially in the late preparatory phase, thanks to the stimulatory effects on the nervous system, typical of power training. Training parameters for a ballistic program are summarized in table 11.3.

Power training of an explosive nature is enhanced when the athlete is physiologically fresh. A well-rested CNS can send more powerful nerve impulses to the working muscles for quick contractions. The opposite is true, however, when the CNS and muscles are exhausted and inhibition is dominant; these conditions prevent the effective involvement of fast-twitch muscle fibers. This shows the problem of having an athlete perform intensive work prior to explosive power training: His or her energy supplies (ATP-CP) are exhausted, sufficient energy is not available, and high-quality work is impossible because fast-twitch fibers fatigue easily and are hardly activated. As a result, the athlete performs movements without vigor.

Table 11.3 Training Parameters for the Ballistic Method

Load	Load that allows projection of the body or implement
Number of exercises	2-6
Number of reps per set	5 or 6
Number of sets per session	2-6
Rest interval	2-3 minutes
Speed of execution	Explosive
Frequency of training	2-4

When using the ballistic method, speed of performance is paramount. Each rep should start dynamically, and the athlete should try to increase the speed constantly as the release or end of the motion approaches. This effort enables the involvement of a higher number of fast-twitch motor units. The critical element here is not the number of reps. The athlete need not perform many reps in order to increase power. Instead, the determining factor is speed of performance, which is dictated by the speed of muscle contraction. Therefore, exercises should be performed only as long as quickness is possible. *Repetitions must be discontinued the moment that speed declines.*

The speed and explosiveness of an exercise are guaranteed only as long as a high number of fast-twitch fibers are involved. When they fatigue, speed decreases. Continuing an activity after speed declines is futile because at this point there is no full activation of fast-twitch motor units, and those that are activated adapt to become slower—an unwanted result for athletes seeking power development. The plasticity of the CNS can work either for or against the objective of training. To be effective, adaptation must lead to the improvement of the athlete's sport performance.

Ballistic training load is dictated by the standard weight of the implements. Medicine balls weigh from 4.5 to 20 pounds (about 2-9 kg), whereas power balls weigh between 2 and 35 pounds (about 1-16 kg).

As in other power-related methods, the number of ballistic exercises must be as low as possible so that the athlete can perform a high number of sets in order to achieve maximum power benefits. Again, exercises should closely mimic technical skills. If such mimicry is not possible, the coach should select exercises that involve the sport's prime movers.

For any explosive power method, the rest interval should be as long as necessary to reach full recovery so that the athlete can repeat the same quality of work in each set. In fact, because most ballistic exercises require a partner, necessity often dictates a short interval between repetitions. For instance, a shot must be fetched, a position taken, and a few preparatory swings made before the shot is heaved back to the first athlete. By that time, some 15 to 20 seconds have elapsed in which the first athlete can rest. For this reason, the number of reps can be higher in ballistic training than in other power training methods.

The frequency per week of using the ballistic method depends on the training phase. In the late preparatory phase, the frequency should be low (1 or 2 sessions); during the conversion phase, it should be higher (2 to 4 sessions). The sport or event must also be considered. The frequency is higher for speed- and power-dominant sports than for sports in which power is of secondary importance. Figure 11.13 shows a sample program combining ballistic and maximum acceleration exercises. This program has been used successfully by players in American football, baseball, lacrosse, soccer, and hockey.

Exercise	WEEK		
	Week 1	Week 2	Week 3*
1. Jump squat and medicine ball chest throw	2 × 5	3 × 5	3 × 5*
2. Medicine ball overhead backward throw	2 × 5	3 × 5	3 × 5*
3. Medicine ball chest throw	2 × 5	3 × 5	3 × 5*
4. Medicine ball overhead forward throw	2 × 5	3 × 5	3 × 5*
5. Medicine ball side throw (each side)	1 × 5	3 × 5	3 × 5*
6. Two-handed shot throw from chest followed by 15-yard (-meter) sprint	3 ×	4 ×	5 ×
7. Push-up followed by 15- yard (-meter) sprint	3 ×	4 ×	5 ×

*With a load heavier than the previous week.

Figure 11.13 Sample program combining ballistic and maximum acceleration exercises.

Power-Resisting Method

This method represents a three-way combination of the isotonic, isometric, and ballistic methods. To help explain this method, here is a description of an exercise. An athlete lies down with knees bent to perform a sit-up. His or her toes are held against the ground by a partner, and the coach stands behind the athlete. The athlete begins the sit-up. When he or she reaches approximately a quarter of hip flexion (135-140 degrees), the coach places his or her palms on the athlete's chest or shoulders, thus stopping the movement. At this point, the athlete is in a maximum static contraction, trying to defeat the resisting power of the coach by recruiting most or all of the possible motor units. After three or four seconds, the coach removes his or her hands, and the maximum static contraction is converted into a dynamic ballistic motion for the rest of the sit-up. The athlete then slowly returns to the starting position and rests for 10 to 20 seconds before performing another rep.

The most important parts of this method are the maximum isometric contraction and the ensuing ballistic action. The ballistic-type motion, with its quick muscle contraction, results in power development. The actions used in this method are similar to those of a catapult machine. The initial isotonic action must be performed slowly. Following the stop, the maximum isometric contraction represents a high pre-tension (loading phase) of the muscles involved. In the case of the sit-up, as the chest or shoulders are released, the trunk is catapulted forward (the ballistic phase). Any other movements that duplicate the previous phases of action can be categorized under the ballistic method with similar effects on power development. In fact, similar power-resisting exercises can be performed for a variety of other movements, such as the following:

- *Pull-up.* The athlete performs an early elbow flexion, at which point the coach or partner stops the action for a few seconds; a dynamic action then follows.
- *Dip.* The athlete performs an early elbow extension, at which point the coach or partner stops the action for a few seconds; a dynamic action then follows.
- *Jump squat with no weights.* The athlete bends the knees, at which point the coach or partner stops the action for a few seconds; a dynamic action then follows.
- *Squat with weights.* Place a first set of safety pins at the height that results in the knee or hip angles at which you want the isometric action to happen (usually a half-squat angle). Place a second set of pins two or three holes below. The athlete

pushes against the pins for two to four seconds, then one or two spotters remove the pins for the dynamic action to follow.

- *Bench press.* Place a bench inside a power rack; place a first set of safety pins in a way that the bar barely touches the chest and a second set one or two holes higher. The athlete pushes against the pins for two to four seconds, then one or two spotters remove the pins for the dynamic action to follow.
- *Trunk rotation with medicine ball held sideways in the hands.* The athlete performs a backward rotation, and as the rotation comes forward the athlete is stopped for two to four seconds; the ballistic action that follows culminates with the release of the ball. The same concept can be applied to most any medicine ball throw.

Another type of power stimulation can be achieved through isotonic weight training by alternating loads (this is also known as the contrast method). The athlete first performs one to three reps with a load of 80% to 90% of 1RM, then immediately performs five or six reps with a low-resistance load of 30% to 50%. The heavy-load reps produce neuromuscular stimulation, allowing the athlete to perform the low-resistance reps more dynamically. This method can be used with a large variety of exercises, from bench pulls to bench presses A note of caution regarding motions that involve knee and arm extensions: Snapping or jerking actions (forced, snapped extensions) should be avoided because they can cause joint damage.

The load for the power-resisting method is related to the exercise performed. For the isometric phase, the contraction should last three or four seconds, or the duration necessary to reach maximum tension. For exercises in which the resistance is provided by a barbell, the load should be 80% to 90% of 1RM for the stimulating phase and 30% to 50% of 1RM for the explosive phase. Exercises should also match the direction of the prime movers' contraction during the sport-specific skills. For maximum power benefit, the number of exercises should be low (2 to 4) so that the athlete can perform a large number of sets (3 to 5).

Power-resisting training can be performed separately or combined with other power training methods. Training parameters for the power-resisting method are summarized in table 11.4.

Table 11.4 Training Parameters for the Power-Resisting Method

Load	Exercise dependent
Number of exercises	2-4
Number of reps per set	3-6
Number of sets per exercise	3-5
Rest interval	2-4 minutes
Speed of execution	Explosive
Frequency per week	1 or 2

Plyometric Method

Since ancient times, athletes have explored a multitude of methods designed to enable them to run faster, jump higher, and throw farther. To achieve such goals, power is essential. Strength gains can be transformed into power only by applying specific power training. Perhaps one of the most successful power training methods is the plyometric method.

Plyometrics employs exercises that elicit the stretch–shortening cycle, or myotatic stretch reflex. These exercises load the muscle in a fast eccentric (lengthening) contraction, which is followed immediately by a concentric (shortening) contraction. Research has demonstrated that if a muscle is quickly stretched before a contraction, it contracts more forcefully and rapidly (Bosco and Komi 1980; Schmidtbleicher 1984; Verkhoshansky 1997; Seiberl et al. 2015). For example, by lowering the center of gravity to perform a takeoff or to swing a golf club, the athlete stretches the muscle rapidly, which results in a more forceful contraction.

Plyometric action relies on the stretch reflex originating in the spinal cord. The main purpose of the stretch reflex is to limit the degree of muscle stretch in order to prevent overstretching. Plyometric movement is based on the reflex contraction of the muscle fibers resulting from the rapid stretching of these same fibers. In fact, when excessive stretching and tearing become a possibility, the stretch receptors send proprioceptive nerve impulses to the spinal cord. The impulses then rebound to the stretch receptors, which produces a braking effect that prevents the muscle fiber from stretching farther, thereby initiating a powerful muscle contraction.

Plyometric exercises work within complex neural mechanisms. Neural adaptations take place in the body's nervous system to enhance both strength and power in athletic training (Sale 1986; Schmidtbleicher 1992; Enoka 2015). In fact, as already stated, neural adaptations can increase the force of a muscle without increasing its size (Dons et al. 1979; Komi and Bosco 1978; Sale 1986; Tesch et al. 1990).

Plyometric training causes muscular and neural changes that facilitate and enhance the performance of more rapid and more powerful movements. The CNS controls muscle force by changing the activity of the muscle's motor units; if greater force generation is required, more motor units are recruited and fired at a higher rate. In this context, an increase in electromyographic recording output following a training program indicates one of three things: more motor units have been recruited, motor units are firing at higher rates, or some combination of these reactions has occurred (Sale 1992). The benefits of plyometric training include increased activation of fast-twitch motor units and, what is more important, a higher rate of firing.

The contractile elements of a muscle are the muscle fibers; however, certain noncontractile parts constitute what is known as the series elastic component. Stretching the series elastic component during eccentric muscle contraction produces elastic potential energy similar to that of a loaded spring. This energy augments the energy generated by muscle fibers. This synergy is visible in plyometric movements. When a muscle is stretched rapidly, the series elastic component is also stretched, and it stores a portion of the load force in the form of elastic potential energy. The recovery of the stored elastic energy occurs during the concentric, or overcoming, phase of muscle contraction triggered by the myotatic reflex.

In plyometric training, a muscle contracts more forcefully and quickly from a prestretched position—and the faster the prestretch, the more forceful the concentric contraction. Correct technique is essential. The athlete must land with the legs slightly bent in order to prevent injury to the knee joints. The shortening contraction should occur immediately after completion of the prestretch phase. The transition from the prestretch phase should be smooth, continuous, and as swift as possible. Increased contact time indicates fatigue induced by repeated reactive training (Gollhofer et al. 1987).

Plyometric training produces the following results:

- quick mobilization of greater innervation activity,
- recruitment of most, if not all, motor units and their corresponding muscle fibers,

- increased firing rate of motor neurons,

- transformation of muscle strength into explosive power,

- development of the nervous system so that it reacts with maximum speed to the lengthening of a muscle, which develops the athlete's ability to shorten (contract) rapidly with maximum force,

- improvement in explosive force with only slight increase in muscle girth due to increase in mean cross-sectional area of fast-twitch fibers (Häkkinen and Komi 1983), which indicates performance enhancement at the neuromuscular level, and

- inhibition of the Golgi tendon organ, which could lead to higher muscle tension and activation at landing, thus producing more powerful muscle contraction—all of which contributes to enhanced power output (Schmidtbleicher 1992).

An athlete can progress faster through the various intensity levels of plyometric training if he or she possesses a good strength training background of several years. Such a background also helps prevent injury. In addition, in the interest of establishing a good base of strength and developing shock-absorbing qualities, one should not dismiss the benefits of introducing children to plyometric exercises. These exercises must be performed over several years, however, and conducted in a manner that respects the principle of progression. Patience and well-planned progression are the key elements of this approach.

A healthy training progression for children first exposes them to low-intensity plyometrics (levels 5 and 4) over several years, say, between the ages of 14 and 16. After this initial period, they can be introduced to more demanding reactive jumps (level 3). Throughout these years of long-term progression, teachers and coaches should teach young athletes the correct plyometric techniques by using the hop and step from the triple jump as the basics of plyometric training.

Plyometric exercises are the subject of some controversy. One area of consideration involves the amount of strength that should be developed before doing plyometrics. Some authors define the safe level as the ability to perform one half squat with a load that is twice one's body weight, but that standard applies only to level 1 plyometrics.

Others address the type of training surface, what equipment to use, and whether additional weights (such as heavy vests and ankle and waist belts) should be worn when performing these exercises. When injury is a concern, and at the start of general preparation, exercises should be performed on a soft surface—either on grass or soft ground or on a padded floor. However, though this precaution may be appropriate for beginners or athletes just starting their preparation, using a soft surface can dampen the stretch reflex; only a hard surface enhances the reactivity of the neuromuscular system. Athletes with an extensive background in sport, strength training, or both should use a hard surface, especially from the specific preparation phase onward.

Plyometric drills should not be performed with barbells, dumbbells, or weighted ankle or waist belts. These weights tend to decrease the reactive ability of the neuromuscular system by slowing down the coupling time (the passage from the eccentric action to the concentric action) and, what is more important, the concentric action itself. Therefore, although such overloading may result in increased strength, it slows the speed of contraction and the rebounding effect. If more eccentric loading is necessary, that can be accomplished by using depth jumps from a high box.

To design a plyometric program properly, coaches and trainers must be aware that the exercises vary in level of intensity and are classified into different groups for better progression. The level of intensity is directly proportional to the height or length of an exercise. High-intensity plyometric exercises, such as depth or drop jumps, result in

MECHANICAL CHARACTERISTICS OF PLYOMETRICS

When an athlete jumps off the ground, much force is required to propel the body mass upward. The athlete must flex and extend the limbs very quickly. Plyometric exercise relies on this quick body action to muster the required power. More specifically, as we have seen, plyometric action relies on the stretch reflex, a protective mechanism that originates in the spinal cord and can be co-opted to increase the power of concentric contraction after a muscle is stretched through eccentric contraction.

When the takeoff leg is planted, the athlete must lower the center of gravity, creating downward velocity. During this amortization (or shock-absorbing) phase, the athlete must produce force to counter the downward motion and prepare for the upward thrusting phase that enables him or her to take off in a different direction. However, a long amortization phase results in loss of power. For example, a long jumper who plants the takeoff leg improperly loses the upward and horizontal velocity required to propel the body forward.

For this reason, the athlete must work toward a shorter and quicker amortization phase, which enables more powerful concentric contraction of the muscle that was stretched during the preceding eccentric contraction (Bosco and Komi 1980). Since force equals mass times acceleration, shortening the amortization phase requires the athlete to exert greater force in order to decelerate the body more quickly. This understanding points out the importance of keeping one's body fat low and one's power-to-weight ratio high. More body mass, and greater downward velocity at impact, require higher average force during the amortization phase.

To maximize jumping ability, one must use the entire body efficiently. For example, when a long jumper or a high jumper lowers the center of gravity before takeoff, he or she reduces the impact of the forces. In addition, upward acceleration of the free limbs (the arms) after the amortization phase increases the vertical forces placed on the takeoff leg. Triple jumpers, for instance, must apply peak force as much as six times their body weight to compensate for the inability to lower their center of gravity during the more upward hopping phase. Long jumpers, on the other hand, can manipulate their bodies more easily just before takeoff. Again, jumpers achieve effective takeoff only if they apply large forces on impact and produce a shorter amortization phase.

Athletes can achieve this quick turnaround only when their neuromuscular system is trained to organize both the relevant kinetic chain and the agonist–antagonist activation and deactivation through a periodized power program. The program should start with lower-impact plyometrics and progress to higher-impact plyometrics aimed at achieving the highest possible jump, regardless of ground contact time and degree of knee and hip flexion (characteristics of the depth jump). After this progression is completed (possibly several times during the career of an athlete), the neuromuscular system is ready to perform shorter ground contact times even when the force to be opposed is higher. However, aiming for short contact time with an ill-prepared athlete results only in a small uncoordinated jump.

Training for the takeoff phase is difficult because few conventional exercises apply. Many jumpers use traditional weight training (e.g., squats), and this work puts a large load on the knee extensors, which over time does provide an adequate strength training base. However, relying only on weight training is problematic because a heavy squat lift is unlikely to be fast enough to use and enhance the elastic qualities of the muscles.

Bounding exercises, on the other hand, can simulate an effective takeoff and improve the athlete's overall jumping ability. Bounding has force–time characteristics similar to those of the takeoff. It also allows athletes to practice resisting heavy loads on the takeoff leg and to exert force in a short time. In addition, bounding exercises involve multijoint movement and facilitate development of the required muscle elasticity.

higher tension in the muscle, which recruits more motor units to perform the action or to resist the pull of gravitational force.

Plyometric exercises can be categorized into two major groups that reflect their degree of impact on the neuromuscular system: low intensity and high intensity. From a more practical viewpoint, plyometric exercises can be divided into five levels of intensity (see table 11.5). This classification can be used to plan effective alternation of training demand throughout the week.

Any plan to incorporate plyometric exercises into a training program should account for the following factors:

- The age and physical development of the athlete
- The skills and techniques involved in plyometric exercises

Table 11.5 Five Intensity Levels of Plyometric Exercise

Intensity	Classification	Exercise	Reps × sets	Reps (or ground contacts) per session	Rest interval (minutes)
1	High intensity	Depth landing: 30-43 in. (75-110 cm)	1-5 × 3-6	3-20	5-8
		Depth jump: >28 inches (70 cm)	1-10 × 2-6	3-40	4-8
		Bounding on one leg (or alternating)	40-100 m (or yd) × 2-4	30-150	3-5
2		Drop jump: 16-24 inches (40-60 cm)	3-10 × 2-6	6-40	3-6
		Hurdles: >24 inches (60 cm)	3-12 × 2-6	6-72	3-5
		Bounding on one leg or alternating	5-30 m (or yd) × 2-6	20-60	3-5
		Speed squat (accentuated eccentric); Jump squat; Kettlebell power swing	3-6 × 2-6	12-24	3-4
3		Hurdles: 16-24 inches (40-60 cm)	6-20 × 2-6	18-80	3-5
4	Low intensity	Box jump: 24-43 inches (60-110 cm)	3-15 × 2-6	12-60	3-5
		Kettlebell swing	10-30 × 2-6	30-180	2-5
5		Low hurdles: <12 inches (30 cm)	6-20 × 3-6	18-80	2-3
		Skipping	10-30 m (or yd) × 7-15	70-250	1-2
		Medicine ball	5-12 × 4-6	20-72	1-3
		Rope	15-50 × 2-6	30-300	1-3

- The principal performance factors of the sport
- The energy requirements of the sport
- The training phase of the annual plan
- For younger athletes, the need to respect methodical progression over a long period (2-4 years), progressing from low intensity (levels 5 and 4), to medium intensity (level 3) and then to high intensity (levels 2 and 1)

Although plyometric exercises are fun, they demand a high level of concentration and are deceptively vigorous and taxing. The lack of discipline to wait for the right moment for each exercise can result in athletes performing high-impact exercises before they are ready. In such cases, the resulting injuries or physiological discomforts are not the fault of the plyometric exercises. Rather, they are the result of the coach's or instructor's lack of knowledge and improper application. The five levels of intensity help coaches design a plan including appropriate exercises that follow a consistent, steady, and orderly progression with appropriate rest intervals.

Progression through the five levels of intensity is achieved over the long term. The two to four years spent incorporating low-impact exercises into the training program of a young athlete are necessary for the progressive adaptation of the ligaments, tendons, and bones. They also allow for the gradual preparation of the shock-absorbing sections of the athlete's body, such as the hips and the spine.

The intensity of plyometric exercises—the amount of tension created in the muscle—depends on the eccentric load of the exercise, which is normally determined by the height from which the exercise is performed. That is why jumps *onto* boxes have a low intensity even when 43-inch (109 cm) boxes are used, because their eccentric load is minimal. Although the height used should be determined strictly by the individual qualities of the athlete, the following general principle applies: The stronger the muscular system is (higher muscular stiffness), the more energy is required to stretch it in order to obtain an elastic effect in the shortening phase. What is optimal height for one athlete may not generate enough stimulation for another.

Ideally, in fact, a force mat (such as the Just Jump System or the SmartJump) or a mobile phone application (for example, MyJump2) should be used to determine the optimal height for the desired power training effect. For instance, the optimal height for a depth jump is the box height that allows the highest rebounding jump, whereas the optimal height for a drop jump is the box height that allows the highest rebounding jump with a ground contact time below 250 milliseconds or the highest RSI (Reactive Strength Index; flight time divided by ground contact time, or the relationship between the reactive jump height and the ground contact time). This distinction means that depth jumps and drop jumps—despite their similar appearance to the untrained eye—not only serve different training objectives but should also be employed at different times during the annual plan. The following information and height information in table 11.14 should be treated only as guidelines.

According to Verkhoshansky (1969), in order to facilitate an athlete's gains in dynamic strength (power), the optimal height for depth jumps for power training of elite level athletes should be between 30 and 43 inches (75-110 cm). Similar findings were reported by Bosco and Komi (1980), who also concluded that above 43 inches (110 cm) the mechanics of the action are changed; in fact, at such heights, the time and energy required to cushion the force of the drop to the ground defeat the purpose of plyometric training. More generally, remember to start your athletes from a lower box and have them progress to a higher box. Most athletes maximize their rebounding jump with a 15- to 20-inch (about 40-50 cm) box, and only the strongest athletes need a 30-inch (75 cm) or more box.

In terms of reps, plyometric drills fall into two categories: single-response and multiple-response. Drills in the first category consist of a single action—such as a high-reactive jump, or a drop jump (level 2)—in which the main purpose is to induce the highest level of tension in the muscles. The objective of such exercises is to develop maximum strength and power.

Multiple-response exercises—such as jumping over multiple medium- (level 3) or low-height (level 4) hurdles and jump squats (level 2) can result in the development of power as well as power endurance.

Often, especially for multiple-response exercises, it is more convenient and practical to equate the number of reps with a distance—for example, 5 sets of 50 meters rather than 5 sets of 25 reps. This approach helps gauge the athlete's neuromuscular readiness as well as his or her progress.

High-quality training requires adequate physiological recuperation between exercises. Often, however, athletes and coaches either pay too little attention to the duration of the rest interval or simply get caught up in the traditions of a given sport, which often dictate that the only rest interval required is the time needed to move from one station to another. This amount of time is inadequate, however, especially considering the physiological characteristics of plyometric training.

Fatigue consists of local fatigue and CNS fatigue. Local fatigue results from depletion of the energy stored in the muscle (ATP-CP, the fuel necessary to perform explosive movements) and the accumulation of lactic acid from reps lasting longer than 10 seconds. During training, athletes also fatigue the CNS, the system that signals the working muscle to perform a given amount of high-quality work. Plyometric training is performed as a result of these nerve impulses, which are characterized by a certain power and frequency. Any high-quality training requires the highest possible levels of contraction power and frequency.

When the rest interval is short (1-2 minutes), the athlete experiences both local and CNS fatigue. The working muscle is unable to remove lactic acid or replenish energy sufficiently to perform the next reps at the same intensity. Similarly, a fatigued CNS is unable to send the powerful nerve impulses necessary to ensure that the prescribed load is performed for the same number of reps and sets before exhaustion sets in. In addition, an exhausted athlete is often just a short step away from injury; therefore, coaches and athletes should pay utmost attention to rest intervals.

As suggested in table 11.5, the appropriate rest interval is a function of the load and the type of plyometric training performed—the higher the exercise intensity, the longer the required rest interval. For maximum-intensity exercises (high-reactive jumps), the rest interval between sets should be three to eight minutes, depending on the athlete's body mass and gender: longer rest intervals for heavier male athletes, and shorter rest intervals for lighter female athletes. The suggested rest interval for intensity level 2 is three to six minutes; for levels 3 and 4, it should be two to five minutes; and for low-impact activities (level 5), it should be one to three minutes.

The type of plyometric training performed by an athlete must be specific to his or her sport. For example, athletes who require a greater degree of horizontal power should engage in more bounding and hopping drills, whereas those whose sports require vertical power should perform vertical jumping exercises. Coaches should also consider the training environment. Many studies have demonstrated that reflexes can be altered or modified using specific training modes (Enoka 1994; Schmidtbleicher 1992), and plyometrics is one form of training that induces particular adaptations in various reflexive actions. However, for the reflexive learning process to be reproduced in the competitive realm, the athlete must be in the same psychological and physiological state as when the reflex adaptation was induced. In other words, the training environment should be a near-perfect replica of the competitive environment.

Sport-Specific Application of Power Training

To reiterate a key point: Power must be developed to meet the needs of a given sport, event, or team position. To further illustrate the need for *specific* application of power, definitive examples are presented in this section. Many elements of the previously described power training methods are also applicable.

Power Endurance

In some sports, athletes must apply a high degree of power repetitively. Examples include sprints in track and field, sprints in swimming, wrestling, and certain team-sport positions, such as American football running back and baseball pitcher.

Sprinting is often misjudged, including the sprinting performed in all team sports that require explosive running (such as American football, basketball, baseball, ice hockey, rugby, soccer, and Australian football). When sprinters cover the classic 100 meters in 10 to 12 seconds, they have trained to perform powerful leg actions throughout the entire race, not just during the start and the following six to eight strides. In a 100-meter race, an athlete takes 48 to 54 strides, depending on stride length; thus, each leg makes 24 to 27 contacts with the ground. In each ground contact, the force applied can be more than twice the athlete's body weight.

In certain sports—American football, rugby, soccer, and Australian football—athletes are often required to repeat a strenuous activity after only a few seconds of game interruption. Similar athletic performances are required in the martial arts, boxing, wrestling, and racket sports. Athletes who compete in such sports need to perform powerful actions over and over. To do so successfully, they need high power output and the ability to repeat it 20 to 30 (or even up to 60) times dynamically and as explosively as possible.

The formula for training power endurance is

$$HV \times HI$$

or high volume (HV) of reps performed explosively, fast, and quickly (at high intensity, or HI) using exercises as close as possible to the motor pattern of sport-specific skills. Athletes with a high level of power endurance are able to avoid a decrease in stride frequency and velocity at the end of a race or have a consistent level of power output throughout a game, depending on what type of power endurance they worked on according to their sporting activity.

Is there a difference between a football player repeating many sprints over the duration of a game and a sprinter maintaining high power output for 50 strides? Yes. Physiologically speaking, the football player is repeating an alactic power activity, often without enough recovery time to refill the ATP-CP stores. As a result, the player enters what we call the lactic power short realm. The sprinter, on the other hand, uses anaerobic alactic (phosphagen) power during the first part of the race (the first 6-8 seconds), then increasingly uses lactic power long when approaching the finish line. For this reason, we say that both the football player and the sprinter need power endurance, yet physiologically their types of power endurance differ from each other.

Power endurance is the determinant abilities in several sports, and maximum strength is a determinant factor in both of these abilities. This section describes the training methodology for developing power endurance in an explosive manner.

Power endurance requires the athlete to apply 30% to 50% of maximum strength both rhythmically and explosively. To train appropriately for developing power endurance, an athlete is required to perform 12 to 30 dynamic reps explosively and nonstop. The needed training can be achieved progressively: start with a low number of reps (10-12) and progress to the sport-specific number of reps—for example, 15 for a 100-meter sprinter or 30 for a 200-meter sprinter.

Early in the conversion phase, the fast-twitch muscle fibers are trained to instantaneously display the highest possible level of power. Parallel with that work, athletes should also increase their quickness of performance for the purpose of increasing the discharge rate of the fast-twitch muscles as much as possible. For power endurance purposes, the fast-twitch fibers are trained to cope with the fatigue and the buildup of lactic acid induced by performing many reps dynamically.

Training is now aimed at developing the endurance component of speed, or specific power moves, typical of the relevant sports. This goal is accomplished by progressively increasing the number of reps or sets. The progression requires the athlete to exert maximum willpower in order to overcome fatigue and reach optimal mental concentration before performing each set. The recommended length of this phase is six to eight weeks; a program any shorter than that is insufficient for achieving the physiological goal of power endurance.

To perform a high number of sets for each prime mover, the number of exercises must be as low as possible (2 to 4, or rarely 5). Each rep of a set must be performed explosively. The rest interval between sets must be three to eight minutes to allow for CNS recovery. During this type of work, athletes experience a high level of lactic acid buildup. This is, in fact, why the number of explosive reps must be high—so that the athlete learns to tolerate the lactic acid buildup and perform successfully in this condition. Without such training, the athlete will not perform successfully during competition. This method also trains the CNS to keep a high frequency of discharge for an extended time despite the resulting muscle fatigue.

Speed of performance must be dynamic and explosive. Unless this rule is strictly observed, power training and power endurance training build muscle mass rather than power; as a result, the outcome is hypertrophy rather than power endurance. Athletes often require a few weeks of power endurance before they can perform 20 to 30 reps explosively and nonstop. In the meantime, they should stop when they become incapable of performing a rep dynamically because at that point power endurance is no longer being trained. Training parameters for power endurance are summarized in table 11.6.

Table 11.6   Training Parameters for the Power Endurance Method

Phase duration	4-6 weeks
Load	30%-50% of 1RM
Number of exercises	2-5
Number of reps per set	12-30
Number of sets per exercise	2 or 3
Rest interval	3-8 minutes
Speed of execution	Explosive
Frequency per week	2 or 3

Figure 11.14 shows a sample four-week training program for a 100-meter sprinter. Figure 11.15 shows a sample four-week training program for a team-sport athlete.

Exercise*	WEEK				Rest interval
	1	**2**	**3**	**4**	
1. Jumping half squat	$\frac{45}{15}$ 2	$\frac{45}{15}$ 3	$\frac{50}{15}$ 2	$\frac{50}{15}$ 3	5–6 min.
2. Heavy kettlebell swing	2×20	3×20	2×20 (heavier kettlebell than weeks 1 and 2)	3×20 (same kettlebell as week 3)	3–4 min.
3. Bench throw	$\frac{45}{15}$ 2	$\frac{45}{15}$ 3	$\frac{50}{15}$ 2	$\frac{50}{15}$ 3	3 min.
4. Lat pull-down (narrow supinated grip)	$\frac{45}{15}$ 2	$\frac{45}{15}$ 3	$\frac{50}{15}$ 2	$\frac{50}{15}$ 3	3 min.
LOADING PATTERN					
		High		High	
	Medium		Medium		

Figure 11.14 Sample four-week training program for a 100-meter sprinter.

*These exercises are the power endurance options of the exercises used during the MxS phase: half squat, reverse leg press, bench press, and heavy lat pull-down.

Exercise	Week 1	Rest intervals between sets and series	Week 2	Rest intervals between sets and series	Week 3	Rest intervals between sets and series	Week 4	Rest intervals between sets and series
1. Jumping half squat	$\frac{45}{12}$ × 3	3 min.	$\frac{45}{15}$ × 4	3 min.	$\frac{50}{12}$ × 3	3 min.	$\frac{50}{15}$ × 4	3 min.
2. Jumping lunge	$\frac{45}{12}$ × 3	3 min.	$\frac{45}{15}$ × 4	3 min.	$\frac{50}{12}$ × 3	3 min.	$\frac{50}{15}$ × 4	3 min.
3. Bench press with accommodating resistance (bands or chains)	$\frac{45}{12}$ × 3	3 min.	$\frac{45}{15}$ × 4	3 min.	$\frac{50}{12}$ × 3	3 min.	$\frac{50}{15}$ × 4	3 min.
4. Lat pull-down (narrow supinated grip)	$\frac{45}{12}$ × 3	3 min.	$\frac{45}{15}$ × 4	3 min.	$\frac{50}{12}$ × 3	3 min.	$\frac{50}{15}$ × 4	3 min.
LOADING PATTERN								
			High				High	
	Medium				Medium			

Figure 11.15 Sample four-week training program for a team-sport athlete.

Landing and Reactive Power

In several sports, landing is not only an important skill but also one that is followed by the performance of another skill—for example, another jump in figure skating or a quick move in another direction in tennis and in many team sports. The athlete must possess both the necessary power to control the landing and the reactive power to quickly perform the next move.

The power required for controlling and absorbing the shock of a landing is related to the height of the jump. For example, a landing after a drop or depth jump from 32 to 40 inches (about 80-100 cm) often loads the ankle joints with six to eight times the athlete's body weight. Similarly, absorbing the shock from a figure skating jump requires the power to handle five to eight times the athlete's body weight. To control such impact forces at the instant of landing, the athlete's muscles must be trained for shock-absorbing power.

Landing involves an eccentric contraction. Without proper training, the athlete lands incorrectly, which produces higher tension with the same amount of muscle fiber activity, thereby placing greater stress on the elastic tissue of the tendons and increasing the risk of injury. To avoid this pitfall, the athlete's training should include eccentric training and plyometrics.

Schmidtbleicher (1992) specified that at the instant of ground contact, athletes experience an inhibitory effect. At the same time, he noted that well-trained athletes cope with impact forces much better than poorly trained athletes do and that the inhibitory effect can be eliminated by drop-jump training. He concluded that the inhibitory mechanisms represent a protective system, especially for novice athletes, meant to shield them from injury.

To enhance landing and reactive power, both concentric and eccentric contractions should be part of an athlete's training. Eccentric strength training and plyometrics, primarily in the form of drop or depth jumps, should mimic the desired landing skill. Drop or depth jumps (also known as reactive jumps) are performed from a raised platform (a box, bench, or chair). The athlete lands in a flexed position (with the knees slightly bent) to absorb the shock. The athlete also lands on the balls of the feet without touching the heels to the ground. This technique is a requirement for most plyometric activities, because touching the ground with the heels indicates that the load is too high for the athlete's extensor muscles.

During the dropping phase, the athlete adopts a ready-to-work position, which enhances the muscles' tension and elastic properties. Upon landing, especially if the athlete is quickly preparing for another action, energy is stored in the elastic elements of the muscle. Upon the ensuing takeoff or quick move in another direction, this readily available energy release summates to the stretching reflex, which recruits more fast-twitch fibers than normal strength training does. This process enables the athlete to perform another quick and explosive action immediately. Reflexes (including the muscle spindle reflex) are trainable, and well-periodized training can improve an athlete's reactive jumps.

Throwing Power

For a pitcher in baseball, a quarterback in American football, or a thrower in track and field, throwing power is generated mostly by fast-twitch muscle fibers. The larger an individual fiber's diameter, the faster it contracts. Similarly, the more fibers a simultaneous contraction involves, the greater the athlete's power to deliver an implement.

Throwers and athletes in sports such as fencing and boxing must develop considerable power in order to accelerate the implement or equipment. These athletes must often overcome the inertia of an implement or a piece of equipment with the greatest possible speed from the beginning of the movement and then increase velocity throughout the movement, especially before the release. To do so, they must apply force that greatly exceeds the resistance of the implement—the more the force exceeds the weight of the implement, the higher the acceleration. Higher acceleration, then, requires a greater difference between the resistance of the implement and the athlete's maximum strength. As a result, athletes whose sport uses throwing power must implement a well-planned MxS and power training phase.

Specific power training for throwing events and movements must focus on the maximum application of force and use the isotonic and ballistic methods. For the isotonic method, the reps (three to eight) need *not* be performed nonstop or at a high rate. In fact, for maximum benefit of explosive contraction in acyclic movements, in which the most fast-twitch fibers are recruited voluntarily at once, athletes should perform one rep at a time while achieving the highest mental concentration before each rep, possibly with an accommodating resistance (barbell plus bands or chains).

Takeoff Power

In many sports, good performance is possible only if the athlete is capable of an explosive takeoff. Examples include jumping events in track and field, ski jumping, volleyball, basketball, soccer, gymnastics, figure skating, and diving. In many cases, takeoff occurs following a short-distance, high-velocity run, during which the muscles prestretch and store energy. At takeoff, this energy is used as an acceleration thrust, producing a powerful jump.

The depth of the crouch needed at the instant of joint flexion depends on muscle fiber makeup as well as on leg power. A deeper crouch requires greater force from the leg extensors. The crouch is a mechanical necessity, though, because it puts the muscles in a state of stretch, giving them a greater distance over which to accelerate for takeoff. The depth of the crouch is proportional to the power of the legs and is usually determined by the muscle fiber make-up of the athlete's lower-body extensor muscles. The higher the percentage of fast-twitch fibers in the extensor muscles of the athlete, the less he or she will

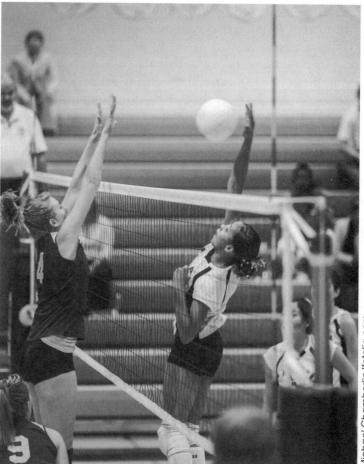

In sports like volleyball, success favors the athlete who is capable of an explosive takeoff.

Michael Chamberlin/fotolia.com

need to flex the knees and hips to perform the reactive jump. If the flexion is too great, the extension (or shortening phase) is performed slowly, and as a result the application of force is slow and the power output of the resulting jump is low, despite its height.

Starting Power

Starting power is an essential and often determinant ability in sports in which the initial speed of action dictates the final outcome. Relevant sports include boxing, karate, fencing, sprinting (the start), and team sports that call for aggressive acceleration from standing. The fundamental physiological characteristic for successful performance in these situations is the ability to start the motion explosively by recruiting the highest possible number of fast-twitch fibers.

In sprinting, starting is performed with the muscles in the prestretched position (both knees and hips bent), from which they can generate greater power than when relaxed or shortened. In this position, the elastic elements of the muscles store kinetic energy that acts like a spring at the sound of the gun. The power used by national-class athletes is very high at the start: 290 pounds (132 kg) for the front leg and 225 pounds (102 kg) for the back leg. Higher starting power enables a more explosive and faster start. Olympic-class sprinters have recorded a starting power of 2 to 2.4 times their own body weight.

In boxing and the martial arts, a quick and powerful start in implementing an offensive skill prevents an opponent from using an effective defensive action. Quick action and powerful starts hinge on the elastic, reactive components of the neuromuscular system. These qualities can be maximized through more specific power training during the conversion phase, which better improves a muscle's stretch reflex and increases the power of the fast-twitch fibers.

Such aspects, which are key to starting a motion quickly and powerfully, can be trained through isotonic, ballistic, and especially maxex and plyometric exercises. They can be performed in a set of repetitive motions or separately. In the latter case, exercises in a set are performed one at a time so that the athlete has enough time to reach maximum mental concentration in order to perform them as explosively as possible. These conditions make it possible to recruit a high number of fast-twitch fibers; consequently, the athlete can perform the action with the greatest power available.

Acceleration Power

In sprinting, swimming, cycling, rowing, and most team sports, performance improvement requires the athlete to develop the ability to accelerate in order to achieve high speed. Doing so requires power. Without power, an athlete cannot perform the required powerful push against the ground in running or overcome water resistance in aquatic sports. Obviously, power is an essential attribute in every sport that requires high acceleration.

In sprinting, for instance, the force applied against the ground is 2 to 2.5 times that of the athlete's body weight. In rowing, the oarsperson must use a constant blade pressure between 100 and 180 pounds (45 and 82 kg) per stroke in order to have a powerful start and maintain high acceleration. And in all sports requiring acceleration power, the relevant forceful action must be performed repetitively and very rapidly. In these situations, more force applied against the ground—or a greater difference between the athlete's maximum strength and the water resistance—enables higher acceleration.

To achieve high acceleration, then, it essential to develop maximum strength. Because this goal is achieved during the MxS phase, the gains must be both maintained and converted to power through specific power training methods. More specifically, the isotonic, ballistic, power-resisting, and plyometric methods can help an athlete apply the series of muscle impulses that activate a great number of fast-twitch fibers at a high rate. Such activation enables the athlete to apply acceleration power at the desired high level.

These methods can be implemented either with a low number of reps (1 to 6) performed explosively and with high frequency, or individually—one rep at a time. In the first case, the goal is repeated displays of cyclic power. In the second case, the goal is to apply the highest amount of power in a single, acyclic attempt in which the elastic–reactive component of strength is less used. Both methods must be used because athletes in sports requiring acceleration power must perform instantaneous powerful actions and do so with high frequency. By applying periodization of strength, athletes increase the likelihood of achieving these effects, as well as reaching peak acceleration power at the right time for major competitions.

Deceleration Power

In several sports, especially racket and team sports, deceleration is as important as acceleration. Team-sport players must be able to accelerate and run as quickly as possible in order to accomplish various goals, such as overtaking an opponent or making oneself available to receive a pass. In some sports—for example, soccer, basketball, lacrosse, and ice hockey—they also need the ability to decelerate quickly, then quickly change their running direction or jump to perform a sport-specific action, such as rebounding an incoming ball. Often, an athlete who can decelerate fast can create a tactical advantage.

Deceleration requires strong legs and good biomechanics; indeed, performing a quick deceleration can require leg force over twice one's body weight. Deceleration is performed through eccentric contraction of the leg muscles. This contraction is facilitated by placing the feet ahead of the center of gravity and leaving the upper body behind it. Muscles developed to decelerate quickly from a fast sprint rely on their elastic properties to amortize and reduce impact forces. The ability to amortize these forces requires power and degrees of knee and hip flexion similar to those needed for absorbing shock while landing.

To train the muscles to decelerate quickly, athletes must employ several methods, such as eccentric contraction and plyometrics. For eccentric contraction, the maximum strength method must be applied with progression from medium to supermaximum loads. For plyometrics, after a few years of normal progression from low- to high-impact exercises, the athlete can use drop or depth jumps from high boxes.

Conversion to Muscular Endurance

Muscle endurance refers to the capacity of an athlete to repeat many (i.e., hundreds) of repetitions against a given resistance for the purpose of maintaining same force application throughout the race. No matter how intensive or comprehensive it is, strength training cannot produce adequate adaptation—or the resulting positive training effect—unless it addresses the specific physiological needs of the chosen sport. Even though most training specialists might agree with this statement, strength-training programs are often inadequate for sports and events in which endurance is a dominant or important component. These programs are still unduly influenced by weightlifting and bodybuilding training methods. However, though doing 20 reps may result in what bodybuilders consider muscular endurance, such a training regimen is grossly inadequate for sports such as mid- and long-distance swimming, rowing, canoeing, boxing, wrestling, cross-country skiing, speedskating, and triathlon—all of which are aerobic endurance dominant.

On the other hand, if an athlete uses only a low-rep strength training program with loads that are submaximal (70% of 1RM) or maximal (well over 80%), the athlete experiences adaptations to such loading in energy supply, recovery, and physiological functioning of the organs and neuromuscular system. As a result, the athlete will achieve increased strength and movement efficiency but not muscular endurance. Such a program, therefore, does not enable optimal performance in endurance-dominant sports.

As we have seen, high-load strength training activates fast-twitch muscle fibers. This fact is well known, accepted, and applied in strength training for sports in which speed and power are the dominant abilities. However, athletic activities of long duration require a different type of training.

During longer-duration sports or events, the pace is often submaximal, and therefore the tension in the muscles is lower. As a result, the CNS first recruits muscle fibers that are specialized and adapted to cope with long-lasting physiological functioning: the slow-twitch (Type I) and the fast-twitch (Type IIA) muscle fibers. As a result of endurance training, the body is better able to use fat as fuel, thus sparing glycogen stores and disposing of and reusing lactic acid more efficiently.

However, these physiological adaptations cannot be accomplished solely by performing the sport. Because the sport-specific training represents a monotonous stimulus, the body is not forced to adapt to a higher level. In other words, for example, continuous rowing might be a sufficient stimulus for improving muscular endurance, but it is not sufficient for increasing sport performance. Instead, athletes should perform strength training with high reps using loads that are low to moderate but higher than what they encounter in their sport-specific activity. This kind of work trains the slow-twitch and fast-twitch muscle fibers to better respond to the dynamics of endurance sports.

Because fatigue seems to occur in stages (Wilmore and Costill 2004), when slow-twitch Type I and fast-twitch Type IIA fibers become exhausted, the powerful fast-twitch Type IIX fibers are recruited to work as well. Therefore, organizing a training program that recruits and maximizes the involvement of all three types of muscle fiber is the best method of enhancing muscular endurance. Athletes in aerobic-dominant sports should do the following.

- Use training methods for muscular endurance of long duration that specifically address the adaptation of the muscle fibers, which are needed during long-duration sporting activities. The better they are trained, the longer they can produce the specific force in long-lasting events.

- Alternate strength training methods for muscular endurance of long duration with methods for power endurance of short duration so that fast-twitch Type IIA and fast-twitch Type IIX fibers are also recruited and, therefore, adapt to the specifics of long-duration activities.

- Use specific endurance training methods—such as long intervals (several reps of 10-30 minutes nonstop) and long-distance training—to adapt the body to effectively use free fatty acid as a fuel and improve cardiovascular efficiency.

- Endurance training also enhances the oxidative capacity of fast-twitch fibers, which increases mitochondria and oxidative enzymes. As a result, the athlete relies more heavily on fat (free fatty acid) for ATP production, the most lasting energy reserve of the body (Wilmore and Costill 2004).

As we have discussed, a strength training program for endurance-dominant sports requires loads that are slightly higher than those encountered in competition. It also requires a high number of reps that approach the duration of the event. Implementing these parameters trains both the nervous system and the metabolic systems of the athlete to cope with the fatigue that is specific to his or her sport. The physiological requirements of training structured in this way closely resemble those of competition. Fortunately, the neuromuscular system is capable of adapting to any type of training.

The importance of maximum strength for endurance-dominant sports increases in proportion to external resistance. For instance, 400-meter swimmers move at a higher velocity than 1,500-meter swimmers. To create the higher velocity, 400-meter swimmers must pull against the water resistance with greater force than 1,500-meter swimmers do. This means that maximum strength is more important for 400-meter swimmers than for 1,500-meter swimmers.

In both cases, however, maximum strength must be improved from year to year if swimmers expect to cover their distance faster. Such improvement is possible only if they improve their specific metabolic endurance and increase the force they use to pull against the water resistance. Only this increased force pushes the body through the water faster. The belief that MxS training makes swimmers slower because of the low velocity of training is a myth. In reality, MxS training is the only way to adapt the athlete's neuromuscular system to recruit more motor units for any sport task, thus providing a strong foundation on which to enhance muscular endurance.

Muscular endurance is best increased through a strength training program that emphasizes a high number of reps performed either explosively or at a steady pace, depending on the specifics of the sport. Both the selected exercises and the number of reps must be geared to produce the desired adaptation to the physiological requirements of the chosen sport or event. Athletes who do not apply adequate training methods during the conversion of maximum strength to muscular endurance cannot expect a positive transfer from training to the competitive environment. For example, a methodology borrowed from bodybuilding or weightlifting, in which 20 reps are considered optimal, will not help an athlete in a sport that requires 200 or more nonstop strokes (such as swimming, rowing, and canoeing) or in marathon running with its 50,000 strides.

However, as in all sport-specific periodization models, the number of reps performed in the sport cannot suddenly appear in the athlete's training schedule. To the contrary, the plan must gradually implement the needed increase in reps (at a specific load). The optimal progression is dictated by the time available for the muscle endurance phase and the target time under tension per set. Similarly, load increases, when necessary, must be between 2.5% and 5% from microcycle to microcycle, because a larger increase can affect the number of reps that the athlete is able to perform.

For endurance sports, aerobic endurance and muscular endurance must be trained at the same time. This requirement can be met either by training the two capabilities on separate days or, sometimes, by combining them in the same training session. In the latter case, muscular endurance should be performed at the end of the session because the specific endurance work often includes technical training. Combined workouts can be limited by fatigue, and if the total work per day must be decreased, the reduction is normally made in the muscular endurance work.

Here are the types of muscular endurance training for various sports.

- *Muscular endurance dynamic (concentric–eccentric).* Cyclic sports (e.g., rowing, swimming, cycling, cross-country skiing, canoeing, kayaking) and certain other sports (e.g., racket sports and boxing)

- *Muscular endurance isometric.* Sports (e.g., sailing and driving) in which the athlete may stay in a specific position (i.e., in isometric contraction) for many minutes

- *Muscular endurance mixed (combining dynamic with isometric).* Grappling, Brazilian jujitsu, shooting, and archery

Because sports can require anywhere from a few seconds to several hours of continuous physical activity, muscular endurance training must address these differences. For best training efficiency, muscular endurance is divided into three types according to the physiological characteristics of endurance sports: muscular endurance of short duration, muscular endurance of medium duration, and muscular endurance of long duration. After studying the following suggested training programs, coaches should feel free to adapt them to their athletes' specific needs and training backgrounds and to the physical environment of their sport.

Muscular Endurance of Short Duration

Sports with a duration between 30 seconds and 2 minutes include certain events in track and field, swimming, canoeing, speedskating, and skiing. In addition, some other sports require intense activity of this duration regularly during a game or match, such as ice hockey, basketball, boxing, and wrestling. During such intense activity, athletes build up a high level of lactic acid—often 12 to 20 millimoles or even more per liter—which shows that the lactic acid energy system is a dominant or at least an important component in the overall performance of that sport or event. Most of these sports require very strong anaerobic capacity as well as very good aerobic power.

One key objective of training for endurance sports is to train athletes to tolerate fatigue; specific strength training should pursue the same goal. As the competitive phase approaches, strength training for muscular endurance short must be designed so that it challenges the athlete's ability to tolerate a high buildup of lactic acid, because the energy sources of muscular endurance of short duration are blood glucose and, in particular, the glycogen stored in the muscles whose anaerobic metabolism determines an accumulation of lactic acid. Through training, the body adapts to tolerate the buildup of lactic acid by an increased expression of proteins responsible for removing lactate through its utilization as an energy substrate source (Billat et al. 2003). This adaptation better prepares the athlete for the vigor of competition and for the fatigue that ultimately affects performance.

Training for muscular endurance of short duration, the athlete develops an oxygen debt. This condition is typical of activities in which the anaerobic energy system prevails. After 60 to 90 seconds of such activity, the heart rate can be as high as 200 beats per minute, and blood lactic acid concentration can be between 12 and 20 millimoles per liter or even higher.

Training for muscular endurance of short duration (MES) involves performing reps explosively at a fast pace. The load is not very high (40% to 60% of 1RM) but reps are performed at high intensity—at or close to the rate in competition. For this reason, athletes should use the fewest possible exercises (2 to 6) to engage the prime movers.

The number of reps can be set precisely, but as in interval training it is more practical to decide the duration of each set—15 to 120 seconds—and the speed of performance—fast but steady. If the number of exercises is low, the athlete can perform three to six sets. The duration and number of sets must be increased progressively.

To elicit the fastest and highest accumulation of lactic acid, the speed of performance must be explosive. In addition, in order to train an athlete to tolerate lactic acid buildup, the rest interval must be such that it enables a high power output in a very acidic environment (3-8 minutes between sets).

Training parameters for MES are given in table 11.7. This approach mimics the event-specific dynamics of lactate accumulation. A general example of MES periodization (e.g., for an 800-meter run, a 200-meter freestyle, or a 1,500-meter skate) is shown in figure 11.16. Figure 11.17 presents a sample six-week program for a national-class 100-meter fly swimmer.

Table 11.7 Training Parameters for Muscular Endurance Short

Phase duration	4-6 weeks
Load	40%-60% of 1RM (according to sport-specific external resistance)
Number of exercises	2-6
Set duration	30-120 seconds (per specific event duration)
Number of sets per exercise	3 or 4 minutes
Rest interval	3-8 minutes
Speed of execution	Explosive
Frequency per week	2

Week 1	Week 2	Week 3	Week 4	Week 5	Week 6
2× (4 × 30 sec.)	3× (3 × 40 sec.)	3× (2 × 60 sec.)	3 × 100 sec.	3 × 110 sec.	3 × 120 sec.

Figure 11.16 General example of MES periodization for a two-minute event.

	WEEK					
Exercise	**1**	**2**	**3**	**4**	**5**	**6**
1. Cable pull while lying on belly (load=50% of 1RM)	2 × (4 × 15 sec.)	3 × (3 × 20 sec.)	4 × (2 × 30 sec.)	3 × 50 sec.	3 × 55 sec.	3 × 60 sec.
2. Medicine ball hold and forward throw while lying on back with arms above head	2 × (4 × 15 sec.)	3 × (3 × 20 sec.)	4 × (2 × 30 sec.)	3 × 50 sec.	3 × 55 sec.	3 × 60 sec.
3. Leg extension (load=50% of 1RM)	2 × (4 × 15 sec.)	3 × (3 × 20 sec.)	4 × (2 × 30 sec.)	3 × 50 sec.	3 × 55 sec.	3 × 60 sec.
4. Cable elbow extension (load=50% of 1RM)	2 × (4 × 15 sec.)	3 × (3 × 20 sec.)	4 × (2 × 30 sec.)	3 × 50 sec.	3 × 55 sec.	3 × 60 sec.
5. Abdominal V-sit	2 × 20	2 × 25	3 × 25	2 × 30	2 × 35	3 × 35
	LOADING PATTERN					
			High			High
		Medium			Medium	
	Low			Low		

Figure 11.17 Sample six-week program for a national-class 100-meter fly swimmer.

Muscular Endurance of Medium and Long Duration

Muscular endurance of medium or long duration is a key factor in improving performance in all sports in which performance time is longer than two minutes. Examples include boxing, wrestling, rowing, swimming (400-1,500 meters), kayaking, canoeing (1,000-10,000 meters), road cycling, cross-country skiing, and biathlon and triathlon running. Training for muscular endurance of medium or long duration can be performed following the principles of interval training of long duration. This training method can also be referred to as extensive interval training because *extensive* implies a high-volume, long-duration type of activity.

The main objective of training for muscular endurance is to increase the athlete's ability to cope with fatigue. Such training improves the athlete's anaerobic and aerobic endurance because it employs a high number of reps—often more than 100. In the early part of a nonstop set with many reps, energy is provided by the anaerobic system. This process produces a buildup of lactic acid that creates physiological and psychological problems for the athlete as he or she attempts to continue the activity. As the athlete overcomes the challenge and continues to work, energy is supplied by the aerobic system. Repetitive muscular endurance training results in a specific adaptation that improves the necessary local aerobic metabolism.

Physiological adaptations promote better oxygen and energy supply and increase the removal of metabolic wastes. For example, repetitive muscular endurance training increases the amount of available glycogen stored both in the muscles and in the liver. Overall, then, muscular endurance training increases physiological efficiency.

Because muscular endurance training employs a relatively low load (around 30%-50% of 1RM), muscles improve their long-term contracting capability without any evident increase in muscle fiber diameter. Only a certain number of motor units are active at one time; the others are at rest and are activated only when and where the contracting fibers become fatigued.

For sports in which muscular endurance represents an important training method, it is also beneficial to improve maximum strength. If the diameter of an individual muscle fiber increases as a result of maximum strength training, a lower number of motor units is required in order to perform a muscular endurance training task. In addition, maximum strength training and plyometric training have been proven to improve movement efficiency. This type of strength reserve created by using fewer units is critical and increases a muscle's capacity to produce work more effectively.

Maximum strength training should not be minimized. To the contrary, within limits, it should be used for all the sports mentioned in this discussion. However, once general preparation is over, doing more than simple maximum strength maintenance provides only negligible benefits for sports of long duration, such as a marathon, and for sports that require less than 30 percent of maximum strength (Hartmann and Tünnemann 1988).

Training for muscular endurance of medium duration (MEM) is suggested for sports in which the duration of competition is between 2 and 8 minutes (events dominated by aerobic power), whereas training for muscular endurance of long duration (MEL) is suggested for sports in which the duration is 8 minutes or longer (events dominated by aerobic capacity). This distinction is necessary because muscular endurance of medium duration has a stronger anaerobic component, whereas muscular endurance of long duration is clearly aerobic. The program designs for each type of muscular endurance are described separately in the following sections because the load, set duration, and speed of execution are also clearly different.

Program Design for Muscular Endurance of Medium Duration

This program is recommended for events that last between 2 and 8 minutes or otherwise require a high level of aerobic power. It can be designed in the form of circuit training or straight sets. The circuit training option is suggested for situations in which it is not possible to practice the sport-specific training with an adequate weekly frequency and therefore the cardiorespiratory adaptations must also be stimulated during the time devoted to training in the gym. The straight-sets approach is suggested for the development of local muscular endurance in longer events; when sets must reach the sport-specific duration; and for sports that require steady power output. It can also be used for intermittent sports. Examples are presented for each of the three options.

The load in training for MEM ranges from 30% to 50% of 1RM (see table 11.8). Throughout the MEM phase, certain parameters are held constant: load, speed of execution, and number of exercises (more for sports in which several muscle groups must be trained, such as wrestling and boxing, and fewer for sports in which either the upper- or lower-body muscle groups prevail, such as speedskating and canoeing). Set duration, however, increases every week or every second week. The program is designed precisely to expose athletes constantly to high levels of fatigue so that they learn to cope with the pain and exhaustion of competition. That is why the rest interval between sets is short, so that the athlete has insufficient time to recover adequately.

Figure 11.18 shows a general example of periodization of MEM (e.g., for 1,500-meter run, 400-meter freestyle swim, 3,000-meter skate, or 1,000-meter kayaking) and figure 11.19 shows a sample MEM program for a wrestler. As shown, the duration and number of reps are increased progressively over a long period. To achieve physiological adaptation in response to such high training, the duration of the conversion phase must be 8 to 10 weeks.

Table 11.8   Training Parameters for Muscular Endurance Medium

Phase duration	8-10 weeks
Load	30%-50% of 1RM (according to sport-specific external resistance)
Number of exercises	4-8
Set duration	2-8 minutes (according to specific event duration)
Number of sets per exercise	3 or 4 minutes
Rest interval	2-3 minutes
Speed of execution	Fast
Frequency per week	2

Week 1	Week 2	Week 3	Week 4	Week 5	Week 6
2 × (4 × 60 sec.)	3 × (3 × 80 sec.)	3 × (2 × 120 sec.)	3 × 200 sec.	3 × 220 sec.	3 × 240 sec.

Figure 11.18   General example of MEM periodization for events lasting about four minutes and requiring steadily high power output.

Circuit training designed for muscular endurance of medium (and long) duration can use a barbell or any other piece of equipment. The advantage of using a barbell is that different limbs can be exercised without stopping to rest, as required in the circuit shown in figure 11.20.

The circuit in figure 11.20 includes eight exercises that, after 9 or 10 weeks, are performed as follows. The athlete places a barbell of 40% of maximum strength on the ground and performs 50 deadlifts. After completing the last rep, the athlete deloads the barbell,

Exercises	WEEK							
	1	2	3	4	5	6	7	8
Zercher squat	2 × 120 sec.	2 × 120 sec.	3 × 120 sec.	3 × 120 sec.	2 × (2 × 60 sec.)	2 × (2 × 60 sec.)	3 × (3 × 40 sec.)	3 × (3 × 40 sec.)
Floor press	2 × 120 sec.	2 × 120 sec.	3 × 120 sec.	3 × 120 sec.	2 × (2 × 60 sec.)	2 × (2 × 60 sec.)	3 × (3 × 40 sec.)	3 × (3 × 40 sec.)
Hip bridge	2 × 120 sec.	2 × 120 sec.	3 × 120 sec.	3 × 120 sec.	2 × (2 × 60 sec.)	2 × (2 × 60 sec.)	3 × (3 × 40 sec.)	3 × (3 × 40 sec.)
Lat machine (neutral narrow grip)	2 × 120 sec.	2 × 120 sec.	3 × 120 sec.	3 × 120 sec.	2 × (2 × 60 sec.)	2 × (2 × 60 sec.)	3 × (3 × 40 sec.)	3 × (3 × 40 sec.)
Barbell curl	2 × 120 sec.	2 × 120 sec.	3 × 120 sec.	3 × 120 sec.	2 × (2 × 60 sec.)	2 × (2 × 60 sec.)	3 × (3 × 40 sec.)	3 × (3 × 40 sec.)
Farmer's walk	2 × 100 sec.	2 × 100 sec.	3 × 80 sec.	3 × 80 sec.	2 × (2 × 60 sec.)	2 × (2 × 60 sec.)	3 × (2 × 40 sec.)	3 × (2 × 40 sec.)

Figure 11.19 A MEM program for a wrestler.

Exercise	NUMBER OF WEEKS			
	3 or 4	3	3	2
Pulley Row	Progressively aim to perform 50–60 reps nonstop per exercise with a load of 30%–50% of 1RM.	Perform 2 exercises nonstop, or 100 reps together (e.g., 50 half squats followed by 50 arm curls); pair the remaining 6 exercises.	Perform 4 exercises nonstop, or 200 reps together. After a rest interval, perform the other 4 exercises in the same manner.	Perform all exercises nonstop (8 exercises × 50 reps = 400 reps nonstop).
Bench press				
Half squat				
Arm curl				
Deadlift				
Bent-over row				
Toe raise				
V-sit				
Rest interval	1 minute between exercises	1–2 minutes between pairs	2 minutes between the groups	1 minute

A similar program can be developed for other sports, such as 400- to 1,500-meter swimming, middle-distance speedskating events, kayaking, and canoeing.

Figure 11.20 Sample MEM circuit for a rower.

lies on the bench, and does 50 bench presses. The athlete then quickly reloads the bar, places the barbell back on the shoulders, and performs 50 half squats. After completing the last squat, the athlete sits on a bench and performs 50 arm curls, then grabs a kettlebell from the ground and performs 50 kettlebell swings. The athlete moves immediately to 50 rowing actions, then once again quickly places the barbell on the shoulders and performs 50 toe raises, which are followed by 50 V-sits performed on the ground. The total number of reps performed in our hypothetical circuit is 400.

The advantage of this method is that the cardiorespiratory system is involved throughout the circuit because training alternates between different muscle groups. This work develops muscular endurance and aerobic endurance—the two crucial abilities for any of the sports discussed in this chapter—which is particularly good when, for instance, the athlete cannot do much specific metabolic training during the macrocycle.

To further clarify the information presented in figure 11.20, coaches should consider the following guidelines.

- The number of reps increases progressively to reach 40 to 60 (or even higher); doing so may take two to three weeks.

- The number of exercises may vary depending on the needs of the sport.

- The number of reps may differ between the first exercises and the last exercises when the latter ones are given lower priority.

- The same exercise can be repeated twice in the same circuit to emphasize the importance of that group of muscles in a given sport.

- The number of exercises may not be the same for the upper and the lower body. This decision should be based on the athlete's strengths and weaknesses and the sport's demands.

- With beginners, the load for a deadlift must be lower (30%-40% of 1RM) and used carefully (employing long-term progression).

- Athletes should maintain a steady speed throughout the circuit, even though they may have the urge to move faster and get the exercise over with.

- Coaches and trainers should set up all needed equipment before training so that the athlete needs as little time as possible to move from one exercise to another, especially in a gym setting. Good choices in such settings include barbell and dumbbell exercises that can be performed in an enclosed space.

- Athletes should perform two exercises nonstop in the second phase, four nonstop in the third phase, and all eight nonstop in the last phase.

- The athlete may need 8 to 10 minutes or longer to perform an eight-exercise circuit nonstop, depending on his or her classification. An even longer circuit can be designed for better improvement of MEL.

- Because both MEM and MEL involve severe physiological demands, this method should be used only by athletes with a strong background in both strength and endurance training (national-class athletes and higher). For a less demanding circuit (for juniors), include only four to six exercises.

- It is best to perform an even number of exercises because of the recommended progression—two exercises performed nonstop, then four, then all eight.

- As an athlete adapts to performing the total number of exercises nonstop during the last phase, the coach can use a stopwatch to monitor improvement. The time required to complete the circuit should decrease as a result of adaptation.

Figure 11.21 This figure shows a suggested MEM program for boxing. This program has to be performed nonstop, from the first to the last exercise, with a steady rhythm, but as fast as possible. The only exception is the jump squat, in which the eccentric phase has to be performed in a fast but controlled fashion to avoid deep knee compression.

For the one-arm standing medicine ball throw, the athlete needs to throw the ball against a solid rebounding wall. The throw must imitate a boxing punch, performed horizontally forward with the other arm being used just as a support, to hold the ball in front of the chest. The weight of the ball can start (depending on the boxer's conditioning) at 6 to 8 pounds (2.7-3.6 kg). The weight should decrease every one or two weeks by one or two pounds. During the last week or two, the ball should weigh 2 to 4 pounds (0.9-1.8 kg).

Because the upper body musculature of a boxer must endure a more anaerobic kind of activity, the duration of the upper-body exercise sets is split. The rest intervals are planned after roughly the duration of a round, then after a progressively longer time, to ensure both a high power output and the development of specific muscular endurance.

Exercise	Week 1	Week 2	Week 3	Week 4
One-arm standing medicine ball chest throw	4×10 reps, 10 sec. rest interval	5×10 reps, 10 sec. rest interval	6×10 reps, 10 sec. rest interval	6×10 reps, 10 sec. rest interval
Jump squat (50% of 1RM)	30 reps	30 reps	30 reps	30 reps
Kettlebell swing	1 min.	1 min.	1.5 min. (lighter kettlebell than in weeks 1 and 2)	1.5 min. (same kettlebell as in week 3)
Within a circuit rest interval	1 min.	1 min.	1 min.	1 min.
One-arm standing medicine ball chest throw	4×10 reps, 10 sec. rest interval	5×10 reps, 10 sec. rest interval	6×10 reps, 10 sec. rest interval	6×10 reps, 10 sec. rest interval
Two-arm standing medicine ball smash-down	4×10 sec., 10 sec. rest interval	5×10 sec., 10 sec. rest interval	6×10 sec., 10 sec. rest interval	6×10 sec., 10 sec. rest interval
Rest interval between circuits	1 min.	1 min.	1 min.	1 min.
Number of circuits	3	3	3 or 4	4 or 5
Total duration of single circuit	8 min.	9 min.	10 min.	10 min.

To prolong the duration of a circuit, add another exercise, such as the abdomen crunch. Professional boxers must progressively use a higher number of circuits to meet the muscular endurance requirements of going 10 or 12 rounds in the ring (e.g., repeat the circuit 5 to 7 times).

Figure 11.21 Sample program for MEM for boxing.

Program Design for Muscular Endurance of Long Duration

Sports of longer duration require a different kind of physiological training. In most of these sports, the athlete applies force against a given resistance—for example, water in swimming, rowing, and canoeing; pedals in cycling (with body weight applied as strength, especially uphill); ice in speed skating; and snow and various terrains in cross-country skiing and biathlon. The dominant energy system in such sports is aerobic capacity, and improved performance is expected to come from increments in both central and peripheral aerobic endurance. Central (cardiovascular) adaptations are addressed mainly by sport-specific training; therefore, strength training must be designed to enhance local muscular endurance.

To increase muscular endurance of long duration, the key training ingredient is a high number of reps performed nonstop. The other training parameters remain constant, as indicated in table 11.9.

Because one training goal of MEL is to enable the athlete to cope with fatigue, the rest interval does not allow full recovery. In fact, only a very short rest (usually 5-10 seconds) is afforded as the athlete changes stations. Similarly, for straight-sets training, only a short rest interval is programmed—again, to prevent a complete muscular recovery—thus further challenging local muscular endurance.

Figure 11.22 shows a typical training program for sports such as triathlon, marathon, kayaking and canoeing (10,000-meter and marathon), long-distance swimming, road cycling, and cross-country skiing. To facilitate monitoring the many minutes of steady work, duration is expressed in minutes rather than number of reps.

The first two exercises can be performed with any combination machine available in a fitness center or a school gymnasium. The last two exercises must be performed using rubber cords, often called elastic cords, which are available in many sporting goods stores. To train long-distance kayakers and canoeists, the elastic cords must be anchored before training so that arm pulls or elbow extensions—typical motions for these two sports—can be performed in a seated position.

The set duration per exercise must be based on the work tolerance and performance level of each athlete. It must also take into consideration the resulting total workout duration. To train muscular endurance of long duration, some have suggested progressing from straight sets to circuits; instead, we suggest progressing from circuits to straight sets in order to further increase local muscular endurance. Here is the reasoning: Circuit training has a greater cardiorespiratory impact than straight sets do. However, long-endurance athletes already have a high level of cardiorespiratory endurance because they devote, on average, 90% of their total annual training time to sport-specific activity. Therefore, their specific strength training must focus on local muscular endurance of the prime movers.

Table 11.9   Training Parameters for Muscular Endurance Long

Phase duration	8-12 weeks
Load	30%-40% of 1RM
Number of exercises	4-6
Number of sets per session	2-4
Rest interval	2 minutes between circuits, 1 minute between sets
Speed of execution	Medium
Frequency per week	2 or 3

Muscular Endurance Isometric

A limited number of sports require athletes to use isometric contraction of long duration during competition. Examples include sailing and motor sports (driving). During training and competition in sailing, the athlete takes a specific position (static in most cases) in which parts of the body perform long-duration isometric contraction. For instance, a sailor may be seated on a side of the board while holding a rope in order to maintain

Exercise	NUMBER OF WEEKS					
	2	**2**	**2**	**2**	**2**	**2 or 3**
Leg press	With a load of 30% of 1RM, do 4 minutes of nonstop work for each exercise.	Do the same work for 7 minutes nonstop per exercise. To maintain proper workout duration, choose between leg presses and arm pulls per circuit (thus do 5 exercises per circuit).	Do 10 minutes of nonstop work of an exercise. To maintain proper workout duration, eliminate the leg presses and arm pulls (thus do 4 exercises per circuit).	Do 6 minutes of nonstop work of an exercise. Take a 1-minute rest, repeat the set, then proceed to the next exercise.	Do 8 minutes of nonstop work of an exercise. Take a 1-minute rest, repeat the set, then proceed to the next exercise. To maintain proper workout duration, only perform one set of leg presses and arm pulls.	Do 10 minutes of nonstop work of an exercise. Take a 1-minute rest, repeat the set, then proceed to the next exercise. To maintain proper workout duration, eliminate the leg press and arm pulls (thus do 4 total exercises).
Arm pull (cords)						
Bench press						
Leg press						
Arm pull (cords)						
Elbow extension (cords)						
Number of circuits completed	3	2	2	—	—	—
Number of sets per exercise	—	—	—	2	2	2
Rest interval between circuits	2 minutes	2 minutes	2 minutes	—	—	—
Rest interval between exercises	—	—	—	1 minute	1 minute	1 minute
Workout duration	76 minutes	72 minutes	82 minutes	84 minutes	84 minutes	84 minutes

A similar concept of training can be applied to other sports, such as long-distance cross-country skiing, kayaking, marathon swimming, and triathlon.

Figure 11.22 Sample MEL training program for an experienced marathon canoeist.

the sail in the most wind-effective position. To do so, the athlete contracts certain parts of the body, such as the abdomen, legs, low back, and arms.

Unlike motor sports, in which specific strength training is performed in the gym, the muscular endurance isometric training for sailing can be performed on the boat or off the boat, as illustrated in the following example. During training, the athlete can use a heavy vest to overload the upper body, creating an additional physiological challenge against the pull of gravity and the centrifugal force during turns. Heavy vests can carry different weights, often as high as 35 pounds (about 16 kg). The scope of training can involve progressively increasing either the weight of the vest or the duration of using it.

Figure 11.23 suggests a progression for using a weighted vest for training in the boat. This progression is only a guideline, applicable as appropriate for the athlete's individual physical capabilities, needs, and training environment. Training for sailing should include a preparatory phase, regardless of whether the sailor lives in a climate that favors year-round training. Figure 11.24 illustrates a suggested strength training program for sailing, in which isometric training is dominant. The angle at which the athlete holds the isometric contraction must be sport-specific. Again, this is only a progression guideline; coaches should adapt it to fit the needs of their athletes, for both sailing and driving.

Weight of vest	10 kg (about 22 lb.)	12 kg (about 26.5 lb.)	15 kg (about 33 lb.)
Duration	2 × 15 min.	3 × 15 min.	4 × 20 min.

Figure 11.23 Sample progression for in-boat use of heavy vests in sailing.

Exercise	WEEK						Rest interval
	1	2	3	4	5	6	
1. Arm pull	5 × 60 sec.	4 × 90 sec.	3 × 120 sec.	2 × 180 sec.	2 × 240 sec.	2 × 240 sec.	1 min.
2. Leg press	5 × 60 sec.	4 × 90 sec.	3 × 120 sec.	2 × 180 sec.	2 × 240 sec.	2 × 240 sec.	2 min.
3. Leg curl	4 × 30 sec.	4 × 45 sec.	2 × 60 sec.	2 × 90 sec.	2 × 120 sec.	2 × 120 sec.	2 min.
4. Back extension	5 × 60 sec.	4 × 90 sec.	3 × 120 sec.	2 × 180 sec.	2 × 240 sec.	2 × 240 sec.	2 min.
5. Bench press	5 × 60 sec.	4 × 90 sec.	3 × 120 sec.	2 × 180 sec.	2 × 240 sec.	2 × 240 sec.	1 min.
6. Roman chair iso crunch	5 × 60 sec.	4 × 90 sec.	3 × 120 sec.	2 × 180 sec.	2 × 240 sec.	2 × 240 sec.	1 min.

Figure 11.24 Sample strength training program for sailing.

Muscular Endurance Using Mixed Contractions Method

Muscular endurance using mixed contractions is specific to certain sports, such as grappling, Brazilian jujitsu, shooting, and archery. The main scope of training for such sports is to expose athletes to mixed-contraction training, such as concentric–isometric–eccentric, in order to ready them for major competition.

Consider pistol shooting, in which the pistol weighs 3 pounds (about 1.4 kg). During competition, the shooter lifts the pistol 20 times, each time holding an isometric contraction of 10 to 15 seconds, with limited rest intervals. Poorly trained athletes have a shaky arm, mostly toward the end of a competition, which is of course far from conducive to high shooting accuracy. Therefore, the scope of training in this sport (see figure 11.25) is to prepare the athlete to lift the pistol at least as many times as needed during competition, using weights greater than the weight of the pistol, for a sport-specific duration of isometric contraction and with sport-specific rest intervals between sets (50 seconds during a final).

Weeks	2	2	2
Weight of dumbbell	1.5 kg (about 3.3 lb.)	2 kg (about 4.4 lb.)	2.5 kg (about 5.5 lb.)
45-degree raise	18 sets x 1 rep	16 sets x 1 rep	14 sets x 1 rep
Isometric contraction duration at specific joint angle	15 sec.	15 sec.	12 sec.
Rest interval between sets	50 sec.	50 sec.	50 sec.

Figure 11.25 Sample progression for mixed concentric–isometric–eccentric training for shooting.

The technical action in pistol shooting is as follows: Lift the pistol from the hip to shoulder level, hold it still for 10 to 15 seconds, shoot, and then lower the pistol to the starting position. The longest shooting round lasts 14 shots. A similar type of action is required in archery, in which the archer performs concentric–isometric contraction against resistance while stretching the bowstring and holding it for a few seconds (5 to 10). The archer then releases the arrow and lowers the bow to prepare for a new attempt.

Mixed martial arts (MMA) also features a mix of eccentric–concentric and isometric contractions during the ground portion of a fight. Such contractions are also needed in grappling and Brazilian jujitsu. As always, these sport-specific strength requirements must be reflected in the athletes' strength training. This need can be met by targeting the prime movers that undergo the isometric contractions either through functional isometrics interspersed with eccentric–concentric exercises or through straight isometric exercises; see figure 11.26.

WORKOUTS 1-3-5**			
Exercise	Sets	Reps	Rest interval
Deadlift	3	1 (75% of 1RM)	2 min.
Bench press	3	2 (75%)	2 min.
Good morning	3	5 (2 reps short to failure)	2 min.
Pull-up with functional isometrics	3	3 (70% of 1RM)	2 min.
Hip bridge	3	3 (70% of 1RM)	2 min.
Radial deviation	2	8	1 min.
Sit-up with weight	2	6	1 min.
WORKOUTS 2-4-6***			
Exercise	Sets	Reps	Rest interval
Isometric kneeling good morning	3	60 sec.	2 min.
Isometric floor press	3	60 sec.	3 min.
One-arm dumbbell row	3	5 (2 reps short to failure)	90 sec.
Front raise	3	8	90 sec.
Standing calf raise	3	8	90 sec.
Iso neck extension on Swiss ball	3	60 sec.	1 min.
Turkish get-up	3	3+3 (L/R)	90 sec.
Farmer's walk	3	60 sec. + 60 sec. (L/R)	90 sec.

*Two-week block before a two-week precompetition taper.

**Workouts 1 and 3 performed in the first week; workout 5 performed in the second week.

***Workout 2 performed in the first week; workouts 4 and 6 performed in the second week.

Figure 11.26 Sample program using mixed concentric–eccentric and isometric training for an MMA, grappling, or Brazilian jujitsu fighter during the competitive phase.

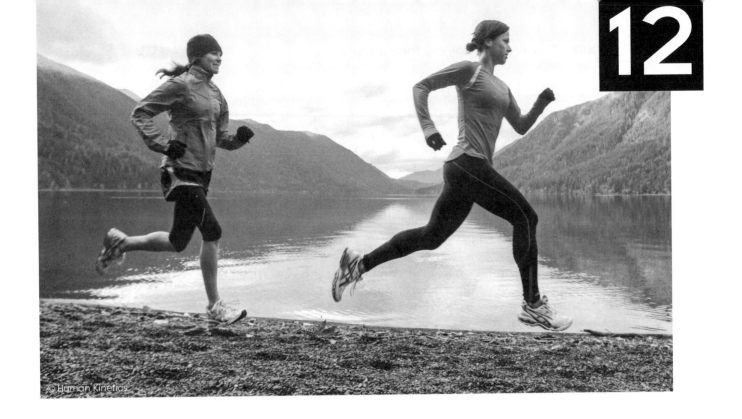

Maintenance, Cessation, and Compensation

Strength training is an important physiological contributor to overall athletic performance. In particular, more explosive skills require more maximum strength and power, and longer activities require more muscular endurance. In both cases, superior performance requires the vital contribution of strength.

The benefits of strength for athletic performance are experienced as long as the neuromuscular system maintains the cellular adaptations induced by training. When strength training is discontinued, the benefits soon decrease as the contractile properties of the muscles diminish. The consequence is the process of detraining—a visible decrease in the contribution of strength to athletic performance. To avoid detraining, athletes must implement sport-specific strength programs during the competitive phase.

Strength training also affects peaking or performing at peak level during the year's main competitions. In several sports, especially power sports, peak performance is often achieved in the early part of the competitive phase. During this time, coaches tend to overlook strength training because specific technical and tactical training become dominant. Unfortunately, this lack of strength training causes decreased performance as the season progresses. In the early part of the season, while strength training remains in effect, the athlete can perform as expected. But when the athlete's ability to contract the muscles powerfully diminishes, so does performance.

According to the theory of periodization of strength, gains in maximum strength during the MxS phase should be transformed into either muscular endurance or power during the conversion phase while maintaining maximum strength levels. Doing so enables athletes to develop the best possible sport-specific strength and equips them with the physiological abilities necessary for strong performance during the competitive phase. This physiological base must be sustained for the athlete to maintain the performance level throughout the competitive phase.

To achieve this, the coach must plan a sport-specific strength maintenance program throughout the competitive phase. Maximum strength is a crucial ingredient for sport-specific strength programs. Many sports require maintenance of some maximum strength during the competitive season, mostly using the low-volume-of-maximum-load method (usually 40%-50% of the volume used for the highest-load microcycle of the maximum strength phase). Gains in maximum strength decline faster if they resulted from a too-short maximum strength phase.

In addition, in many sports, the only type of strength training performed is event-specific power training. Maximum strength training is often overlooked, and gains are therefore short-lived. Another methodological error occurs when strength training is done only during the preparatory phase; in that case, strength gains deteriorate as the competitive phase progresses and approaches its peak.

With all of this in mind, coaches should not question *whether* to prescribe strength maintenance training during the competitive phase but rather *how* to do so. They must keep in mind the dominant ability of the sport and carefully consider what types of strength the athlete needs to maintain. Most sports require some elements of maximum strength, power, and muscular endurance. The most important decision, therefore, is not which of the three to maintain but in what proportion—and how best to integrate them into training.

Athletes in power sports must maintain both maximum strength and power. Because these abilities cannot be substituted for each other—rather, they are complementary—one

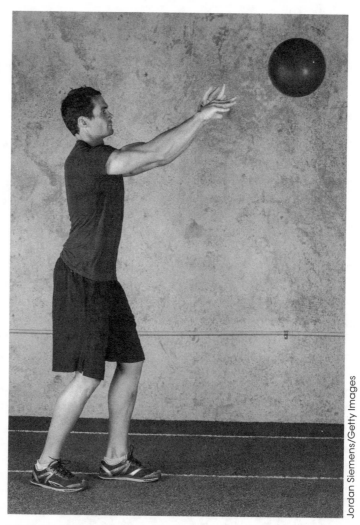

Jordan Siemens/Getty Images

Medicine ball training can help athletes maintain power.

should not be maintained at the expense of the other. For instance, throwers in track and field and linemen in American football must maintain maximum strength during the competitive phase with a roughly equal proportion of maximum strength and power. Most athletes in team sports should maintain maximum strength, power, and either power endurance or muscular endurance, depending on the position they play. For endurance sports, however, the ratio between maximum strength and muscular endurance depends both on the duration of the event and on which energy system is dominant. For the majority of endurance sports, muscular endurance is the dominant component of strength.

The proportion of different types of strength to maintain also depends on the duration of the competitive phase. The longer this phase, the more important it is to maintain some elements of maximum strength, because this type of strength is an important component of both power and muscular endurance. Overlooking this fact results in the detraining of maximum strength, which affects both power and muscular endurance. Table 12.1 shows the proportions of different types of strength to be maintained during the competitive phase for various sports and positions.

The same training methods suggested in earlier chapters should be applied during the maintenance phase. What differs during this phase is not the methodology but the volume of strength training as compared with the volume of technical, tactical, and other training. During this phase, the strength maintenance program should be subordinate to other types of training. The athlete should use the lowest number of exercises (2 to 4, or 6 for some multiplanar sports) to address the prime movers. With this approach, the athlete expends the least possible energy for maintenance of strength, leaving the majority of energy for technical and tactical training.

The one to three strength training sessions per week during the competitive phase should be as short as possible. Indeed, a good maintenance program can often be accomplished in 20 to 30 minutes. Of course, the frequency of strength training sessions also depends on the competition schedule. If no competitions are scheduled on the weekend, then a microcycle may include two (or perhaps three) strength training sessions. If a game or competition is planned on the weekend, then one (or perhaps two) short strength training sessions can be planned.

Table 12.1 Strength Proportions for the Competitive Phase

Sport or event	Maximum strength %	Power %	Power endurance %	Muscular endurance %
Athletics				
Sprinting	40	40	20	—
Jumping	30	70	—	—
Throwing	50	50	—	—
Baseball				
Pitcher	40	40	20	—
Field player	20	70	10	—
Basketball	20	60	20	—
Biathlon	—	—	20	80
Boxing	20	20	30	30

(continued)

Table 12.1 *(continued)*

Sport or event	Maximum strength %	Power %	Power endurance %	Muscular endurance %
Canoeing, kayaking				
500 m	40	30	20	10
1,000 m	20	20	20	40
10,000 m	—	—	20	80
Cycling				
Track 200 m	40	40	20	—
4,000 m pursuit	10	30	20	40
Diving	30	70	—	—
Fencing	20	50	30	—
Field hockey	—	40	20	40
Figure skating	40	40	20	—
Football (American)				
Linemen	50	50	—	—
Linebackers	30	50	20	—
Running backs	30	50	20	—
Wide receivers	30	50	20	—
Defensive backs	30	50	20	—
Tailbacks	30	40	20	10
Football (Australian)	30	40	20	10
Ice hockey	20	40	30	10
Martial arts	—	60	30	10
Rowing	20	—	20	60
Rugby	30	40	30	—
Skiing				
Alpine	40	30	30	—
Nordic	—	—	20	80
Soccer				
Goalie	40	60	—	—
Field positions	30	50	20	—
Speedskating				
Sprinting	30	50	20	—
Distance	—	10	20	70
Swimming				
Sprinting	40	40	20	—
Middle distance	10	10	20	60
Long distance	—	—	20	80
Tennis	10	50	30	10
Volleyball	40	50	10	—
Water polo	10	20	20	50
Wrestling	20	20	20	40

The number of sets is also usually low (one to four), depending on whether the athlete is training for power endurance or for muscular endurance. For power and maximum strength, a range of two to four sets is possible because the number of reps is usually low. The rest interval should be longer than usual so that the athlete can recover almost entirely during the break. The intent of the maintenance phase is not to create fatigue but to stabilize performance and maintain high power output. For muscular endurance training, only one or two sets should be performed because the number of reps is higher. For muscular endurance medium training during the competitive phase, the set duration should not exceed one minute; for muscular endurance long, it should not exceed six minutes.

The planning for each microcycle of a maintenance program depends on the type of strength being sought. For power training, athletes should perform exercises that enhance explosiveness by using resistance close to that encountered in competition. Two types of resistance are suggested: increased load and decreased load. Increased-load training involves using a resistance slightly higher than that of competition; it enhances both maximum strength and power. Exercises of this type should be specific to the prevailing skills of the particular sport. This type of exercise is suggested mostly for the early part of the competitive phase as a transition from maximum strength to power. Decreased-load training, on the other hand, involves using a resistance below that encountered in competition. It enhances explosiveness and should prevail in the phase prior to major competition.

Both types of load increase the ability to recruit a high number of fast-twitch muscle fibers and improve coordination of the muscles involved. More generally, if the competitive phase is longer than five months, athletes should dedicate at least 25% of the total work to the maintenance of maximum strength because the detraining of maximum strength negatively affects sport-specific strength.

Variations of Loading Pattern for the Competitive Phase

Strength training is not a rigid process. On the contrary, programs should be flexible and adapted to the athlete's well-being and training progress, to the requirements of the sport, and to the competition schedule. The content of a training session must be planned to match the overall intensity or demand of sport-specific elements in that session and should take into account the proximity of the competition or game. The examples suggested in this section assume that strength training is performed following specific work on technique and tactics and drills for speed and specific endurance. Consequently, the athlete has little time or energy to spare, and strength training must be short and sport specific.

The following guidelines explain in some detail the loading parameter of strength and power maintenance sessions throughout the competitive microcycle. Descriptions are provided for heavy-, medium-, and low-load sessions and for certain other general considerations.

- A heavy-load or heavy-demand strength training session lasts 20 to 30 minutes. It trains maximum strength or a combination of maximum strength and power. Athletes perform four or five total exercises specifically for the prime movers. Strength is trained with a load of 70% to 80% of 1RM (and sometimes up to 90%, depending on the exercise type and the sport) as fast and dynamically as possible while maintaining good technique. Athletes perform 1 to 3 reps in 2 to 4 sets with a rest interval of two to three minutes between sets.

273

- A medium-load strength training session also lasts 20 to 30 minutes. It trains maximum strength, power, or a combination of the two. Athletes perform a total of three or four exercises. For strength, they use a load of 60% to 70% of 1RM. They perform 3 to 5 explosive reps in 2 or 3 sets with a rest interval of two to three minutes between sets.

- A low-load strength training session lasts 15 to 30 minutes. It trains maximum strength, power, or a combination of the two. Athletes perform two or three total exercises and explosively move a load of 50% to 60% of 1RM. They perform 1 to 6 reps over 2 or 3 sets with a rest interval of two to three minutes between sets.

- Rest intervals should be adjusted according to the number of exercises and the volume of the set to fit within the allotted training time, but generally a longer rest interval is advisable.

- Strength and power exercises that work the same muscle groups can be paired in jump-set fashion to save training time yet allow sufficient time for recovery between two sets of the same exercise.

The following sections present several practical examples of loading pattern dynamics for both individual and team sports during competitive-phase microcycles.

Individual Sports

Figure 12.1 shows a suggested strength training plan for athletes in the competitive phase of speed and power sports (e.g., sprinting, jumping, and throwing events in track and field; 50-meter swimming; the martial arts; fencing). For the first two or three days following competition, the objective of training is regeneration. Only two strength training sessions are planned, both later in the week, and the first is of low intensity.

The only time strength training is challenging is during week 2. The third week involves peaking for competition again, so only two strength training sessions are planned, and the second one is of low intensity. To ensure that the Wednesday session is of low demand, the rest intervals between 2 or 3 sets of strength and power training should be long (3-4 minutes) for full regeneration. In addition, the number of reps per set should be far from failure (e.g., 3-6 reps at 50% of 1RM, 2-5 reps at 55%, or 1 or 2 reps at 60%). This approach prevents residual fatigue that could affect the athlete's performance in the upcoming competition.

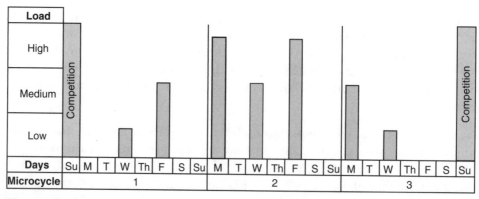

Figure 12.1 Suggested plan for strength training (and loading magnitude) for a speed- and power-dominant sport in which competitions occur three weeks apart.

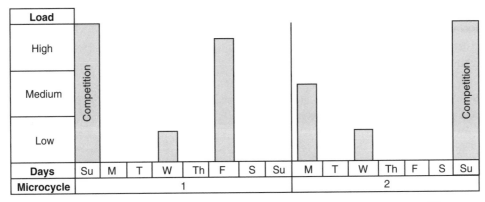

Figure 12.2 Suggested strength training schedule for an athlete whose competitions occur two weeks apart.

Figure 12.2 addresses similar concerns for an athlete whose competitions occur two weeks apart. When designing such a plan, coaches should allow two or three days of regenerative low-intensity training following the first competition. Training must then involve low intensity again on the last two or three days before the next competition in order to facilitate peaking.

Weekly competition in individual sports is far from ideal, simply because the more that athletes compete the less time they have for training. During peri-

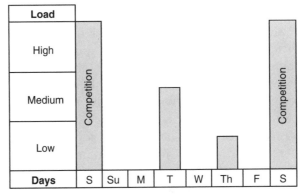

Figure 12.3 Suggested strength training schedule for sports in which weekly competition is the norm.

ods marked by weekly competition, especially when fatigue is high, most coaches look for training elements to cut, and unfortunately strength training is often the first to go. Coaches should instead lower the volume of specific training and keep general training higher in order to compensate for specific physiological systems fatigue.

For sports in which weekly competition is the norm, figure 12.3 illustrates a strength training plan that can be altered to accommodate high levels of fatigue. Coaches should keep in mind, however, that planning too many training cycles amid weekly competition produces a predictable outcome: overtraining, with its ensuing loss of speed and power.

Team Sports

Without negating the importance of specific endurance, power is the dominant ability for most team sports. To avoid detraining of power, a maintenance program must be planned throughout the competitive phase. The examples presented in this section address two competitive schedules: one game per week and two games per week. These examples are valid for college baseball, college basketball, volleyball, American football, ice hockey, field hockey, Australian football, soccer, rugby, lacrosse, and water polo.

Despite the various pressures faced by a team—such as the need for more technical or tactical training and the team's rank in league standings—the coach must find the time, and athletes must find the energy, to work on maintaining strength and power. In fact, the longer the competitive phase the more important it is to maintain power. Figure 12.4

suggests a plan for a cycle with a game scheduled every Saturday, but it can be adjusted for any other day of the week. A strength training session of medium demand is proposed for Tuesday. If an athlete's level of fatigue is higher than expected, the overall demand can be reduced by using a low load.

Even for team sports with two games per week, it is possible to implement a maintenance program for strength training. However, the program should be limited to one or two sets of three exercises at 50% to 70% of 1RM, or a maximum of 20 minutes (see figure 12.5).

Strength training programs look quite different for athletes in some sports, such as linemen in American football, throwers in track and field, and heavy-weight boxers and wrestlers. The suggested program for such athletes lasts 60 to 75 minutes. The strength sought is made up of 40% to 50% maximum strength and 50% to 60% power. Athletes perform four to six exercises as explosively as possible using a load of 70% to 80% of 1RM. They perform 3 to 6 reps over 3 to 6 sets with a rest interval of three to four minutes between sets.

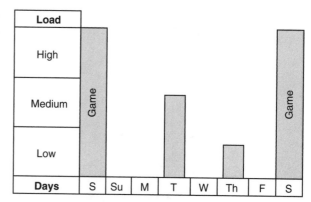

Figure 12.4 Suggested strength training schedule for a team sport involving a game every weekend.

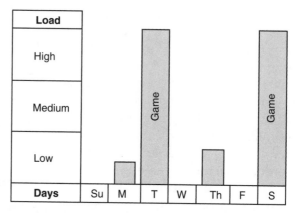

Figure 12.5 Suggested maintenance program for strength training for a team sport involving two games per week.

For team-sport athletes who perform many jumps during training and games (e.g., in basketball or volleyball), plyometric training should be reduced to a minimum as compared with the end of the preparatory phase. This reduction alleviates strain on the athlete's legs throughout the season.

The strength maintenance program should end 3 to 14 days before the most important competition of the year so that athletes can use all of their energy to achieve their best possible performance. The longer cessation phase is especially indicated for those sports in which speed is fundamental (e.g., track events, non-contact or low-contact martial arts, and soccer).

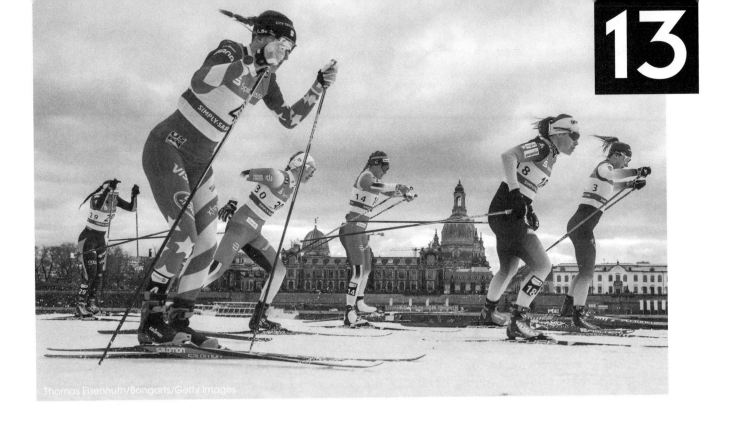

Thomas Eisenhuth/Bongarts/Getty Images

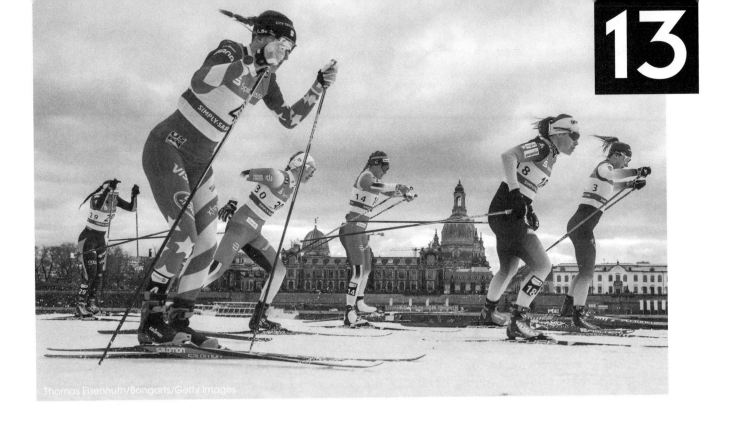

Peaking for Maximum Performance

Many coaches and athletes consider peaking to be akin to a heavenly favor. In reality, however, the ability to peak for competition represents nothing more than a strategy that you design by manipulating load variables to reach physical and psychological supercompensation before an important event. The performance inconsistencies we often witness may depend on the training that the athlete does during the preparatory period; on the ratio between volume, intensity, and recovery during preparation; or on the number of competitions in which the athlete takes part.

The following sequencing is essential for an athlete's ability to peak for competition.

1. Train to compete.
2. Recover and regenerate before starting to train again.
3. Train for the next competition.
4. Manipulate load variables to supercompensate and reach peak performance during the next competition.

We can define *peak status* as a *temporary athletic shape status*—maintainable for two or three weeks at most—that is marked by maximal psychological and physiological efficiency and an optimal level of technical and tactical preparedness.

From a psychological point of view, peaking is a state of readiness for action with intense emotional arousal. The objective aspects of peaking from a psychological point of view manifest themselves as a capacity for quicker and more efficient adaptation to the stress of competition.

Tapering Methodology

The dynamics of the peaking microcycles allow athletes to face the most important competition of the year at the top of their psychophysical energy. Together, these microcycles represent an unloading macrocycle referred to as the taper macrocycle. They are used in most sports—particularly in individual sports—regardless of the annual plan structure (mono-, bi-, or tri-cycle) in order to reach peak performance. During the taper, the training load is gradually reduced, both to eliminate the fatigue induced by the preceding training period and to maintain or enhance the positive adaptations elicited by that training.

The taper macrocycle has a maximum duration of three weeks in order to avoid detraining of physiological systems that are key to performance. This is unlike the tradition in some sports, such as swimming, which uses a five- to six-week taper with a reduction of training volume and its simultaneous intensification that might elicit subpar performance when performance counts the most.

Athletes who do not peak with a two-week taper, or who have a delayed peak right after the most important competition of the year, might be slow or biphasic responders, so they would need a three-week taper.

On the other hand, most athletes who are not in an overreaching status respond quickly to the unloading period and begin to become detrained by the third week. Because an overreaching status is precisely a status of high internal load, we can claim that the fundamental factor in determining taper duration is the athlete's internal load status three weeks before the most important competition of the year. Other factors, such as body weight, sex, weekly training hours, and load-reduction strategy of choice, influence the way the taper is planned. Some general rules about the taper are summarized in table 13.1.

Of course, even the type of load reduction strategy used during the taper relates to the total load of the pre-taper macrocycle (and thus to the internal load). A high-load pre-taper macrocycle that led to an overreaching status calls for a quicker load reduction, such as the fast-decay exponential taper in the case of a three-week duration or the step taper in the case of a two-week duration. On the other hand, a pre-taper macrocycle with a lower load may call for a slower reduction of the load (slow-decay exponential taper or linear taper) or a reduction of the taper length to 7 to 10 days rather than 14. Faced with these options, coaches must use their experience, along with the information provided in this chapter, to decide whether the unloading period will be longer or shorter and whether the load reduction will be slower or quicker.

Taper Guidelines

As a starting point for establishing the ideal taper for each athlete, we suggest using an exponential taper of two weeks with a volume reduction of 60%, preceded by a three-week macrocycle of high-intensity training. Again, the training factors that can be manipulated during the taper to reduce the athlete's internal load are intensity, volume, and frequency of training.

Table 13.1   Factors Affecting Duration of the Precompetition Unloading Period

CHARACTERISTICS		EFFECT OVER THE DURATION OF THE TAPER
Body weight	High	More lasting
	Low	Less lasting
Gender	Male	More lasting with less time dedicated to strength maintenance*
	Female	Less lasting with more time dedicated to strength maintenance*
Load of pre-taper macrocycle	High	More lasting
	Low	Less lasting
Load-reduction strategy during taper	Linear	More lasting
	Step	Less lasting
Weekly training hours	High	More lasting (>15 hours)
	Low	Less lasting (<10 hours)

*This is because male athletes dissipate fatigue more slowly and retain strength longer.

Intensity Manipulation

Several studies have demonstrated that the intensity used during the taper is fundamentally important both to maintaining the adaptations induced by the athlete's previous training and to stimulating additional adaptations (Hickson et al. 1985; Shepley et al. 1992; Convertino et al. 1981; Mujika 1998; Bosquet et al. 2007; McNeely and Sandler 2007). More specifically, intensity is reduced by an average of only 5% to 10%.

The highest reduction percentage should be reached only in the last days of the taper. In addition, recent computer simulations suggest that the most reduced level of intensity reduction should be reached four days before the event and that intensity should be increased again by using medium and medium-high intensities during the last three days in order to stimulate further adaptations without affecting the elimination of fatigue (Thomas, Mujika, and Busso 2009).

Volume Manipulation

One study has shown that training adaptations obtained in 10 weeks can be maintained for an additional 28 weeks with a reduction of volume ranging from 30% to 60% (Graves et al. 1988). In addition, several studies of elite athletes have reported positive effects on performance with a reduction of maximum volume during the taper ranging from 40% to 85%; the most important improvements came with a reduction in the range of 40% to 60% (Houmard et al. 1989; McConell et al. 1993; Martin et al. 1994; Rietjens et al. 2001; Mujika et al. 1995; Shepley et al. 1992; Bosquet et al. 2007). As shown in table 13.2, the percentage of volume reduction throughout the taper is determined by several factors, including taper duration, residual internal fatigue, and type of load reduction.

Frequency Manipulation

Part of the reduction in volume that is needed in order to reach peaking form can be obtained by reducing the number of weekly training sessions. This practice is recommended only for speed and power sports, however, especially if alactic-dominant. In all

Table 13.2   Factors Affecting Training Volume in the Precompetition Unloading Period

	CHARACTERISTIC	EFFECT ON TAPER VOLUME
Load of pre-taper macrocycle	High	Greater reduction
	Low	Smaller reduction
Taper duration	Short	Greater reduction
	Long	Smaller reduction
Type of load reduction	Linear	Higher mean volume Lower final volume
	Step	Lower mean volume Higher final volume

other circumstances, we suggest reducing the volume of each session, especially in sports with an elevated technical aspect (e.g., swimming, rowing, cross-country skiing, kayaking, gymnastics) and for high-level athletes in general.

It is a common practice in high-level team sports to plan two or three days off from training either during the first week of the taper or between the first and second weeks. This approach is taken because team-sport athletes usually enter the taper period before tournaments or cup finals in an overreaching state due to the long competitive season. For this reason, for professional and national teams, sports medicine practitioners are strongly advised to check athletes' testosterone-to-cortisol ratio and CPK levels (possibly checking them throughout the season for comparison). The results give strength and conditioning coaches more information to use in establishing training load during the taper for each player.

As shown in table 13.3, the progressive decrease in volume and intensity of all training activities during the competitive phase—as well as the increased use of recovery techniques—helps athletes replenish energy stores, achieve supercompensation, relax mentally, and build motivation to attain their best possible results in the competition targeted for peak performance. The strategy presented in the table must be applied for the duration of the tapering period to ensure maximum neuromuscular benefits prior to major competition. During this time, the focus shifts to recovery and regeneration through proper rest, nutrition, supplementation, and soft-tissue therapies (e.g., deep massage, myofascial release). In terms of training, this is a time to reap the benefits of well-planned preparation and competitive periods.

Peaking and Neuromuscular Potentiation

Many successful coaches use periodization of training, tapering, and methods of neuromuscular system potentiation to help their athletes achieve peak performance. This section discusses how coaches can induce peak performance by using two special training techniques: post-activation potentiation and post-contraction sensory discharge. These methods are geared to develop maximum tension in the muscle, but maximum tension is difficult to achieve in a practical setting. Effective techniques for stimulating the neuromuscular system and promoting maximum motor unit recruitment include training with heavy loads, performing high-impact plyometrics, and implementing isometric contrac-

Table 13.3 Training and Recovery Strategies and Benefits During the Taper

	STRATEGIES	BENEFITS
Dynamics of volume	• Decrease total distance or duration by 40% to 60%. • Decrease number of reps. • Increase rest interval to full recovery. • Don't introduce new exercises.	• Achieve supercompensation of all physiological systems. • Increase readiness of the neuromuscular system. • Facilitate replenishment of energy stores.
Dynamics of intensity	• Reduce intensity by 5% to 10% for power sports and 20% to 30% for endurance sports, especially in the first week. • Raise intensity a few days before competition.	
Neuromuscular stimulation	Use the neuromuscular system potentiation methods described in this chapter.	• Induce prepeaking neuromuscular state. • Increase recruitment of fast-twitch muscle fibers. • Increase discharge rate of fast-twitch muscle fibers. • Maximize arousal of the neuromuscular system. • Increase reactivity of the neuromuscular system.
Recovery methods	• Use soft-tissue management techniques (e.g., deep massage, myofascial release). • Control heart rate variability values to ensure proper recovery dynamics. • Control sleep quality (e.g., use the Sleep as Android app to wake at ideal time). • Use psychological relaxation, motivation, and visualization techniques (e.g., hypnosis, which can induce a deep state of relaxation and faster nervous system recovery). • Ensure proper nutrition and sport-specific food supplementation.	• Improve soft-tissue compliance and joint mobility. • Increase readiness of the neuromuscular system. • Relax mentally. • Increase confidence. • Increase arousal. • Replenish energy stores. • Sustain maximal power output throughout competition.

tions. Increased motor unit recruitment heightens an athlete's force development, which can then be applied to power activities.

Considering their specific physiological benefits, these techniques are suggested mostly for speed and power sports—for example, sprinting, jumping, and throwing in track and field; the martial arts; short events in water sports (e.g., diving, swimming sprints); track cycling; and speedskating. On the other hand, neuromuscular system potentiation methods are *not* suggested for long-lasting events (e.g., soccer) and even more emphatically not for sports in which the aerobic system is dominant, because the benefits to the sport-specific performance would be negligible if present at all.

The greatest challenge faced by coaches and trainers lies in applying systematic laboratory research to athletic training. Following intense isometric contractions or electrical stimulation causing a summation of twitches up to a tetanus state, any further stimulation would elicit a maximal twitch force (Enoka 2002), yet even strong concentric actions can elicit a potentiation (Gullich and Schmidtbleicher 1996; Chiu et al. 2003; Rixon, Lamont, and Bemben 2007).

Maximal twitch force, or post-activation potentiation, can be maintained for about 8 to 12 minutes before returning to control levels (Enoka 2002). When heavy eccentric–concentric exercises (over 80% of 1RM) are used, such as those presented in figure 13.1, a further potentiation—post-activation potentiation—appears after 6 to 7 hours and can last up to 24 hours. For this reason, such exercises can be used either on the morning of competition or the day before.

Post-contraction sensory discharge, on the other hand, is a physiological mechanism that can be applied right before competition. Brief and intense episodes of activity 5 to 20 minutes prior to the competition can be used to heighten the athlete's neural contribution to subsequent movements that occur in sport (Enoka 2002). For instance, highly trained sprinters often perform 1 or 2 sets of 2 to 4 reps of explosive plyometric (level 2 or 3) exercises 5 to 10 minutes prior to a race. This activity increases the muscle spindle discharge (Enoka 2002) and the subsequent neural drive to the prime movers. That is why short and intense activities lasting mere seconds harness greater power output for the movement that follows.

Post-activation potentiation is smaller in the slow-twitch muscle fibers than in the fast-twitch fibers (O'Leary, Hope, and Sale 1998; Hamada et al. 2000), which explains the important application of post-activation potentiation to speed and power sports, for which the activation of fast-twitch fibers is paramount. Furthermore, warm muscle elicits higher post-activation potentiation than cold muscle does (Gossen, Allingham, and Sale 2001). Therefore, proper warm-up not only prevents injury but should also increase the

Exercise	Load (% of 1RM)	Reps	RI (min.)	Load (% of 1RM)	Reps	RI (min.)	Load (% of 1RM)	Reps	RI (min.)
Quarter squat	100*	3	4	110*	3	6	120*	3	4
Walking lunge	80	2+2 (R+L)	4	80	2+2 (R+L)	4	—	—	—
Bench press	75	3	3	82.5	3	—	—	—	—

RI = rest interval; R+L = right plus left

*Of full squat 1RM

Figure 13.1 Neuromuscular potentiation session for use on the morning of a race by a 60-meter, 100-meter, or 200-meter sprinter.

force-generating capability of muscle. In addition, through a process of adaptation, as the force-generating capacity of a muscle increases, so does the post-activation potentiation.

Strength Training During the Transition Phase

Following a lengthy period of hard work and stressful competition—during which an athlete's determination, motivation, and will are tested—the athlete experiences a high degree of physiological and psychological fatigue. Although muscular fatigue may disappear in a few days, fatigue of the central nervous system and the psyche (as observed in an athlete's behavior) can last much longer.

The more intensive the training and the more competitions athletes are exposed to, the greater their fatigue will be. Under such conditions, they would have difficulty beginning a new yearly training cycle; therefore, before starting another season of training, they must rest, both physically and psychologically. When the new preparatory phase does begin, they should be completely regenerated and ready to participate in training. In fact, following a successful transition phase, they should feel a strong desire to train again.

The transition phase—often inappropriately referred to as the "off-season"—serves as a link between two annual plans. Its major objectives are psychological rest, relaxation, and biological regeneration, as well as maintenance of an acceptable level of general physical preparation. This phase has a different duration depending on the level of the athlete: a beginner or junior athlete might have a short three- or four-week transition phase, whereas an experienced Olympic athlete, at the end of a quadrennial Olympic cycle, might take up to eight weeks of transition phase. This is possible because of the level of stress and residual fatigue experienced by the Olympians throughout the Olym-

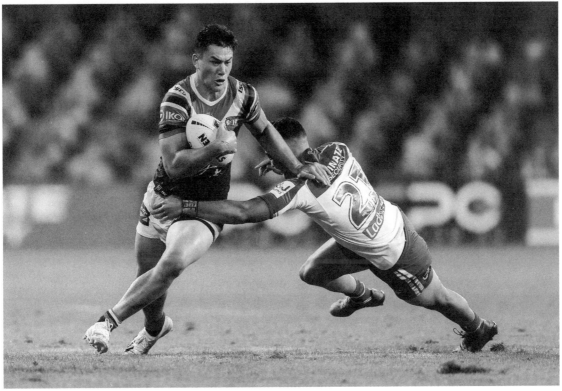

Mark Metcalfe/Getty Images

The transition phase allows for psychological rest and physical relaxation after a grueling season.

pic year, and because of their ability to regain fitness and specific skills once their new preparation has started. A lower-level athlete who has a long transition, though, will detrain, visibly losing most of his or her fitness.

To maintain a decent level of fitness, athletes should train two or three times a week during the transition phase, and at least one workout should be used for strength training. Less effort is required to maintain at least 50% of the previous fitness level than to redevelop it from zero. In fact, an athlete who starts from zero after the transition phase has experienced a great deal of detraining. The phenomenon of detraining of strength has been documented since the 1960s. Hettinger (1966) found that muscles can lose up to 30% of their strength capacity in one week of immobilization. Although that is an extreme case, a wealth of similar findings is contained in exercise physiology and strength training books, and coaches can expect a great loss of muscle strength after just two weeks of complete inactivity.

During transition, athletes should also perform compensation work to involve muscle groups that receive little attention throughout the preparatory and competitive phases. This means paying attention to the antagonist muscles and the stabilizers. For example, these two muscle groups can be activated in a dedicated 20- to 30-minute session after any informal physical training (e.g., a pickup game or recreational play). The program can be relaxed, and athletes can work at their own pace for as long as they desire. The program need not be stressful. In fact, stress is undesirable during transition. Forget the formal program with its specific load, tempo, specific numbers of reps and sets, and rest intervals. For once, athletes should do as they please.

References

Aagaard, P. and Andersen, J.L. 2011. Effects of resistance training on endurance capacity and muscle fiber composition in young top-level cyclists. *Scandinavian Journal of Medicine and Science in Sports* 21 (6): e298-307.

Aagaard, P., Simonsen, E.B., Anderson, J.L., Magnusson, S.P., and Halkaer-Kristensen, K. 1994. Moment and power generation during maximal knee extensions performed at low and high speeds. *European Journal of Applied Physiology* 89: 2249-57.

Abbruzzese, G., Morena, M., Spadavecchia, L., and Schieppati, M. 1994. Response of arm flexor muscles to magnetic and electrical brain stimulation during shortening and lengthening tasks in man. *Journal of Physiology—London* 481: 499-507.

Adams, T.M., Worlay, D., and Throgmartin, D. 1987. The effects of selected plyometric and weight training on muscular leg power. *Track and Field Quarterly Review* 87: 45-7.

Adlercreutz, H., et al. 1986. Effect of training on plasma anabolic and catabolic steroid hormones and their response during physical exercise. *International Journal of Sports Medicine.* 7 (1): 27-8.

Ahtiainen, J.P., et al. 2011. Recovery after heavy resistance exercise and skeletal muscle androgen receptor and insulin-like growth factor-I isoform expression in strength trained men. *Journal of Strength and Conditioning Research* 25 (3): 767-77.

American College of Sports Medicine. 2000. Joint position statement of the American College of Sports Medicine, American Dietetic Association, and Dietitians of Canada on nutrition and athletic performance. *Medicine and Science in Sports and Exercise* 32 (12): 2130-45.

Andersen, J.L., and Aagaard, P. 2000. Myosin heavy chain IIX overshoot in human skeletal muscle. *Muscle Nerve* 23 (7): 1095-1104.

Andersen, J.L., Klitgaard, H., and Saltin, B. 1994. Myosin heavy chain isoforms in single fibres from m. vastus lateralis of sprinters: Influence of training. *Acta Physiologica Scandinavica* 151 (2): 135-42.

Andersen, L.L., et al. 2005. Changes in the human muscle force-velocity relationship in response to resistance training and subsequent detraining. *Journal of Applied Physiology* 99 (1): 87-94.

Andersen, L.L., et al. 2010. Early and late rate of force development: Differential adaptive responses to resistance training? *Scandinavian Journal of Medicine and Science in Sports* 20 (1): e162-69.

Anderson, K., and Behm, D.G. 2004. Maintenance of EMG activity and loss of force output with instability. *Journal of Strength and Conditioning Research* 18: 637-40.

Anderson, K., Behm, D.G., and Curnew R.S. 2002. Muscle force and neuromuscular activation under stable and unstable conditions. *Journal of Strength and Conditioning Research* 16: 416-22.

Appell, H.J. 1990. Muscular atrophy following immobilization: A review. *Sports Medicine* 10 (1): 42-58.

Armstrong, R.B. 1986. Muscle damage and endurance events. *Sports Medicine* 3: 370-81.

Armstrong, R.B., Warren, G.L., and Warren, J.A. 1991. Mechanics of exercise-induced muscle fiber injury. *Sports Medicine* 12 (3): 184-207.

Ashton-Miller, J.A., Wojtys, E.M., Huston, L.J., and Fry-Welch, D. 2001. Can proprioception be improved by exercise? *Knee Surgery Sports Traumatology Arthroscopy* 9 (3): 128-36.

Asmussen, E., and Mazin, B. 1978. A central nervous system component in local muscular fatigue. *European Journal of Applied Physiology* 38: 9-15.

Åstrand, P.O., and Rodahl, K. 1985. *Textbook of work physiology.* New York: McGraw-Hill.

Atha, J. 1984. Strengthening muscle. *Exercise and Sport Sciences Reviews* 9: 1-73.

Augustsson, J., Thomeé, R., Hornstedt, P., Lindblom, J., Karlsson, J., and Grimby, G. 2003. Effect of pre-exhaustion exercise on lower extremity muscle activation during a leg press exercise. *Journal of Strength and Conditioning Research* 17 (2): 411-16.

References

Babraj, J.A., et al. 2005. Collagen synthesis in human musculoskeletal tissues and skin. *American Journal of Physiology—Endocrinology and Metabolism* 289 (5): E864-69.

Baker, D., Nance, S., and Moore, M. 2001. The load that maximizes the average mechanical power output during explosive bench press throws in highly trained athletes. *Journal of Strength and Conditioning Research* 15 (1): 20-4.

Baker, D. 1995. Selecting the appropriate exercises and loads for speed-strength development. *Strength and Conditioning Coach* 3 (2): 8-16.

Baker, D.G., and Newton, R.U. 2007. Change in power output across a high-repetition set of bench throws and jump squats in highly trained athletes. *Journal of Strength and Conditioning Research* 21 (4): 1007-11.

Balsom, P.D., Wood, K., Olsson, P., and Ekblom, B. 1999. Carbohydrate intake and multiple sprint sports: With special reference to football. *International Journal of Sport Medicine* 20: 48-52.

Bangsbo, J. 1994. Energy demands in competitive soccer. *Journal of Sports Sciences* 12 Spec No: S5-12.

———. 1999. Science and football. *Journal of Sports Sciences* 17 (10): 755-6.

Bangsbo, J., Iaia, F.M., and Krustrup, P. 2007. Metabolic response and fatigue in soccer. *International Journal of Sports Physiology and Performance* 2 (2): 111-27.

Banister E.W., Carter J.B., and Zarkadas, P.C. 1999. Training theory and taper: Validation in triathlon athletes. *European Journal of Applied Physiology and Occupational Physiology* 79 (2): 179-86.

———. 1995. Modelling the effect of taper on performance, maximal oxygen uptake, and the anaerobic threshold in endurance triathletes. *Advances in Experimental Medicine and Biology* 393: 179-86.

Baroga, L. 1978. Contemporary tendencies in the methodology of strength development. *Educatie Fizica si Sport* 6: 22-36.

Bazyler, C.D., Sato, K., Wassinger, C.A., Lamont, H.S., and Stone, M.H. 2014. The efficacy of incorporating partial squats in maximal strength training. *Journal of Strength and Conditioning Research* 28 (11): 3024-32.

Behm, D., and Sale, D.G. 1993. Intended rather than actual movement velocity determines velocity-specific training response. *Journal of Applied Physiology* 74: 359-68.

Beliard, S.M., Chaveau, M., Moscatiello, T., Cross, F., Ecarnot, F., and Becker, F. 2015. Compression garments and exercise: No influence on pressure applied. *Journal of Sports Science & Medicine* March 14 (1): 75-83.

Belli, A., Kyröläinen, H., and Komi, P.V. 2002. Moment and power of lower limb joints in running. *International Journal of Sports Medicine* 23 (2): 136-41.

Bennet, W.M., and Rennie, M.J. 1991. Protein anabolic actions of insulin in the human body. *Diabetic Medicine* 8: 199-207.

Berardi, J., and Andrews, R. 2009. *Nutrition: The complete guide.* Carpinteria, CA: International Sports Science Association.

Bergeron, G. 1982. Therapeutic massage. *Journal of the Canadian Athletic Therapists Association* Summer: 15-17.

Bergstrom, J., Hermansen, L., Hultman, E., and Saltin, B. 1967. Diet, muscle glycogen and physical performance. *Acta Physiologica Scandinavica* 71: 140-50.

Besier, T.F., Lloyd, B.G., Cochrane, J.L., and Ackland, T.R. 2001. External loading of the knee joint during running and cutting maneuvers. *Medicine and Science in Sports and Exercise* 33: 1168-75.

Bigland-Ritchie, B., Johansson, R., Lippold, O.C.J., and Woods, J.J. 1983. Contractile speed and EMG changes during fatigue of sustained maximal voluntary contractions. *Journal of Neurophysiology* 50 (1): 313-24.

Billat, V.L., Flechet, B., Petit, B., Muriaux, G., and Koralsztein, J.P. 1999. Interval training at $\dot{V}O_2$max: Effects on aerobic performance and overtraining markers. *Medicine and Science in Sports and Exercise* 31 (1): 156-63.

Billat, V.L., Petot, H. Karp, J.R., Sarre, G., Morton, R.H., and Mille-Hamard, L. 2013. The sustainability of $\dot{V}O_2$max: Effect of decreasing the workload. *European Journal of Applied Physiology* 113 (2): 385-94.

Billat, V.L., Sirvent, P., Py, G., Koralsztein, J.P., and Mercier, J. 2003. The concept of maximal lactate steady state: A bridge between biochemistry, physiology and sport science. *Sports Medicine* 33 (6): 407-26.

Biolo, G., Fleming, R.Y.D., and Wolfe, R.R. 1995. Physiologic hyperinsulinemia stimulates protein synthesis and enhances transport of selected amino acids in human skeletal muscle. *Journal of Clinical Investigation* 95: 811-19.

Biolo, G., Tipton, K.D., Klein, S., and Wolfe, R.R. 1997. An abundant supply of amino acids enhances the metabolic effect of exercise on muscle protein. *American Journal of Physiology* 273: E119-22.

Biolo, G., Williams, B.D., Fleming, R.Y.D., and Wolfe, R.R. 1999. Insulin action on muscle protein kinetics and amino acid transport during recovery after resistance exercise. *Diabetes* 48: 949-57.

Bishop, N.C., Blannin, A.K., Rand, L., et al. 1999. Effect of carbohydrate and fluid intake on the blood leukocyte responses to prolonged cycling. *International Journal of Sports Medicine* 17: 26-27.

Bishop, N.C., Blannin, A.K., Walsh, N.P., and Gleeson, M. 2001. Carbohydrate beverage ingestion and neutrophil degranulation responses following cycling to fatigue at 75% of $\dot{V}O_2$max. *International Journal of Sports Medicine* 22: 226-31.

Bloomquist, K., et al. 2013. Effect of range of motion in heavy load squatting on muscle and tendon adaptations. *European Journal of Applied Physiology* 8: 2133-61.

Bogdanis, G.C., Nevill, M.E., Boobis, L.H., and Lakomy, H.K. 1996. Contribution of phosphocreatine and aerobic metabolism to energy supply during repeated sprint exercise. *Journal of Applied Physiology* 80: 876-84.

Bompa, T. 1965a. Periodization of strength. *Sports Review* 1: 26-31.

———. 1965b. Periodization of strength for power sports. International Conference on Advancements in Sports Training, Moscow.

———. 1977. Characteristics of strength training for rowing. International Seminar on Training in Rowing, Stockholm.

———. 1983. *Theory and methodology of training.* Dubuque, IA: Kendall/Hunt Publishing Company.

———. 1993. *Periodization of strength: The new wave in strength training.* Toronto: Veritas.

———. 1999. *Periodization: Theory and methodology of training.* 4th ed. Champaign, IL: Human Kinetics.

Bompa T.O. 2006. *Total training for coaching team sports: A self help guide.* Toronto. Sport Books Publisher.

Bompa, T., and Claro, F. 2008. *Periodization in rugby.* Aachen, Germany: Meyer & Meyer Sport.

Bompa T., Hebbelinck, M., and Van Gheluwe, B. 1978. A biomechanical analysis of the rowing stroke employing two different oar grips. The XXI World Congress in Sports Medicine, Brasilia, Brazil.

Bompa, T.O. 2005. *Treinando atletas de deporto colectivo.* São Paulo, Brazil: Phorte Editora.

Bompa, T.O. 2016. Strength training and injury prevention, Sports Science Congress, Bucharest, Romania.

Bompa, T.O., and Buzzichelli, C.A. 2018. *Periodization: Theory and methodology of training.* 6th ed. Champaign, IL: Human Kinetics.

Bompa, T.O., and Haff, G.G. 2009. *Periodization: Theory and methodology of training.* 5th ed. Champaign, IL: Human Kinetics.

Bonen, A. 2001. The expression of lactate transporters (MCT1 and MCT4) in heart and muscle. *European Journal of Applied Physiology* 86 (1): 6-11.

Bonen, A., and Belcastro, A. 1977. A physiological rationale for active recovery exercise. *Canadian Journal of Applied Sports Sciences* 2: 63-64.

Borsheim, E., Cree, M.G., Tipton, K.D., Elliott, T.A., Aarsland, A., and Wolfe, R.R. 2004. Effect of carbohydrate intake on net muscle protein synthesis during recovery from resistance exercise. *Journal of Applied Physiology* 96 (2): 674-78.

Bosco, C., and Komi, P.V. 1980. Influence of countermovement amplitude in potentiation of muscular performance. In *Biomechanics VII proceedings*, 129-35. Baltimore: University Park Press.

Bosquet, L., Montpetit, J., Arvisais, D., and Mujika, I. 2007. Effects of tapering on performance: A meta-analysis. *Medicine and Science in Sports and Exercise* 39 (8): 1358-65.

Brooks, G.A., Brauner, K.T., and Cassens, R.G. 1973. Glycogen synthesis and metabolism of lactic acid after exercise. *American Journal of Physiology* 224: 1162-66.

Brooks, G.A., and Fahey, T. 1985. *Exercise physiology: Human bioenergetics and its application.* New York: Wiley.

Brooks, G.A., Fahey, T.D., and White, T.P. 1996. *Exercise physiology: Human bioenergetics and its applications.* 2nd ed. Mountainview, CA: Mayfield.

Broughton, A. 2001. *Neural mechanisms are the most important determinants of strength adaptations.* Proposition for debate. School of Physiotherapy, Curtin University.

Brughelli, M., Cronin, J. and Chaouachi, A. 2011. Effects of running velocity on running kinetics and kinematics. *Journal of Strength and Conditioning Research* 25 (4): 933-39.

Bührle, M. 1985. *Grundlagen des maximal-und Schnellkraft Trainings.* Schorndorf: Hofmann Verlag.

References

Bührle, M., and Schmidtbleicher, D. 1981. Komponenten der maximal-und Schnellkraft-Versuch einer Neustrukturierung auf der Basis empirischer Ergebnisse. *Sportwissenschaft* 11: 11-27.

Burd, N.A., et al. 2010. Low-load high-volume resistance exercise stimulates muscle protein synthesis more than high-load low-volume resistance exercise in young men. *PLOS ONE* 5 (8): e12033.

Burkes, L.M., Collier, G.R., and Hargreaves, M. 1998. Glycemic index—A new tool in sport nutrition? *International Journal of Sport Nutrition* 8 (4): 401-15.

Burkett, B. 2018. *Applied sport mechanics.* 4th ed. Champaign, IL: Human Kinetics.

Campos, J., Poletaev, P., Cuesta, A., Pablos, C., & Carratalà. 2006. Kinematical analysis of the snatch in elite male junior weightlifters of different weight categories. *Journal of Strength and Conditioning Research*, 20 (4): 843-50.

Caraffa, A., Cerulli, G., Projetti, M., Aisa, G., and Rizzo, A. 1996. Prevention of anterior cruciate ligament injuries in soccer. A prospective controlled study of proprioceptive training. *Knee Surgery, Sports Traumatology, Arthroscopy* 4 (1): 19-21.

Chen, J.L., et al. 2011. Parasympathetic nervous activity mirrors recovery status in weightlifting performance after training. *Journal of Strength and Conditioning Research* 25 (6): 1546-52.

Chiu, L.Z., et al. 2003. Postactivation potentiation response in athletic and recreationally trained individuals. *Journal of Strength and Conditioning Research* 17 (4): 671-77.

Cinique, C. 1989. Massage for cyclists: The winning touch? *The Physician and Sportsmedicine* 17 (10): 167-70.

Clark, N., 1984. The training table: Recovering from exhaustive workouts. *Strength and Conditioning Journal* 6 (6): 36-37.

Colado, J.C., et al. 2011. The progression of paraspinal muscle recruitment intensity in localized and global strength training exercises is not based on instability alone. *Archives of Physical Medicine and Rehabilitation* 92 (11): 1875-83.

Compton, D., Hill, P.M., and Sinclair, J.D. 1973. Weight-lifters' blackout. *Lancet* 302 (7840): 1234-37.

Conlee, R.K. 1987. Muscle glycogen and exercise endurance: A twenty-year perspective. *Exercise and Sport Sciences Reviews* 15: 1-28.

Convertino, V.A., Keil, L.C., Bernauer, E.M., and Greenleaf, J.E. 1981. Plasma volume, osmolality, vasopressin, and renin activity during graded exercise in man. *Journal of Applied Physiology* 50 (1): 123-28.

Conwit, R.A. et al. 2000. Fatigue effects on motor unit activity during submaximal contractions. *Archives of Physical Medicine and Rehabilitation* 81 (9): 1211-16.

Coombes, J.S., and Hamilton, K.L. 2000. The effectiveness of commercially available sports drinks. *Sports Medicine* 29 (3): 181-209.

Councilman, J.E. 1968. *The science of swimming.* Englewood Cliffs, NJ: Prentice Hall.

Coutts, A., Reaburn, P., Piva, T.J., and Murphy, A. 2007. Changes in selected biochemical, muscular strength, power, and endurance measures during deliberate overreaching and tapering in rugby league players. *International Journal of Sports Medicine* 28 (2): 116-24.

Coyle, E.F. 1999. Physiological determinants of endurance exercise performance. *Journal of Science and Medicine in Sport* 2 (3): 181-89.

Coyle, E.F., Feiring, D.C., Rotkis, T.C., Cote, R.W., Roby, F.B., Lee, W., and Wilmore, J.H. 1991. Specificity of power improvements through slow and fast isokinetic training. *Journal of Applied Physiology: Respiratory Environment Exercise Physiology* 51 (6): 1437-42.

Cramer, J.T., et al. 2005. The acute effects of static stretching on peak torque, mean power output, electromyography, and mechanomyography. *European Journal of Applied Physiology* 93 (5-6): 530-39.

Crameri, R.M., et al. 2004. Enhanced procollagen processing in skeletal muscle after a single bout of eccentric loading in humans. *Matrix Biology* 23 (4): 259-64.

D'Amico, A., and Morin, C. 2011. Effects of myofascial release on human performance: a review of the literature. *Semantic Scholar.* Corpus ID 26560281.

Davis, J., Jackson, D.A., Broadwell, M.S., Queary, J.L., and Lambert, C.L. 1997. Carbohydrate drinks delay fatigue during intermittent, high-intensity cycling in active men and women. *International Journal of Sports Nutrition* 7 (4): 261-73.

Davis, R.M., Welsh, R.S., De Volve, K.L., and Alderson, N.A. 1999. Effects of branched-chain amino acids and carbohydrate on fatigue during intermittent, high-intensity running. *International Journal of Sports Medicine* 20 (5): 309-14.

De Luca, C.J., and Erim, Z. 1994. Common drive of motor units in regulation of muscle force. *Trends in Neuroscience* 17: 299-305.

De Luca, C.J., LeFever, R.S., McCue, M.P., and Xenakis, A.P. 1982. Behaviour of human motor units in different muscles during linearly varying contractions. *Journal of Physiology—London* 329: 113-28.

de Salles, B.F., et al. 2010. Strength increases in upper and lower body are larger with longer inter-set rest intervals in trained men. *Journal of Science and Medicine in Sport* 13 (4): 429-33.

Devine, K.L., LeVeau, B.F., and Yack, H.J. 1981. Electromyographic activity recorded from an unexercised muscle during maximal isometric exercise of the contralateral agonists and antagonists. *Physical Therapy* 6 (6): 898-903.

Doessing, S., and Kjaer, M., 2005. Growth hormone and connective tissue in exercise. *Scandinavian Journal of Medicine and Science in Sports* 15 (4): 202-10.

Dons, B., Bollerup, K., Bonde-Petersen, F., and Hancke, S. 1979. The effects of weight lifting exercise related to muscle fibre composition and muscle cross-sectional area in humans. *European Journal of Applied Physiology* 40: 95-106.

Dorado, C., Sanchis-Moysi, J., and Calbet, J.A., 2004. Effects of recovery mode on performance, O_2 uptake, and O_2 deficit during high-intensity intermittent exercise. *Canadian Journal of Applied Physiology* 29 (3): 227-44.

Dudley, G.A., and Fleck, S.J. 1987. Strength and endurance training: Are they mutually exclusive? *Sports Medicine* 4: 79-85.

Ebbing, C., and Clarkson, P. 1989. Exercise-induced muscle damage and adaptation. *Sports Medicine* 7: 207-34.

Edge, J., Bishop, D., Goodman, C., and Dawson, B. 2005. Effects of high- and moderate-intensity training on metabolism and repeated sprints. *Medicine and Science in Sports and Exercise* 37 (11): 1975-82.

Edgerton, R.V. 1976. Neuromuscular adaptation to power and endurance work. *Canadian Journal of Applied Sports Sciences* 1: 49-58.

Ekstrand, J., Waldén, M., and Hägglund, M. 2004. Risk for injury when playing in a national football team, *Scandinavian Journal of Medicine and Science in Sports* 14 (1): 34-8.

Eliassen, W., Saeterbakken, A.H., and van den Tillart, R. 2018. Comparison of bilateral and unilateral squat exercises on barbell kinematics and muscle activation. *International Journal of Sports Physical Therapy* Aug: 13 (5): 871-81.

Enoka, R. 1996. Eccentric contractions require unique activation strategies by the nervous system. *Journal of Applied Physiology* 81 (6): 2339-46.

Enoka, R.M. 1994. *Neuromechanical basis of kinesiology.* 2nd ed. Champaign, IL: Human Kinetics.

———. 2002. *Neuromechanics of human movement.* 3rd ed. Champaign, IL: Human Kinetics.

———. 2015. *Neuromechanics of human movement.* 4th ed. Champaign, IL: Human Kinetics.

Enoka, R.M., and Stuart, D.G. 1992. Neurobiology of muscle fatigue. *Journal of Applied Physiology* 72 (5): 1631-38.

Evangelista, P. 2010. Principles of Strength Training, a presentation for the Tudor Bompa Institute - Italia. Ciccarelli Editore.

Evertsen, F., Medbo, J.I., Jebens, E.P., and Gjovaag, T.F. 1999. Effect of training on the activity of five muscle enzymes studied in elite cross-country skiers. *Acta Physiologica Scandinavica* 167 (3): 247-57.

Fabiato, A., and Fabiato, F. 1978. The effect of pH on myofilaments and the sarcoplasmic reticulum of skinned cells from cardiac and skeletal muscle. *Journal of Physiology* 276: 233-55.

Fahey, T.D. 1992. How to cope with muscle soreness. *Powerlifting USA* 15 (7): 10-11.

Fama, B.J., and Bueti, D.R. 2011. The acute effect of self-myofascial release on lower extremity plyometric performance. Theses and Dissertations. Paper 2. Sacred Heart University.

Farrow, D., Young, W., and Bruce, L. 2005. The development of a test of reactive agility for netball: A new methodology. *Journal of Science and Medicine in Sport* 8 (1): 52-60.

Febbraio, M.A., and Pedersen, B.K. 2005. Contraction-induced myokine production and release: Is skeletal muscle an endocrine organ? *Exercise and Sport Sciences Reviews* 33 (3): 114-19.

References

Ferret, J.M., and Cotte, T. 2003. Analyse des differences de preparation medico sportive de l'Equipe de France de football pour le coupes du monde 1998 et 2002, Lutter contre le Dopage en géran la recuperation physique, Publications de l'Université de Saint-Etienne 23-26.

Fitts, R.H., and Widrick, J.J. 1996. Muscle mechanics: Adaptations with exercise-training. *Exercise and Sport Sciences Reviews* 24: 427-73.

Fleck, S.J., and Kraemer, W.J. 1996. *Periodization breakthrough.* New York: Advanced Research Press.

Forslund, A.H., et al. 2000. The 24-h whole body leucine and urea kinetics at normal and high protein intake with exercise in healthy adults. *American Journal of Physiology* 278: E857-67.

Fox, E.L. 1984. *Sports physiology.* New York: CBS College.

Fox, E.L., Bowes, R.W., and Foss, M.L. 1989. *The physiological basis of physical education and athletics.* Dubuque, IA: Brown.

Franchi, M.V., Reeves, N.D., and Narici, M.V. 2017. Skeletal muscles remodeling in response to eccentric a concentric loading: Morphological, molecular and metabolic adaptation. *Frontiers in Physiology* 8: 447.

Frank, C.B. 1996. Ligament injuries: Pathophysiology and healing. In *Athletic injuries and rehabilitation,* edited by J.E. Zachazewski, D.J. Magee, and W.S. Wilson, 9-26. Philadelphia: Saunders.

Friden, J., and Lieber, R.L. 1992. Structural and mechanical basis of exercise-induced muscle injury. *Medicine in Science and Sports Exercise* 24: 521-30.

Fritzsche, R.G., et al. 2000. Water and carbohydrate ingestion during prolonged exercise increase maximal neuromuscular power. *Journal of Applied Physiology* 88 (2): 730-37.

Fry, R.W., Morton, R., and Keast, D. 1991. Overtraining in athletics. *Sports Medicine* 2 (1): 32-65.

García-Fernández, P., Guodemar-Pérez, J., Ruiz-López, M., Rodríguez-López, E.S. and Hervás-Pérez, J.P. 2017. Injury rate in professional soccer players within the community of Madrid: A comparative, epidemiological cohort study among the first, second and second B divisions. *Journal of Physiotherapy and Physical Rehabilitation 2* (152). http://doi.org/10.4172/2573-0312.1000152

Garhammer, J. 1989. Weightlifting and training. In *Biomechanics of sport,* edited by C.L. Vaughn, 169-211. Boca Raton, FL: CRC Press.

Gauron, E.F. 1984. *Mental training for peak performance.* New York: Sports Science Associates.

Gibala, M.J., MacDougall, J.D., Tarnopolsky, M.A., Stauber, W.T., and Elorriaga, A. 1995. Changes in human skeletal muscle ultrastructure and force production after acute resistance exercise. *Journal of Applied Physiology* 78 (2): 702-8.

Godfrey, R.J., et al. 2003. The exercise-induced growth hormone response in athletes. *Sports Medicine* 33: 599-613.

Goldberg, A.L., Etlinger, J.D., Goldspink, D.F., and Jablecki, C. 1975. Mechanism of work-induced hypertrophy of skeletal muscle. *Medicine and Science in Sports and Exercise* 7: 185-98.

Goldspink, G. 2005. Mechanical signals, IGF-I gene splicing, and muscle adaptation. *Physiology* 20: 232-38.

———. 2012. Age-related loss of muscle mass and strength. *Journal of Aging Research* 2012. https://doi.org/10.1155/2012/158279

Gollhofer, A., Fujitsuka, P.A., Miyashita, N., and Yashita, M. 1987. Fatigue during stretch-shortening cycle exercises: Changes in neuro-muscular activation patterns of human skeletal muscle. *Journal of Sports Medicine* 8: 30-47.

Gollnick, P., Armstrong, R., Saubert, C., Piehl, K., and Saltin, B. 1972. Enzyme activity and fibre composition in skeletal muscle of untrained and trained men. *Journal of Applied Physiology* 33 (3): 312-19.

González-Badillo, J.J., et al. 2014. Maximal intended velocity training induces greater gains in bench press performance than deliberately slower half-velocity training. *European Journal of Sport Science* 15: 1-10.

Gorostiaga, E.M., Navarro-Amézqueta, I., Calbet, J.A., Hellsten, Y., Cusso, R., Guerrero, M., Granados, C., González-Izal, M., Ibañez, J., and Izquierdo, M. 2012. Energy metabolism during repeated sets of leg press exercise leading to failure or not. *PLOS One* 7 (7): e40621.

Gossen, R.E., Allingham, K., and Sale, D.G. 2001. Effect of temperature on post-tetanic potentiation in human dorsiflexor muscles. *Canadian Journal of Physiology and Pharmacology* 79: 49-58.

Goto, K., et al. 2004. Muscular adaptations to combinations of high- and low-intensity resistance exercises. *Journal of Strength and Conditioning Research* 18 (4): 730-37.

Goto, K., et al. 2007. Effects of resistance exercise on lipolysis during subsequent submaximal exercise. *Medicine and Science in Sports and Exercise* 39 (2): 308-15.

Graves, J.E., et al. 1988. Effect of reduced training frequency on muscular strength. *International Journal of Sports Medicine* 9 (5): 316-19.

Gregg, R.A., and Mastellone, A.F. 1957. Cross exercise: A review of the literature and study utilizing electromyographic techniques. *American Journal of Physical Medicine* 38: 269-80.

Grizard, J., et al. 1999. Insulin action on skeletal muscle protein metabolism during catabolic states. *Reproduction Nutrition Development* 39 (1): 61-74.

Gullich, A., and Schmidtbleicher, D. 1996. MVC-induced short-term potentiation of explosive force. *New Studies in Athletics* 11 (4): 67-81.

Haff, G.G, et al. 2000. Carbohydrate supplementation attenuates muscle glycogen loss during acute bouts of resistance exercise. *International Journal of Sport Nutrition and Exercise Metabolism* 10: 326-39.

Hagberg, et al. 1979. Effect of training on hormonal responses to exercise in competitive swimmers. *European Journal of Applied Physiology and Occupational Physiology* 41 (3): 211-19.

Hainaut, K., and Duchateau, J. 1989. Muscle fatigue: Effects of training and disuse. *Muscle & Nerve* 12: 660-69.

Haiyan, L., et al. 2011. Macrophages recruited via CCR2 produce insulin-like growth factor-1 to repair acute skeletal muscle injury. *FASEB Journal* 25 (1): 358-69.

Häkkinen, K. 1986. Training and detraining adaptations in electromyography. Muscle fibre and force production characteristics of human leg extensor muscle with special reference to prolonged heavy resistance and explosive-type strength training. *Studies in Sport, Physical Education and Health* 20. Jyväskylä, Finland: University of Jyväskylä.

————. 1989. Neuromuscular and hormonal adaptations during strength and power training. *Journal of Sports Medicine and Physical Fitness* 29 (1): 9-26.

Häkkinen, K., and Komi, P. 1983. Electromyographic changes during strength training and detraining. *Medicine and Science in Sports and Exercise* 15: 455-60.

Häkkinen, K., and Pakarinen, A. 1993. Acute hormonal responses to two different fatiguing heavy-resistance protocols in male athletes. *Journal of Applied Physiology* 74 (2): 882-87.

Hall, E., Bishop, D., and Gee, T. 2016. Effect of Plyometric training on handspring vault performance and functional power in youth female gymnasts. PloS one. 11. e0148790. 10.1371/journal.pone.0148790.

Hamada, T., et al. 2000. Post activation potentiation, fiber type, and twitch contraction time in human knee extensor muscles. *Journal of Applied Physiology* 88 (6): 2131-37.

Hameed, M., et al. 2008. Effects of eccentric cycling exercise on IGF-I splice variant expression in the muscles of young and elderly people. *Scandinavian Journal of Medicine and Science in Sports* 18 (4): 447-52.

Hamlyn, N., et al. 2007. Trunk muscle activation during dynamic weight-training exercises and isometric instability activities. *Journal of Strength and Conditioning Research* 21 (4): 1108-12.

Harre, D., ed. 1982. *Trainingslehre*. Berlin: Sportverlag.

————. 2005. *Teoria dell' allenamento*. Roma, Società Stampa Sportiva.

Harrison, B.C., et al. 2011. IIb or not IIb? Regulation of myosin heavy chain gene expression in mice and men. *Skeletal Muscle* 1 (1): 1-5.

Hartmann, J., and Tünnemann, H. 1988. *Fitness and strength training*. Berlin: Sportverlag.

Hartmann, H., et al. 2012. Influence of squatting depth on jumping performance. *Journal of Strength and Conditioning Research* 26 (12): 3243-61.

Hassell, A.L, Lindsted, S., and Nishikawa, K.C. 2017. Physiological mechanisms of eccentric contraction and its applications: a role for the giant titin protein. *Frontiers in Physiology* 9 (8): 70.

Hawley, J.A., Tipton, K.D., and Millard-Stafford, M.L. 2006. Promoting training adaptations through nutritional interventions. *Journal of Sports Sciences* 24 (7): 709-21.

Hay, J.G. 1993. *The biomechanics of sports techniques*. Englewood Cliffs, NJ: Prentice Hall.

Healey, K.C., et al. 2014 The effects of myofascial release with foam rolling on performance. *Journal of Strength and Conditioning Research* 28 (1): 61-68.

Hellebrand, F., and Houtz, S. 1956. Mechanism of muscle training in man: Experimental demonstration of the overload principle. *Physical Therapy Review* 36: 371-83.

References

Hellebrandt, F.A., Parrish, A.M., and Houtz, S.J. 1947. Cross education: The influence of unilateral exercise on the contralateral limb. *Archive of Physical Medicine* 28: 78-84.

Helms, Eric. 2010. *Effects of Training-Induced Hormonal Changes on Muscular Hypertrophy*. 3dmusclejourney.com/resources/Effects_of_Training-Induced_Hormonal_Changes_on_Muscular_Hypertrophy_by_Eric_Helms.pdf.

Henneman, E., Somjen, G., and Carpenter, D.O. 1965. Functional significance of cell size in spinal motoneurons. *Journal of Neurophysiology* 28: 560-80.

Hennig, R., and Lomo, T. 1987. Gradation of force output in normal fast and slow muscle of the rat. *Acta Physiologica Scandinavica* 130: 133-42.

Hessel, A.L., Lindstedt, S.L., and Nishikawa, K.C., 2017. Physiological mechanism of eccentric contraction and its application: A role for the giant titin protein. *Frontiers in Physiology* 9 (8): 70.

Hermansen, L., and Vaage, O. 1977. Lactate disappearance and glycogen synthesis in human muscle after maximal exercise. *American Journal of Physiology* 233 (5): E422-29.

Hettinger, T. 1966. *Isometric muscle training*. Stuttgart: Georg Thieme Verlag.

Hettinger, T., and Müler, E. 1953. Muskelleistung and Muskel Training. *Arbeitsphysiologie* 15: 111-26.

Hickson, R., et al. 1985. Reduced training intensities and loss of aerobic power, endurance, and cardiac growth. *Journal of Applied Physiology* 58: 492-99.

Hickson, R.C., Dvorak, B.A., Corostiaga, T.T., and Foster, C. 1988. Strength training and performance in endurance-trained subjects. *Medicine and Science in Sports and Exercise* 20 (2) (Suppl.): 586.

Hody, S., Croisier, J.L., Bury, T., Register, B., and Leprince, P. 2019. Eccentric muscle contractions: Risks and benefits. *Frontiers in Physiology* 3 (10): 536.

Hoff, J., Gran, A., and Helgerud, J. 2002. Maximal strength training improves aerobic endurance performance. *Scandinavian Journal of Medicine and Science in Sports* 12 (5): 288-95.

Hoffman, J.R., Ratamess, N.A., Tranchina, C.P., Rashti, S.L., Kang, J., and Faigenbaum, A.D. 2010. Effect of a proprietary protein supplement on recovery indices following resistance exercise in strength/power athletes. *Amino Acids* 38 (3): 771-78.

Hornberger, T.A., et al. 2006. The role of phospholipase D and phosphatidic acid in the mechanical activation of mTOR signaling in skeletal muscle. *Proceedings of the National Academy of Science of the United States of America* 103 (12): 4741-46.

Hortobagyi, T., Hill, J., Houmard, A., Fraser, D., Lambert, J., and Israel, G. 1996. Adaptive responses to muscle lengthening and shortening in humans. *Journal of Applied Physiology* 80 (3): 765-72.

Houmard, J.A., Kirwan, J.P., Flynn, M.G., and Mitchell, J.B. 1989. Effects of reduced training on submaximal and maximal running responses. *International Journal of Sports Medicine* 10: 30-33.

Houmard, J.A. 1991. Impact of reduced training on performance in endurance athletes. *Sports Medicine* 12 (6): 380-93.

Howard, J.D., Ritchie, M.R., Gater, D.A., Gater, D.R., and Enoka, R.M. 1985. Determining factors of strength: Physiological foundations. *National Strength and Conditioning Journal* 7 (6): 16-21.

Hubbard, T.J., et al. 2004. Does cryotherapy hasten return to participation? A systematic literature review. *Journal of Athletic Training* 39 (1): 88-94.

Hultman, E., and Sjoholm, H. 1983. Energy metabolism and contraction force of skeletal muscle in-situ during electrical stimulation. *Journal of Physiology* 345: 525-32.

International Olympic Committee. 2010. *Consensus Statement on Sport Nutrition*. olympic.org/Documents/Reports/EN/CONSENSUS-FINAL-v8-en.pdf

Israel, S. 1972. *The acute syndrome of detraining*. Berlin: GDR National Olympic Committee. 2: 30-35.

Ivy, J., and Portman, R. 2004. *Nutrient timing*. Laguna Beach, CA: Basic Health Publications.

Ivy, J.L, et al. 2003. Effect of carbohydrate-protein supplement on endurance performance during exercise of varying intensity. *International Journal of Sport Nutrition and Exercise Metabolism* 13: 42-49, 52-56, 338-401.

Izquierdo, M., et al. 2006. Differential effects of strength training leading to failure versus not to failure on hormonal responses, strength and muscle power increases. *Journal of Applied Physiology* 100: 1647-56.

Jacobs, I., Esbornsson, M., Sylven, C., Holm, I., and Jansson, E. 1987. Sprint training effects on muscle myoglobin, enzymes, fibre types, and blood lactate. *Medicine and Science in Sports and Exercise* 19 (4): 368-74.

Janssen, P. 2001. *Lactate threshold training*. Champaign, IL: Human Kinetics.

Jezova, D., et al. 1985. Plasma testosterone and catecholamine responses to physical exercise of different intensities in men. *European Journal of Applied Physiology and Occupational Physiology* 54 (1): 62-66.

Johns, R.J., and Wright, V. 1962. Relative importance of various tissues in joint stiffness. *Journal of Applied Physiology* 17: 824.

Jorgensen, J.O., et al. 2003. Exercise, hormones and body temperature: Regulation and action of Gh during exercise. *Journal of Endocrinological Investigation* 26 (9): 38-42.

Kandarian, S.C., and Jackman, R.W. 2006. Intracellular signaling during skeletal muscle atrophy. *Muscle & Nerve* 33 (2): 155-65.

Kanehisa, J., and Miyashita, M. 1983. Effect of isometric and isokinetic muscle training on static strength and dynamic power. *European Journal of Applied Physiology* 50: 365-71.

Kannus, P., Alosa, D., Cook, L., Johnson, R.J., Renstrom, P., Pope, M., Beynnon, B., Yasuda, K., Nichols, C., and Kaplan, M. 1992. Effect of one-legged exercise on the strength, power and endurance of the contralateral leg: A randomized, controlled study using isometric and concentric isokinetic training. *European Journal of Applied Physiology* 64 (2): 117-26.

Karlsson, J., and Saltin, B. 1971. Diet, muscle glycogen and endurance performance. *Journal of Applied Physiology* 31 (2): 203-6.

Kawamori, N., et al. 2013. Relationships between ground reaction impulse and sprint acceleration performance in team sport athletes. *Journal of Strength and Conditioning Research* 27 (3): 568-73.

Kerksick, C., et al. 2008. International society of sport nutrition position stand: Nutrient timing. *Journal of the International Society of Sport Nutrition* 5: 17.

King, I. 1998. *How to Write Strength Training Programs.* Toowong (AUS): Kings Sport Publishing. 123.

Kjaer, M., et al. 2005. Metabolic activity and collagen turnover in human tendon in response to physical activity. *Journal of Musculoskeletal and Neuronal Interactions* 5 (1): 41-52.

Kjaer, M., et al. 2006. Extracellular matrix adaptation of tendon and skeletal muscle to exercise. *Journal of Anatomy* 208 (4): 445-50.

Komi, P.V., and Bosco, C. 1978. Utilization of stored elastic energy in leg extensor muscles by men and women. *Medicine and Science in Sports and Exercise* 10 (4): 261-65.

Komi, P.V., and Buskirk, E.R. 1972. Effect of eccentric and concentric muscle conditioning on tension and electrical activity of human muscle. *Ergonomics* 15 (4): 417-34.

Kraemer, W.J., and Ratamess, N.A. 2005. Hormonal responses and adaptations to resistance exercise and training. *Sports Medicine* 35: 339-61.

Kraemer, W.J., Ratamess, N.A., Volek, J.S., Häkkinen, K., Rubin, M.R., French, D.N., Gómez, A.L., et al. 2006. The effects of amino acid supplementation on hormonal responses to resistance training overreaching. *Metabolism* 55 (3): 282-91.

Kyröläinen, H., Avela, J., and Komi, P.V. 2005. Changes in muscle activity with increasing running speed. *Journal of Sports Sciences* 23 (1): 1101-9.

Kugler, A., Kruger-Franke, M., Reininger, S., Trouillier, H.H., and Rosemeyer, B. 1996. Muscular imbalance and shoulder pain in volleyball attackers. *British Journal of Sports Medicine* 30 (3): 256-59.

Kuipers, H., and Keizer, H.A. 1988. Overtraining in elite athletes: Review and directions for the future. *Sports Medicine* 6: 79-92.

Kuoppasalmi, K., and Adlercreutz, H. 1985. Interaction between anabolic and catabolic steroid hormones in muscular exercise. *Exercise Endocrinology.* Berlin: de Gruyter: 65-98.

Kyröläinen, H., et al. 2001. Biomechanical factors affecting running economy. *Medicine and Science in Sports and Exercise* 33 (8): 1330-37.

Lamb, D.R. 1984. *Physiology of Exercise: Responses and Adaptations.* 2nd ed. New York: MacMillan.

Langberg, H., et al. 2007. Eccentric rehabilitation exercise increases peritendinous type I collagen synthesis in humans with Achilles tendinosis. *Scandinavian Journal of Medicine and Science in Sports* 17: 61-66.

Lange, L. 1919. *Über functionelle Anpassung.* Berlin: Springer Verlag.

Latash, M.L. 1998. *Neurophysiological basis of movement.* Champaign, IL: Human Kinetics.

La Torre, A., et al. 2010. Acute effects of static stretching on squat jump performance at different knee starting angles. *Journal of Strength and Conditioning Research* 24 (3): 687-94.

References

Laubach, L.L. 1976. Comparative muscle strength of men and women: A review of the literature. *Aviation, Space, and Environmental Medicine* 47: 534-42.

Lee, M., and Carroll, T. 2007. Cross-education: Possible mechanisms for the contralateral effects of unilateral resistance training. *Sports Medicine* 37 (1): 1-14.

Lemon, P.W., et al. 1997. Moderate physical activity can increase dietary protein needs. *Canadian Journal of Applied Physiology* 22: 494-503.

Lephart, S.M., Ferris, C.M., Riemann, B.L., Myers, J.B., and Fu, F.H. 2002. Gender differences in strength and lower extremity kinematics during landing. *Clinical Orthopaedics and Related Research* 402: 162-69.

Liu, Y., et al. 2008. Response of growth and myogenic factors in human skeletal muscle to strength training. *British Journal of Sports Medicine* 42 (12): 989-93.

MacDonald, G.Z., et al. 2013. An acute bout of self-myofascial release increases range of motion without a subsequent decrease in neuromuscular performance. *Journal of Strength and Conditioning Research* 27 (3): 812-21.

MacDougall, J.D., Tuxen, D., Sale, D.G., Moroz, J.R., and Sutton, J.R. 1985. Arterial blood pressure response to heavy resistance exercise. *Journal of Applied Physiology* 58 (3): 785-90.

Mallinson, J.E., Taylor, T., Teodosiu, D.C., Clark, R.B., Constantin, D., Franchi, M.V. Narici, M.V., Auer, D., and Greenhaff, P.L. 2020. Longitudinal hypertrophic and transcriptional responses to high-load eccentric–concentric vs concentric training in males. *Scandinavian Journal or Medicine and Science in Sports,* 00:1-15.

Marsden, C., Meadows, J.F., and Merton, P.A. 1971. Isolated single motor units in human muscle and their rate of discharge during maximal voluntary effort. *Journal of Physiology—London* 217: 12P-13P.

Martin, D.T, Scifres, J.C., Zimmerman, S.D, and Wilkinson, J.G. 1994. Effects of interval training and a taper on cycling performance and isokinetic leg strength. *International Journal of Sports Medicine* 15: 485-91.

Martuscello, J., Nuzzo, J.L. Ashley, C.D., Campbell, B.I., Orriola, J.J., and Mayer, J.M. 2012. Systematic review of core muscle electromyographic activity during physical fitness exercises. *Journal of Strength and Conditioning Research* 27 (6): 1684-98.

Mathews, D.K., and Fox, E.L. 1976. *The physiological basis of physical education and athletics.* Philadelphia: Saunders.

Matveyev, L. 1965. *The Problem of Periodization of Sport Training.*

Maughan, R.J., Goodburn, R., Griffin, J., Irani, M., Kirwan, J.P., Leiper, J.B., MacLaren, D.P., McLatchie, G., Tsintsas, K., and Williams, C. 1993. Fluid replacement in sport and exercise—A consensus statement. *British Journal of Sports Medicine* 27 (1): 34-35.

McConell, G.K., Costill, D.L., Widrick, J.J., Hickey, M.S., Tanaka, H., and Gastin, P.B. 1993. Reduced training volume and intensity maintain capacity but not performance in distance runners. *International Journal of Sports Medicine* 14: 33-37.

McDonagh, M., and Davies, C.T.M. 1984. Adaptive response of mammalian skeletal muscle to exercise with high loads. *European Journal of Applied Physiology* 52: 139-55.

McMaster, D.T, Gill, N., Cronin, J., and McGuigan, M. 2013. The development, retention, and decay rates of strength and power in elite rugby union, rugby league, and American football: A systematic review. *Sports Medicine* 43 (5): 367-84.

McNeely, E., and Sandler, D. 2007. Tapering for endurance athletes. *Strength and Conditioning Journal* 29 (5): 18-24.

Micheli, L.J. 1988. Strength training in the young athlete. In *Competitive sports for children and youth,* edited by E.W. Brown and C.E. Branta, 99-105. Champaign, IL: Human Kinetics.

Miller, B.F., et al. 2005. Coordinated collagen and muscle protein synthesis in human patella tendon and quadriceps muscle after exercise. *Journal of Physiology* 567 (Pt 3): 1021-33.

Mizner, R.L., Stevens, J.E., and Snyder-Mackler, L. 2003. Voluntary activation and decreased force production of the quadriceps femoris muscle after total knee arthroplasty. *Physical Therapy* 83 (4): 359-65.

Moeller, F., et al. 1985. Duration of stretching effect on range of motion in lower extremities. *Archives of Physical Medicine and Rehabilitation* 66: 171-73.

Mohr, M., Krustrup, P., and Bangsbo, J. 2005. Fatigue in soccer: A brief review. *Journal of Sports Sciences* 23 (6): 593-99.

Morgan, R.E., and Adamson, G.T. 1959. *Circuit weight training.* London: Bell.

Morin, J.B. 2011. Technical ability of force application as a determinant factor of sprint performance. *Medicine and Science in Sports and Exercise* 43 (9): 1680-88.

Morin, J.B., et al. 2012. Mechanical determinants of 100-m sprint running performance. *European Journal of Applied Physiology* 112 (11): 3921-30.

Moritani, T. 1992. Time course of adaptations during strength and power training. In *Strength and power in sport*, edited by P.V. Komi, 266-78. Champaign, IL: Human Kinetics.

Moritani, T., and deVries, H.A. 1979. Neural factors versus hypertrophy in the time course of muscle strength gain. *American Journal of Physical Medicine* 58 (3): 115-30.

Mujika, I. 1998. The influence of training characteristics and tapering on adaptation in highly trained individuals: A review. *International Journal of Sports Medicine* 19: 439-46.

———. 2009. *Tapering and peaking for optimal performance*. Champaign, IL: Human Kinetics.

Mujika, I., Chatard, J.C., Busso, T., Geyssant, A., Barale, F., and Lacoste, L. 1995. Effects of training on performance in competitive swimming. *Canadian Journal of Applied Physiology* 20 (4): 395-406.

Mujika, I., and S. Padilla. 2000. Detraining: Loss of training-induced physiological and performance adaptation. *Sports Medicine* 30 (3): 145-154.

Mujika, I., Padilla, S., and Pyne, D. 2002. Swimming performance changes during the final 3 weeks of training leading to the Sydney 2000 Olympic Games, *International Journal of Sports Medicine* 23 (8): 582-87.

Nardone, A., Romanò, C., and Schieppati, M. 1989. Selective recruitment of high-threshold human motor units during voluntary isotonic lengthening of active muscles. *Journal of Physiology* 409: 451-71.

Nelson, A.G., Arnall, D.A., Loy, S.F., Silvester, L.J., and Conlee, R.K. 1990. Consequences of combining strength and endurance training regimens. *Physical Therapy* 70 (5): 287-94.

Nelson, A.G., et al. 2005. Acute effects of passive muscle stretching on sprint performance. *Journal of Sports Sciences* 23 (5): 449-54.

Newsholme, E. 2005. *Keep on running: The science of training and performance*. Hoboken, NJ: Wiley.

Newton, R., Murphy, A., Humphries, B., Wilson, G., Kraemer, W., and Häkkinen, K. 1996. Influence of load and stretch shortening cycle on the kinematics, kinetics and muscle activation that occurs during explosive bench press throws. *European Journal of Applied Physiology* 75: 333-42.

Newton, R., Kraemer, W., Häkkinen, K., Humphries, B., and Murphy, A. 1996. Kinematics, kinetics and muscle activation during explosive upper body movements. *Journal of Applied Biomechanics* 12: 31-43.

Nicholson, G., Bennett, T.D., Bissas, A. and Merlino, S. 2019. *Biomechanical Report for the IAAF World Indoor Championships 2018: High Jump Men*. Birmingham, UK: International Association of Athletics Federations.

Noakes, T.D., et al. 2005. From catastrophe to complexity: A novel model of integrative central neural regulation of effort and fatigue during exercise in humans: Summary and conclusions. *British Journal of Sports Medicine* 39: 120-24.

Nummela, A., et al. 2007. Factors related to top running speed and economy. *International Journal of Sports Medicine* 28 (8): 655-61.

Nuzzo, J.L. 2008. Trunk muscle activity during stability ball and free weight exercises. *Journal of Strength and Conditioning Research* 22 (1): 95-102.

Okamura, K., et al. 1997. Effect of amino acid and glucose administration during post-exercise recovery on protein kinetics in dogs. *American Journal of Physiology* 272: E1023-30.

O'Leary, D.D., Hope, K., and Sale, D.G. 1998. Influence of gender on post-tetanic potentiation in human dorsiflexors. *Canadian Journal of Physiology and Pharmacology* 76: 772-79.

Owino, V., et al. 2001 Age-related loss of skeletal muscle function and the inability to express the autocrine form of insulin-like growth factor-1 (MGF) in response to mechanical overload. *FEBS Letters* 505 (2): 259-63.

Ozolin, N.G. 1971. *Athlete's training system for competition*. Moscow: Phyzkultura i sports.

Petibois, C., and Deleris, G. 2003. Effects of short and long-term detraining on the metabolic response to endurance exercises. *International Journal of Sports Medicine*, 24: 320-325.

Piehl, K. 1974. Time course for refilling of glycogen stores in human muscle fibres following exercise-induced glycogen depletion. *Acta Physiologica Scandinavica* 90: 297-302.

Pincivero, D.M., and Campy, R.M. 2004. The effects of rest interval length and training on quadriceps femoris muscle. Part I: Knee extensor torque and muscle fatigue. *Journal of Sports Medicine and Physical Fitness* 44 (2): 111-18.

References

Pincivero, D.M., Lephart, S.M., and Karunakara, R.G. 1997. Effects of rest interval on isokinetic strength and functional performance after short-term high intensity training. *British Journal of Sports Medicine* 31 (3): 229-34.

Ploutz, L., et al. 1994. Effect of resistance training on muscle use during exercise. *Journal of Applied Physiology* 76: 1675-81.

Power, K., et al. 2004. An acute bout of static stretching: Effects on force and jumping performance. *Medicine and Science in Sports and Exercise* 36 (8): 1389-96.

Powers, S.K., Lawler, J., Dodd, S., Tulley, R., Landry, G., and Wheeler, K. 1990. Fluid replacement drinks during high intensity exercise: Effects on minimizing exercise-induced disturbances in homeostasis. *European Journal of Applied Physiology and Occupational Physiology* 60 (1): 54-60.

Pyne, D.B., et al. 2009. Peaking for optimal performance: Research limitations and future directions. *Journal of Sports Sciences* 27 (3): 195-202.

Raglin, J.S. 1992. Anxiety and sport performance. *Exercise Sports Science Review* 20: 243-74.

Ranieri, F., and Di Lazzaro, V. 2012. The role of motor neuron drive in muscle fatigue. *Neuromuscular Disorders* 22 (3): S157-61.

Rasmussen, R.B., and Phillips, S.M. 2003. Contractile and nutritional regulation of human muscle growth. *Exercise and Sport Sciences Reviews* 31 (3): 127-31.

Ready, S.L., Seifert, J., and Burke, E. 1999. Effect of two sport drinks on muscle tissue stress and performance. *Medicine and Science in Sports and Exercise* 31 (5): S119.

Reid, P.J., Oliver, J.L., De Ste Croix, M.B.A., Myer, G.D., and Lloyd, R.S. 2018. An audit of injuries in six English professional soccer academies. *Journal of Sports Sciences* 3: 13.

Reilly, T., and Ekblom, B. 2005. The use of recovery methods post-exercise. *Journal of Sports Sciences* 23 (6): 619-27.

Rennie, M.J., and Millward, D.J. 1983. 3-methylhistidine excretion and the urinary 3-methylhistidine/creatinine ratio are poor indicators of skeletal muscle protein breakdown. *Clinical Science* 65: 217-25.

Rhea, M.R., et al. 2009. Alterations in speed of squat movement and the use of accommodated resistance among college athletes training for power. *Journal of Strength and Conditioning Research* 23 (9): 2645-50.

Rietjens, G.J., Keizer, H.A., Kuipers, H., and Saris, W.H. 2001. A reduction in training volume and intensity for 21 days does not impair performance in cyclists. *British Journal of Sports Medicine* 35 (6): 431-34.

Rixon, K.P., Lamont, H.S., and Bemben, M.G. 2007. Influence of type of muscle contraction, gender, and lifting experience on postactivation potentiation performance. *Journal of Strength and Conditioning Research* 21 (2): 500-05.

Robinson, J.M., et al. 1995. Effects of different weight training exercise/rest intervals on strength, power, and high intensity exercise endurance. *Journal of Strength and Conditioning Research* 9 (4): 216-21.

Roemmich, J.N., and Rogol, A.D. 1997. Exercise and growth hormone: Does one affect the other? *Journal of Pediatrics* 131: S75-80.

Roig, M., O'Brien, K., Murray, G.R., McKinnon, P., Shadgan, B., and Reid, W.D. 2009. The effects of eccentric versus concentric resistance training on muscle strength and mass in healthy adults: A systematic review with meta-analysis. *British Journal of Sports Medicine* 43 (8): 556-68.

Roman Suarez, I. 1986. *Levantamiento de pesas—Periodo competitivo*. La Habana, Cuba: Editorial Científico-Técnica.

Rønnestad, B.R., and Mujika, I. 2013. Optimizing strength training for running and cycling endurance performance: A review. *Scandinavian Journal of Medicine and Science in Sports* 24 (4): 603-12.

Roschel, H., et al. 2011. Effect of eccentric exercise velocity on akt/mtor/p70(s6k) signaling in human skeletal muscle. *Applied Physiology Nutrition and Metabolism* 36 (2): 283-90.

Sahlin, K. 1986. Metabolic changes limiting muscular performance. *Biochemistry of Exercise* 16: 86-98.

Sale, D. 1986. Neural adaptation in strength and power training. In *Human muscle power*, edited by L. Jones, L.N. McCartney, and A. McConias, 289-304. Champaign, IL: Human Kinetics.

———. 1992. Neural adaptations to strength training. In *Strength and power in sport*, edited by P.V. Komi, 249-65. Oxford: Blackwell Scientific.

Sale, D.G., MacDougall, J.D., Jakobs, I., and Garner, S. 1990. Interaction between concurrent strength and endurance training. *Journal of Applied Physiology* 68 (1): 260-70.

Saltin, B. 1973. Metabolic fundamentals in exercise. *Medicine and Science in Sports* 5: 137-46.

Samuel, M.N., et al. 2008. Acute effects of static and ballistic stretching on measures of strength and power. *Journal of Strength and Conditioning Research* 22 (5): 1422-28.

Santa Maria, D., Gryzbinski, P., and Hatfield, B. 1985. Power as a function of load for a supine bench press exercise [Abstract]. *National Strength and Conditioning Association Journal* 6: 58.

Sariyildiz, M., et al. 2011. Cross-education of muscle strength: Cross-training effects are not confined to untrained contralateral homologous muscle. *Scandinavian Journal of Medicine and Science in Sport* 21 (6): e359-64.

Schanzer, W. 2002. *Analysis of non-hormonal nutritional supplements for anabolic-androgenic steroids.* www.olympic.org/Documents/Reports/EN/en_report_324.pdf.

Schillings, M.L., et al. 2000. *Central and peripheral aspects of exercise-induced fatigue.* med.uni-jena.de/motorik/pdk/schillings.pdf.

Schmidtbleicher, D. 1984. *Sportliches Krafttraining und motorische Grundlagenfoschung.* In W. Berger, V. Dietz, A. Hufschmidt, R. Jung, K.-H. Mauritz, and D. Schmidtbleicher, *Haltung und Bewegung beim Menschen*, 155-88. Berlin: Springer.

———. 1992. Training for power events. In *Strength and power in sport*, edited by P.V. Komi, 381-95. Oxford, UK: Blackwell Scientific.

Schmidtbleicher, D., et al. 2014. Long-term strength training effects on change-of-direction sprint performance. *Journal of Strength and Conditioning Research* 28 (1): 223-31.

Schoenfeld, B.J. 2012. Does exercise-induced muscle damage play a role in skeletal muscle hypertrophy? *Journal of Strength and Conditioning Research* 26 (5): 1441-53.

Seiberl, W., Power, G.A., Herzog, W., and Hahn, D. 2015. The stretch-shortening cycle (SSC) revisited: Residual force enhancement contributes to increased performance during fast SSCs of human m. abductor policis. *Physiological Reports* May 3 (5): e12401.

Shepley, B., MacDougall, J.D., Cipriano, N., Sutton, J.R., Tarnopolsky, M.A., and Coates, G. 1992. Physiological effects of tapering in highly trained athletes. *Journal of Applied Physiology* 72: 706-11.

Sirotic, A.C., and Coutts, A.J. 2007. Physiological and performance test correlates of prolonged, high-intensity, intermittent running performance in moderately trained women team sport athletes. *Journal of Strength and Conditioning Research* 21 (1): 138-44.

Sjøgaard, G., et al. 1985. Water and ion shifts in skeletal muscle of humans with intense dynamic knee extension. *American Journal of Physiology* 248 (2 pt 2): R190-96.

Söderman, K., Wener, S., Pietila, T., Engstrom. B., and Alfredson, H. 2000. Balance board training: Prevention of traumatic injuries of the lower extremities in female soccer players? A perspective randomized intervention study. *Knee Surgery, Sports Traumatology, Arthroscopy* 8 (6): 356-63.

Staley, C. 2005. *Muscle logic.* Emmaus, PA: Rodale Press.

Stanek, J.M. 2015. The effectiveness of compression socks for athletic performance and recovery. *Journal of Sports Rehabilitation* 26: 109-14.

Staron, R.S., Hagerman, F.C., and Hikida, R.S. 1981. The effects of detraining on an elite power lifter. *Journal of Neurological Sciences* 51: 247-57.

Stickford, A.S., Chapman, R.F., Johnston, J.D., and Stager, J.M. 2015. Lower leg compression, running mechanics and economy in elite distance runners. *International Journal of Sports Physiology and Performance* 10 (1): 76-83.

Stone, M.H., and O'Bryant, H.S. 1984. *Weight training: A scientific approach.* Minneapolis: Burgess.

Stone, M., O'Bryant, H., Garhammer, J., McMillan, J., and Rozenek. R. 1982. A theoretical model of strength training. *National Strength & Conditioning Association Journal* 4(4): 36-39.

Stone, M.H., Stone, M., and Sands, W.A. 2007. *Principles and practice of resistance training.* Champaign, IL: Human Kinetics.

Sullivan, K.M., et al. 2013. Roller-massager application to the hamstrings increases sit-and-reach range of motion within five to ten seconds without performance impairments. *International Journal of Sports Physical Therapy* 8 (3): 228-36.

Takagi, R., et al. 2011. Influence of icing on muscle regeneration after crush injury to skeletal muscles in rats. *Journal of Applied Physiology* 110 (2): 382-88.

References

Takarada, Y., et al. 2000. Rapid increase in plasma growth hormone after low-intensity resistance exercise with vascular occlusion. *Journal of Applied Physiology* 88 (1): 61-5.

Taylor, J.L., Todd, G., and Gandevia, S.C. 2006. Evidence for a supraspinal contribution to human muscle fatigue. *Clinical and Experimental Pharmacology and Physiology* 33 (4): 400-5.

Terjung, R.L., and Hood, D.A. 1986. Biochemical adaptations in skeletal muscle induced by exercise training. In *Nutrition and aerobic exercise*, edited by D.K. Layman, 8-27. Washington, DC: American Chemical Society.

Tesch, P. 1980. Muscle fatigue in man. *Acta Physiologica Scandinavica Supplementum* 480: 3-40.

Tesch, P., Sjšdon, B., Thorstensson, A., and Karlsson, J. 1978. Muscle fatigue and its relation to lactate accumulation and LDH activity in man. *Acta Physiologica Scandinavica* 103: 413-20.

Tesch, P.A., and Larsson, L. 1982. Muscle hypertrophy in bodybuilders. *European Journal of Applied Physiology and Occupational Physiology* 49 (3): 301-6.

Tesch, P.A., Thorsson, A., and Kaiser, P. 1984. Muscle capillary supply and fiber type characteristics in weight and power lifters. *Journal of Applied Physiology* 56: 35-38.

Tesch, P.A., Dudley, G.A., Durvisin, M.R., Hather, M., and Harris, R.T. 1990. Force and EMG signal patterns during repeated bouts of concentric and eccentric muscle actions. *Acta Physiologica Scandinavica* 138: 263-271.

Thacker, S.B., Stroup, D.F., Branche, C.M., Gilchrist, J., Goodman, R.A., and Porter Kelling, E. 2003. Prevention of knee injuries in sports. A systematic review of literature. *Journal of Sports Medicine and Physical Fitness* 43 (2): 165-79.

Thomas, L., Mujika, I., and Busso, T. 2009. Computer simulations assessing the potential performance benefit of a final increase in training during pre-event taper. *Journal of Strength and Conditioning Research* 23 (6): 1729-36.

Thorstensson, A. 1977. Observations on strength training and detraining. *Acta Physiologica Scandinavica* 100: 491-93.

Tipton, K.D., Ferrando, A.A., Phillips, S.M., Doyle Jr., D., and Wolfe, R.R. 1999. Postexercise net protein synthesis in human muscle from orally administered amino acids. *American Journal of Physiology* 276: E628-34.

Tipton, K.D., and Wolfe, R.R. 2001. Exercise, protein metabolism, and muscle growth. *International Journal of Sport Nutrition and Exercise Metabolism* 11 (1): 109-32.

———. 2004. Protein and amino acid for athletes. *Journal of Sports Science* 22 (1): 65-79.

Trinity, J.D., et al. 2006. Maximal mechanical power during a taper in elite swimmers. *Medicine and Science in Sports and Exercise*, 38 (9): 1643-49.

Tucker, C.B., Bissas, A. and Merlino, S. 2019. Biomechanical Report for the IAAF World Indoor Championships 2018: Long Jump Men. Birmingham, UK: International Association of Athletics Federations.

Van Cutsem, M., Duchateau, J., and Hainaut, K. 1998. Changes in single motor unit behaviour contribute to the increase in contraction speed after dynamic training in humans. *Journal of Physiology* 513: 295-305.

Van Someren, K.A. 2006. The physiology of anaerobic endurance training. In *The Physiology of Training*, edited by G. Whyte., 88. London: Elsevier.

Verkhoshansky, Y.L.V. 1969. Perspectives in the improvement of speed-strength preparation of jumpers. *Yessis Review of Soviet Physical Education and Sports* 4 (2): 28-29.

———. 1997. *Tutto sul metodo d'urto*. Roma, Società Stampa Sportiva.

von Lieres, H.C. Wilkau, G.I.., Bezodis, N.E., Simpson, S., and Bezodis, I.N. 2020. Phase analysis in maximal sprinting: An investigation of step-to-step technical changes between the initial acceleration, transition and maximal velocity phases. *Sports Biomechanics* 19 (2): 141-156. DOI: 10.1080/14763141.2018.1473479

Wade, A.J., Broadhead, M.W., Cady, E.B., Llewelyn, M.E., Tong, H.N., and Newham, D.J. 2000. Influence of muscle temperature during fatiguing work with the first dorsal interosseous muscle in man: A 31P-NMR spectroscopy study. *European Journal of Applied Physiology* 81 (3): 203-9.

Wathen, D. 1994. Agonist-antagonist ratios for slow concentric isokinetic movements. In *Essentials of strength training and conditioning*, edited by T.R. Baechle. Champaign, IL: Human Kinetics.

Wee, J., et al. 2005. GH secretion in acute exercise may result in post-exercise lipolysis. *Growth Hormone & IGF Research Journal* 15 (6): 397-404.

Weir, J.P., et al. 2006. Is fatigue all in your head? A critical review of the central governor model. *British Journal of Sports Medicine* 40 (7): 573-86.

Welsh, R.S., Davis, J.M., Burke, J.R., and Williams, H.G. 2002. Carbohydrates and physical/mental performance during intermittent exercise to fatigue. *Medicine and Science in Sports and Exercise* 34 (4): 723-31.

Wester, J.U., Jespersen, S.M., Nielsen, K.D., and Neumann, L. 1996. Wobble board training after partial sprains of the lateral ligaments of the ankle: A prospective randomized study. *Journal of Orthopaedic and Sports Physical Therapy* 23 (5): 332-36.

Wayard, P.G., et al. 2000. Faster top running speeds are achieved with greater ground forces, not more rapid leg movements. *Journal of Applied Physiology* 89 (5): 1991-99.

White, J.P., et al. 2013. Testosterone regulation of Akt/mTORC1/FoxO3a signaling in skeletal muscle. *Molecular and Cellular Endocrinology* 365 (2): 174-86.

Wiemann, K., and Tidow, G. 1995. Relative activity of hip and knee extensors in sprinting—Implications for training. *New Studies in Athletics* 10 (1): 29-49.

Wigernaes, I., Hostmark, A.T., Stromme, S.B., Kierulf, P., and Birkeland, K. 2001. Active recovery and post-exercise white blood cell count, free fatty acids and hormones in endurance athletes. *European Journal of Applied Physiology* 84 (4): 358-66.

Willems, T., Witvrouw, E., Verstuyft, J., Vaes, P., and De Clercq, D. 2002. Proprioception and muscle strength in subjects with a history of ankle sprains and chronic instability. *Journal of Athletic Training* 37 (4): 487-93.

Wilmore, J., and Costill, D. 2004. *Physiology of sport and exercise.* 3rd ed. Champaign, IL: Human Kinetics.

Wilmore, J.H., and Costill, D.L. 1988. Training for sport and activity. In *The physiological basis of the conditioning process.* Dubuque, IA: Brown.

Wilmore, J.H., Parr, R.B., Girandola, R.N., Ward, P., Vodak, P.A., Barstow, T.J., Pipes, T.V., Romero, G.T., and Leslie, P. 1978. Physiological alterations consequent to circuit weight training. *Medicine and Science in Sports and Exercise* 10: 79-84.

Wojtys, E.M., Huston, L.J., Taylor, P.D., and Bastian, S.D. 1996. Neuromuscular adaptations in isokinetic, isotonic, and agility training programs. *American Journal of Sports Medicine,* Mar-Apr 1996; 24 (2): 187-92.

Wojtys, E.M., Huston, L.J., Schock, H.J., Boylan, J.P., and Ashton-Miller, J.A. 2003. Gender differences in muscular protection of the knee in torsion in size-matched athletes. *Journal of Bone and Joint Surgery—American Volume* 85-A (5): 782-89.

Woo, S.L.-Y., An, K.-N., Arnoczky, S.P., Wayne, J.S., Fithian, D.C., and Myers, B.S. 1994. Anatomy, biology and biomechanics of tendon, ligament, and meniscus. In *Orthopaedic basic science,* edited by S.R. Simon, 45-87. Park Ridge, IL: American Academy of Orthopaedic Surgeons.

Wright, J.E. 1980. Anabolic steroids and athletics. *Exercise and Sport Sciences Reviews* 8: 149-202.

Wysotchin, 1976. Die muskelentspannung von sprintern. *Die Lehre der Leichtathletik.* 19: 593-596.

Yamaguchi, T., et al. 2006. Acute effect of static stretching on power output during concentric dynamic constant external resistance leg extension. *Journal of Strength and Conditioning Research* 20 (4): 804-10.

Yarasheski, K.E., et al. 1992. Effect of growth hormone and resistance exercise on muscle growth in young men. *American Journal of Physiology* 262(3 Pt.1): E261-7.

Yessis, M. 1990. *Soviet training methods.* New York: Barnes & Noble.

Zatsiorsky, V.M. 1995. *Science and Practice of Strength Training.* Champaign, IL: Human Kinetics.

Zawadzki, K.M., Yaspelkis, B.B., and Ivy, J.L. 1992. Carbohydrate-protein complex increases the rate of muscle glycogen storage after exercise. *Journal of Applied Physiology* 72: 1854-59.

Zehnder, M., Rico-Sanz, J., Kühne, G., and Boutellier, U. 2001. Resynthesis of muscle glycogen after soccer-specific performance examined by 13C-magnetic resonance spectroscopy in elite players. *European Journal of Applied Physiology* 84 (5): 443-47.

Zeller, B.L., McCrory, J.L., Kibler, W.B., and Uhl, T.L. 2003. Differences in kinematics and electromyographical activity between men and women during the single-legged squat. *American Journal of Sports Medicine* 31 (3): 449-56.

Zhang, P., et al. 2007. Signaling mechanisms involved in disuse muscle atrophy. *Medical Hypotheses* 69 (2): 310-21.

Zhou, S. 2003. Cross-education and neuromuscular adaptations during early stage of strength training. *Journal of Exercise Science and Fitness* 1 (1): 54-60.

Zijdewind, I., and Kernell, D. 2001. Bilateral interactions during contractions of intrinsic hand muscles. *Journal of Neurophysiology* 85 (5): 1907-13.

Index

Note: The italicized *f* and *t* following page numbers refer to figures and tables, respectively.

Index

Index

Index

About the Authors

Tudor O. Bompa, PhD, revolutionized Western training methods when he introduced his groundbreaking theory of periodization in his native Romania in 1963. He has personally trained 11 Olympic medalists (including 4 gold medalists) and has served as a consultant to coaches and athletes worldwide.

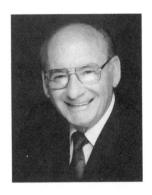

Bompa's books on training methods, including *Theory and Methodology of Training: The Key to Athletic Performance* and *Periodization*, have been translated into 19 languages and used in more than 180 countries for training athletes and for educating and certifying coaches. Bompa has been invited to speak about training in 46 countries and has been awarded certificates of honor and appreciation from such prestigious organizations as the Ministry of Culture of Argentina, the Australian Sports Council, the Spanish Olympic Committee, the National Strength and Conditioning Association (2014 Alvin Roy Award for Career Achievement), and the International Olympic Committee.

A member of the Canadian Olympic Association and the Romanian National Council of Sports, Bompa is a professor emeritus of York University, where he began teaching training theories in 1987. In 2017, Bompa was awarded the honorary title of *doctor honoris causa* in his home country of Romania.

Carlo A. Buzzichelli is a PhD candidate at the Superior Institute of Physical Culture and Sports of Havana (Cuba). He is a professional strength and conditioning coach; the director of the International Strength and Conditioning Institute; a consultant for Olympic track and field athletes in Cuba, Italy, and the Philippines; an adjunct professor of theory and methodology of training at the University of Milan (Italy); and a member of the President's Advisory Council of the International Sports Sciences Association (ISSA). Buzzichelli has held seminars and lectures at various universities and sport institutes worldwide and was an invited lecturer at the 2012 International Workshop on Strength and Conditioning in Trivandrum

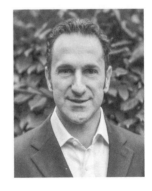

(India), the 2015 Performance Training Summit in Beijing (China), the 2016 International Workshop on Strength and Conditioning in Bucharest (Romania), the 2017 Track and Field National Team Coaches Forum in Havana (Cuba), the 2018 Philippines Academy of Rehabilitation Medicine Conference in Manila (Philippines), the 2018 International Conference on Football Science in Florence (Italy), the 2018 International Conference on Combat Sports Strength and Conditioning in Warsaw (Poland), and the 2019 International Workshop on Strength and Conditioning in Gwalior (India).

Buzzichelli's coaching experience includes the 2002 Commonwealth Games; the 2003, 2017, and 2019 World Track and Field Championships; and the 2016 Summer Olympics. As a strength and conditioning coach for team sports, his three senior teams in two different sports (volleyball and soccer) have achieved a total of five promotions in five seasons. As a coach of individual sports, Buzzichelli's athletes have won more than 50 medals at national championships in four sports (track and field, swimming, Brazilian jiujitsu, and powerlifting), set 10 national records in powerlifting and track and field, and won 15 medals at international competitions. In 2015, Buzzichelli coached two Italian champions in two different sports; in 2016, two of his athletes earned international titles in two different combat sports.

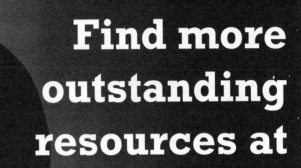
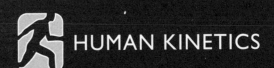

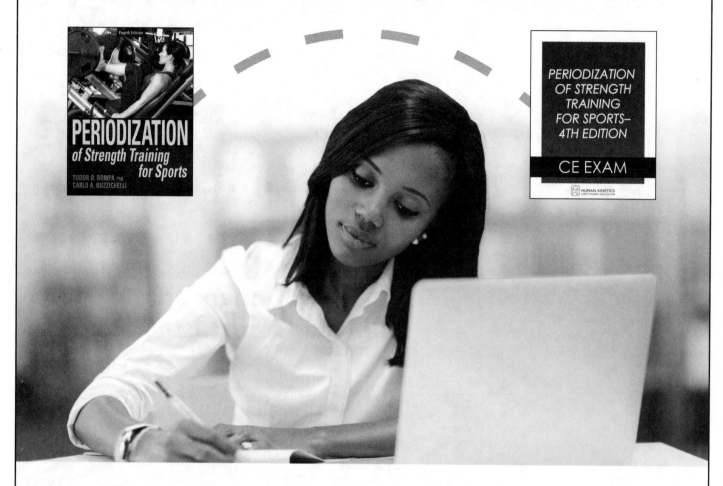
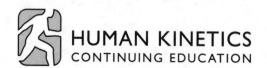